A Therapist's Guide
to Pediatric Assessment

A Therapist's Guide to Pediatric Assessment

Edited by
Linda King-Thomas, M.H.S., O.T.R.
Bonnie J. Hacker, M.H.S., O.T.R.

Developmental Therapy Associates
Durham, North Carolina

Little, Brown and Company
Boston/Toronto

Library of Congress Catalog Card No. 87–81450

ISBN 0-316-49372-4

Printed in the United States of America

RRD VA

Contents

Contributing Authors

Georgia A. DeGangi, M.S., O.T.R.
Clinical Instructor, Department of Pediatrics, Georgetown University School of Medicine and Health Sciences, Washington

Betty N. Gordon, Ph.D.
Assistant Professor, Department of Psychology, University of North Carolina at Chapel Hill

Bonnie J. Hacker, M.H.S., O.T.R.
Private Practice, Developmental Therapy Associates, Durham, North Carolina

Cathee J. Huber, R.N., M.N.
Associate Professor, School of Nursing, and Chief Nursing Specialist, Clinical Center for the Study of Development and Learning, University of North Carolina at Chapel Hill

Linda King-Thomas, M.S.H., O.T.R.
Private Practice, Developmental Therapy Associates, Durham, North Carolina

Patricia B. Porter, Ph.D.
Assistant Professor, Medical Allied Health Professions, and Director of Clinical Programs, Clinical Center for the Study of Development and Learning, University of North Carolina at Chapel Hill

Joan C. Rogers, Ph.D.
Professor of Occupational Therapy, School of Health Related Professions, and Assistant Professor of Psychiatry, University of Pittsburgh School of Medicine; Program Director of Occupational Therapy, Geriatric Psychiatry and Behavioral Neurology Module, Western Psychiatric Institute and Clinic, University of Pittsburgh

Victoria Shea, Ph.D.
Clinical Assistant Professor, Department of Psychiatry, University of North Carolina at Chapel Hill

Shelley Stowers, M.P.H., O.T.R.
Occupational Therapy Consultant, Columbia Outreach Motor Services, Portland, Oregon

Patricia O. Towle, Ph.D.
Assistant Professor, Department of Psychiatry and Human Behavior, New York Medical College, Valhalla

Preface

Therapists have long recognized that careful assessment techniques and adequate measurement tools are necessary to appropriately evaluate the pediatric population. This book was conceived as the result of a need identified by North Carolinian occupational therapists for more information on clinical assessment tools used in the evaluation of children. Tests commonly used in practice come from a variety of sources, and a comprehensive listing and review was not available to assist therapists in making appropriate selections. Furthermore, few therapists had developed skills in critically analyzing the tests they were using and yet were in the position of making judgments based on the results of these tests. It was this impetus that provided the foundation for this book.

The editors of this text are committed to the concept of providing quality therapeutic services to children, services that are dependent on both careful use of evaluation tools and an understanding of the assessment process. Readers of this book are demonstrating their professional responsibility by taking a critical look at the evaluation tools currently available, understanding their strengths and limitations, and then making informed decisions on what tools are appropriate to use as part of the assessment process for a particular child. Because this assessment process involves consideration of many aspects of the child's development, tests commonly used by occupational therapists, physical therapists, speech and language pathologists, and psychologists were included. As skilled clinicians we have an obligation to the children with whom we work to understand the implications of test findings from other professionals and to be able to integrate relevant information into the assessment process for a particular child.

The editors extend thanks and appreciation to Henry, Elizabeth, Jordan, Erin, and Daniel, all of whom provided support and endured long hours of absenteeism for this book to be completed, and to the occupational therapists in North Carolina who voiced the need.

L.K-T.
B.J.H.

Pediatric Assessment

I

Pediatric assessment is a skilled professional responsibility that should not be assumed lightly. Decisions regarding not only intervention, but also classification and placement, are made as a result of assessment of a child's development. Furthermore, parental expectations and a child's feelings of self-worth and competence can often be influenced, positively or negatively, by the findings of an evaluation.

Part I provides information regarding the skills and considerations that therapists must be aware of in order to provide responsible assessment. Chapter 1 "The Assessment Process" explores concepts of pediatric assessment, including standardized test administration and ecological evaluation of the child in his or her environment. Chapter 2 "Responsibilities of the Examiner" helps the reader examine more closely the professional responsibility required in assessment. Considerations include assessment purpose and technical adequacy as well as legal and ethical issues. Chapter 3 "Selection of Evaluation Instruments" guides the reader in the psychometric evaluation of norm-referenced and criterion-referenced standardized tests. Chapter 4 "Use of Standardized Tests with the Physically Handicapped" considers the implications of adapting tests for children with verbal and motoric limitations and offers guidelines for use. Specific reviews of commonly used standardized pediatric evaluation tools are found in Part II.

The Assessment Process

Cathee J. Huber
Linda King-Thomas

Assessing the development of children is an important skill needed by parents, educators, and health professionals. Parents are interested in learning what to expect as their children grow and develop, and in knowing whether physical or cognitive problems requiring intervention are present. Educators and school personnel are interested in determining appropriate classroom placement and in obtaining necessary intervention services. Health professionals are interested in promoting physical and mental health, and in preventing problems that compromise good health or make poor health unnecessarily worse.

DEFINITION OF ASSESSMENT

Assessment is the complex and individually specific process of gathering information in order to identify areas of strengths and weaknesses and to interpret the findings for effective program planning. The actual testing of the child is only one component of the assessment process. Other methods of gathering information include (1) obtaining histories from parents, teachers, and other professionals involved with the child and (2) observing the child in his or her environment. *Comprehensive assessment* of a child requires consideration of the interplay between the child and the environment. Viewing both the child and the environment as a single unit has been identified as *ecological assessment* [4].

ECOLOGICAL ASSESSMENT

The ecological assessment process provides a structured means of broadening the data-gathering aspect of assessment to include the child's environment. In addition to standardized testing, the assessment process places equal importance on information gathered from interviews, questionnaires, checklists, and observations of the child in his or her environment, thus providing a broader perspective of the child's functioning. This approach is particularly useful for the multihandicapped and severely developmentally delayed child, since standardized tests are often not available for this population [4].

The environment is viewed as having influence on the child's behavior and performance. For example, a hyperactive child may perform better in a structured classroom with an understanding teacher. A child with delayed expressive language and poor vocabulary may perform better in a home environment that encourages the use of language and provides the proper feedback for vocabulary building. The relationships of the child with others, whether parents, teachers, or caregivers, also becomes an important consideration. Listening attentively during interviews to obtain an idea of the perception of the child's functional abilities can provide valuable information. For example, the handicapped child may be further handicapped by unrealistic expectations, denial of dysfunction, or lack of opportunities. Changes in the child's environment also become part of the strategies for intervention. For example, parent education classes, smaller classroom size, behavior modification programs, and suggested toys and activities might be strategies used to change a child's environment [4].

A team approach is used for ecological assessment, with team communication early in the process. Team members might include a physician, nurse, special educator, teacher, psychologist, occupational therapist, physical therapist, speech and language therapist, audiologist, or nutritionist, depending on the facility completing the evaluation. Team planning *before* diagnosis can help refine the referral questions and determine specific areas for evaluation. Preliminary avenues for intervention can also be explored [4].

An inexpensive screening device to identify children early is very desirable. "When children are not identified until school age, much valuable information may have been lost" [4]. The screening results also provide necessary information to the team for diagnostic planning before the evaluation. Early identification and treatment results in more effective and less expensive intervention [7].

COMPONENTS OF ASSESSMENT

The assessment process involves (1) investigating the reason for referral, (2) gathering historical information, (3) selecting the appropriate screening or evaluation tool, (4) administering and scoring the test or tests, (5) synthesizing the results of the tests and other information that has been obtained, (6) interpreting the findings, (7) effectively communicating the results orally or in writing (or both), and (8) providing directions, suggestions, or individual program plans (individualized education program [IEP], treatment plan) to assist in the appropriate use of results for intervention [5]. Although the process appears to be a rather straightforward series of events, it is in fact more circular (like a

spiral moving closer to an end goal). Synthesis of information and data gathering helps to further delineate the referral question, change the selection of tests, or add tests until finally all the information is gathered and synthesized for the interpretation of results. Methods of gathering information include obtaining histories, recording observations of the child, and administering tests.

Histories

Information obtained from gathering histories about a child and his or her performance in various environments (e.g., school, home) can be invaluable in the evaluation process. Interviews and questionnaires can be used to obtain a picture of past and current behaviors. Important information to be obtained may include the following:

1. Familial history including incidence of developmental or learning problems in family members and familial characteristics (e.g., handedness, slow speech acquisition).
2. Birth history including information regarding pregnancy and delivery, such as length of pregnancy, ease of delivery, and complications in the prenatal and perinatal period.
3. Medical history including any remarkable incidences in the postnatal period, hospitalizations, medications, medical diagnoses, and status of vision and hearing.
4. Developmental history including motor, language, and self-help developmental milestones; failure to progress; or loss of skills.
5. Play history including types of play activities or games, social skills with peers, self-esteem status, interests and hobbies.
6. Educational history including current grade level, repeating of grades, preschool experience, strengths and weaknesses, special education or related services, behaviors in the classroom.
7. Home history including daily routine and

experiences for the child, responsibilities in the home, siblings or relatives living in the home, behaviors in the home.

The use of this information in the assessment process helps to validate the test findings outside of the one-to-one testing situation and provides a functional interpretation of the test results. Assessment information is also gathered through direct observation of the child in familiar environments.

Observations

Observations, when used properly, are a non-biased reporting method of the child's interaction with the environment, either animate (e.g., a teacher or classmate) or inanimate (e.g., monkey bars or a history lesson). A proper recording procedure is needed for the observation to be objective, complete, and reliable. The three major categories of observation recordings are (1) recording the rate of behavior (frequency and/or duration), (2) using a checklist or rating scale, and (3) reporting a specific behavioral event in an anecdotal fashion [4].

The *rate of behavior* method is frequently used to obtain baseline data and to assist in developing programming goals for a behavior management problem. If a behavior is intermittent, such as getting up from the classroom seat inappropriately or noncompliance with an activity, the number of occurrences or frequency during a designated period of time is recorded. If a behavior is continuous, such as completing a written assignment or working independently, the duration of that behavior within a designated time period is recorded. The baseline data provide clear information about a given behavior, and progress can be objectively measured [4].

A checklist or rating scale can be completed by a parent, teacher, or consistent caregiver in order to obtain information about positive and negative behaviors. A *checklist* is a collection of behaviors that tend to occur more often in children with a specific disability. For example, a checklist of behaviors attempting to identify tactile defensiveness (an avoidance or discomfort with touch) might include a dislike for textured foods; refusal to walk barefoot in the grass or sand; discomfort with light or unexpected touch; difficulty with toothbrushing, hairwashing, or cutting; avoidance of ''messy'' activities such as finger painting; and/or insistence on wearing long sleeves and long pants in hot weather.

Rating scales are similar to checklists but provide more qualitative data. A rating system usually involves a number scale to rate the quality, degree, or frequency of a behavior [4]. A typical example of a rating system is 5 = always, 4 = often, 3 = sometimes, 2 = rarely, 1 = never. Behaviors such as hyperactivity, aggression, and withdrawal are frequently observed with a checklist or rating scale.

An *anecdotal record* of a specific event is the third category of a behavioral observation. This method involves direct observation by the reporter. The style of recording the event should be brief and objective, with no interpretation or judgment of the behavior in the record. The specifics of the time, date, place, and event or activity being observed should be included [4]. An anecdotal record of a classroom observation might include work habits, conversations with peers or teachers, or the need for assistance and clarification of an assignment. The time and effort needed to properly record the observations and maintain objectivity often make this method of information gathering seem impractical. However, the information obtained from observations can be invaluable in the assessment process to bridge the gap between actual test performance and performance in the environment. For example, the child who maintains good attention in a one-to-one testing situation, yet who cannot remain focused in a group situation, needs to have a synthesis of information from histories and observations in conjunction with more formal testing (1) to properly address the problem of attention and (2) to plan strategies for intervention.

Histories and observations of the child provide the necessary information about child-environment interactions. Appendix A includes three samples of questionnaires that combine both history and checklist methods of data gathering.

Testing

Tests can be divided into two major areas: screening and evaluation. *Screening* provides preliminary information which indicates whether a need for further testing exists; *evaluation* offers a clear delineation of strengths and weaknesses, which may offer a diagnosis, identify the need for intervention, and provide guidelines for appropriate goal-directed intervention. Screenings can be done on an individual basis or in a large group such as a prekindergarten screening program administered by the public schools. Diagnostic evaluation is always completed on an individual basis.

Screening

Children with severe handicapping conditions are generally identified by concerned parents, family members, or professionals by 2 years of age. However, mild or moderate handicaps are often not identified until later, perhaps when the child enrolls in a preschool program or public school. Screening is a way of examining large numbers of children in a presumably normal population. Screenings can actually be thought of as a method of prevention. The three levels of intervention are primary, secondary, and tertiary. *Primary prevention* refers to the prevention of the occurrence of disease or disability. Generally, public health professionals and physicians are involved at this level by providing immunizations against childhood diseases (measles, polio) and by reducing the socioeconomic factors of poverty and malnutrition which may have an impact on health (e.g., the ingestion of

lead paint contributing to mental retardation). *Secondary prevention* refers to the early detection of a problem that has not yet developed obvious symptoms and for which help has not yet been spontaneously sought. Pediatric screening is a form of secondary prevention. The vision and hearing screenings provided in public schools, the Denver Developmental Screening Test often administered routinely in the physician's office at a given age, or large-scale developmental screening administered by public schools before children enter kindergarten are common examples of secondary prevention. *Tertiary prevention* refers to the identification and treatment of a problem after recognizable symptoms have appeared. Evaluation might be considered a form of tertiary prevention since the identification of specific areas for intervention frequently occurs after a comprehensive evaluation. Examples might include administration of an intelligence test to identify cognitive abilities or a specific language test to identify receptive language abilities [3, 7].

The primary purpose of a pediatric screening is to identify the presence, or possible presence, of deviations from normal growth and development as early as possible.

Screening is the acquiring of preliminary information about characteristics which may be significant to the health, education, and well-being of the individual and which are relevant to his life tasks. The means of data collection must be appropriate and reasonable with regard to the economics of time, money, and resources for dealing with large numbers of persons [1].

By focusing on the acquisition of preliminary information that may be significant to the health, education, or well-being of a child, pediatric screening can be used both to identify potential problems and to provide anticipatory guidance to parents. *Anticipatory guidance* is a means of educating parents about the expected stages of normal growth and development as well as the appropriate play activities and toys needed to promote development and learning. In addition, the early identification of difficulties can be cost-effective. Ulrey states, ''There is ample evidence that identification and treatment of children during the preschool period is cost-effective and reduces subsequent special education and special service costs during the school age period'' [7].

Screening should never be considered more than the initial step in the process of providing preventive health care to children. It can never be considered diagnostic and must be part of a program in which there is a well-defined plan for using the acquired information. A good program provides anticipatory guidance for parents and caretakers when the child's screening tests results are normal (negative) (Fig. 1-1). In addition, this program provides for rescreening and/or in-depth evaluation when the child's screening results are abnormal (positive). It must be emphasized that screening tests are designed only to collect preliminary information about a potential problem. They must never be used as a substitute for an appropriate diagnostic test.

Fig. 1-1. Components of the process of developmental screening.

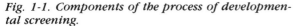

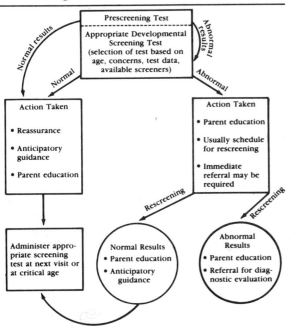

SELECTION OF APPROPRIATE SCREENING TESTS. Screening test selection should be based on carefully thought-out standards. Standards for screening test selection may be even more important than those for evaluation instrument selection because, theoretically at least, so many decisions (e.g., need or lack of need for evaluation) are based on briefer tests and, therefore, a more limited amount of information. With recent interest in early identification of developmental problems, many screening tests have been developed. These tests are not of uniform quality, and it is the responsibility of the professional using them to determine which ones are actually capable of accomplishing their stated purpose. Determination of how well a screening test meets the following set of criteria will help to answer that question:

1. *Acceptability.* Screening tests must be acceptable to all who will be affected by them, including the children and families screened, the professional who will receive resulting referrals, and the community as a whole.
2. *Simplicity.* Screening tests should be relatively easy to teach, learn, and administer.
3. *Cost.* The cost of a screening test includes cost of the equipment, preparing and paying personnel, the cost of inaccurate results, personal costs to the individual being screened (e.g., loss of school time), and the total cost of the test in relation to the benefits of early detection.
4. *Appropriateness.* Appropriateness of screening tests is based on the prevalence of the problem in the population under consideration (i.e., similarity of demographic and standardization characteristics).
5. *Reliability (precision).* Screening tests must be capable of yielding consistent results, both in repeated trials and when administered by different examiners. Evidence of reliability studies should be present in the screening manuals.
6. *Validity (accuracy).* Screening tests must be capable of giving a true measure of the be-

havior, skill, or characteristic being tested. Evidence of validation studies should be present in screening test manuals. Aspects of validity particularly important to screening include screening test validity (percentage of agreement with criterion test), sensitivity (ability to identify abnormal as abnormal), specificity (ability to identify normal as normal), rates of over- and underreferral, and predictive validity of positive and negative findings.

Once the appropriate screening test has been selected and administered, and the need for further evaluation identified, the appropriate follow-up should occur (Fig. 1-2). Sometimes the examiner administering the screening tool will be the same person administering the in-depth evaluation. More commonly, however, the results of the screening test may be used to refer the child to the appropriate professional(s) in order to obtain the needed diagnostic and treatment services. Familiarity with the available screening tests and discussion with referring agencies will help to expedite appropriate referrals for more in-depth evaluation.

Evaluation

Evaluation identifies strengths and weaknesses of a child in regard to developmental norms and expectations. The findings may result in a diagnosis, identify the need for intervention, and provide the foundation for developing goal-directed intervention. Diagnosis can be thought of as the art of distinguishing one disease (or one aspect of a developmental or learning problem) from another. It is the process of accurate documentation of the presence or absence of abnormality.

Whenever possible, diagnosis includes determination of the *reason* or *cause* for presence of the abnormality in question. Developmental abnormalities can include problems in physical (including musculoskeletal or neuromuscular), nutritional, cognitive, social, language, educa-

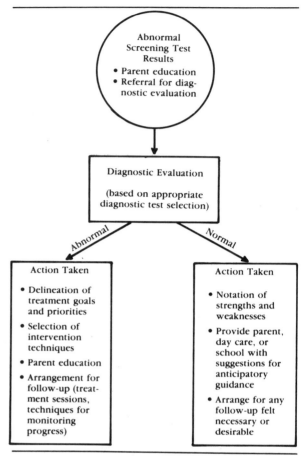

Fig. 1-2. Components of the process of diagnostic testing.

tional, or environmental areas. Whether or not the definitive cause of the problem can be identified, accurate documentation of its presence is the only way in which appropriate intervention can be determined. Quality of life for children with developmental or learning problems is highly dependent on appropriate intervention. Thus, the end result of pediatric evaluation should be the establishment of specific appropriate goals to guide intervention.

Two major types of evaluation tests include norm-referenced tests and criterion-referenced tests. Both provide valuable information for different purposes. *Norm-referenced tests* provide scores that can be compared with a standardized comparable population. This comparison results in the identification of similarities or differences in the individual child's performance and that of a standardized group. These tests are most commonly used for diagnosis. However, test results are meaningful only when the child is similar to the comparison population. For example, it would be totally inappropriate to use a verbal intelligence test to measure the cognition of a deaf or hearing-impaired child.

Caution must be exercised when interpreting the test scores of a handicapped child's performance from a test that has been normed on a nonhandicapped population. Issues involved in testing the physically handicapped child are addressed in Chapter 4. Although norm-referenced tests are useful in identifying the presence or absence of a handicap or delay and the degree of the handicap or delay, they may provide little information about programming [7]. The criterion-referenced tests provide useful information for program planning, creating needed bridges between diagnosis and educational intervention. The criterion-referenced test describes the child's current functioning and provides guidelines regarding what future skills should be emerging. The components needed to perform a skill or task are frequently included in a criterion-referenced test. Therefore, the sequence of the skills and not the age level becomes most important. Frequently, however, both types of evaluation tests must be used to properly diagnose the child and provide programming strategies.

SELECTION OF APPROPRIATE EVALUATION TESTS. The best way to ensure that the evaluation test of choice is capable of revealing characteristics indicating presence or absence of the problem of interest is to examine it against a set of standards for development of such tests. Some objective judgments about the quality of the test can then be made.

The Standards for Educational and Psychological Tests by the American Psychological Association provides a set of standards for systematic analysis of educational and psychological diagnostic tests [1]. These standards are also intended to apply to ". . . any assessment procedure, assessment device or assessment aid, that is, to any systematic basis for making inference about characteristics of people" [1]. The standards are written so that desirable properties of diagnostic tests are outlined, allowing consideration of each test by test users and developers alike. Consideration of these properties by test users generally leads to selection of the tests and procedures most suited to the desired use.

These standards were written to apply to standardized tests. However, the same general categories can be useful to practitioners who must rely in part on nonstandardized tests and procedures. For example, tests used by occupational and physical therapists include items for which the quality as well as the presence of a movement must be evaluated. It is more difficult to standardize how quality of movement is to be judged than to determine whether or not a movement is present. Obviously, nonstandardized tools are necessary in the practices of various health professionals. Still, it must be remembered that use of any diagnostic tool contributes to decisions affecting the lives of trusting clients. Systematic analysis, to the degree possible, of both standardized and nonstandardized tests and procedures, according to the criteria outlined in *The Standards for Educational and Psychological Tests,* is highly desirable [1].

REVIEW

An ecological method of assessment ensures the most comprehensive picture of a child, the environment of that child, and the child-environment interaction. Intervention strategies are uniquely designed for the child-environment interactions. Gathering information from testing, observations, and interviews provides the necessary information for a meaningful intervention plan. These procedures require the skills and judgment of a trained professional.

The importance of professional accountability in pediatric assessment should never be underestimated. Each person participating in selection and application of standardized or non-standardized screening or diagnostic tests must be constantly aware of the potential effects of the decisions they will be making. Children's lives can be positively or negatively affected by the results, depending on the validity and interpretation of findings. The issue of professional accountability is addressed in greater depth in Chapter 2.

REFERENCES

1. American Psychological Association, American Educational Research Association, and National Council on Measurement in Education. Standards for Educational and Psychological Tests (rev. ed.). Washington, D.C.: American Psychological Association, 1974.

2. Frankenburg, W. K., and Camp, B. *Pediatric Screening Tests.* Springfield, Ill.: Thomas, 1974.

3. Lessler, K. Health and education screening of school-age children—Definition and objectives. *Am. J. Public Health* 62 : 191, 1972.

4. Milliken, R. K., and Buckley, J. J. *Assessment of Multihandicapped and Developmentally Disabled Children.* Rockville, Md.: Aspen Systems, 1983.

5. Shea, V. Overview of the Assessment Process. In C. S. Newmark (ed.), *Major Psychological Assessment Instructions.* Rockleigh, N.J.: Allyn & Bacon, 1985.

6. Stangler, S., Huber, C., and Routh, D. *Screening Growth and Development of Preschool Children: A Guide for Test Selection.* New York: McGraw-Hill, 1980.

7. Ulrey, G. The Screening Assessment and Intervention of Children with Developmental Disabilities. In S. I. Pfeiffer (ed.), *Clinical Child Psychology: An Introduction to Theory, Research, and Practice.* Orlando, Fla.: Grune & Stratton, 1985.

Responsibilities of the Examiner

Linda King-Thomas

The responsibilities of the examiner in the assessment process should not be taken lightly. The decisions based on the test results can have a tremendous impact both positively and negatively on the lives of a child and his or her family. The practitioner who is competent in assessing developmental and learning difficulties and who can identify the proper programming needs must be skilled in several areas. Assessment is a complex process requiring knowledge of child development as well as principles of test measurement [8]. Being informed as to when a particular skill should be achieved by the child provides a basis from which to judge the quality of a response, whether it be sentence length, problem-solving strategies, or balance reactions. An understanding of tests, informal measurements, and psychometric principles is important in making the best possible selection of assessment tools for the individual child's needs.

A first area of skill development relates to the *specialized training* often required to adequately administer a test in a standardized manner and to accurately interpret the test results [8]. In addition to individual test results, the assessment process should also gather information from (1) parent, child, and teacher interviews, (2) observations of the child in a nonstructured, nontesting environment, and (3) evaluation of the environment (home and school) in which the child is functioning. This information then needs to be integrated and synthesized with the test results and the initial referral question to achieve a meaningful and valid end product [12].

A second area of skill development for the ex-aminer is the ability to *successfully report* (either in writing or orally) evaluation findings. The overuse of jargon and technical terminology and the lack of explanation of test scores reported in standard deviations, percentile ranks, and stanine scores does not result in a meaningful interpretation of the assessment for parents, physicians, or other professionals [12].

A third area of skill development (beyond the scope of this text) is the *successful implementation* of the programming recommendations and the effective use of service delivery models.

For the examiner to be responsible in his or her role as an evaluator in the assessment process, four considerations must be integrated into the clinical practice of assessment: (1) purpose(s) of the assessment, (2) technical adequacy of the assessment, (3) legal issues, and (4) ethical issues [8].

PURPOSE

The purpose of an assessment can generally be divided into two major areas: (1) identification and classification and (2) programming for intervention and remediation. Several state and federal agencies have been involved in identifying and classifying children with special needs both before and after 1975, when Public Law (Pub. L.) 94-142, the Education for All Handicapped Children Act, was passed. Pub. L. 94-142 states that children who have been identified and are labeled as eligible based on an assessment can receive special education and related services (e.g., occupational therapy, physical therapy, speech and language therapy, audiology, psychology, recreation). Children with special needs can fall under several labels: autistic, academically gifted, hearing impaired, mentally handicapped, multihandicapped, orthopedically impaired, other health impaired, pregnant, seriously emotionally handicapped, specific learning disabilities, speech and/or language impaired, and visually impaired [10]. Pub. L. 94-142 ensures that the intervention and remediation needs of special children as they relate to educational programming are met by the public schools.

Classification of children based on an assessment can be useful in other ways. When conducting research on the etiology of problems or on the effectiveness of intervention and remediation programs, proper classification of the research population is essential. When organizing public or private service agencies that focus on a specific disease or disability, a means of identifying who might be served by the agency is important. When conducting a needs assessment and planning services for a community, children need to be categorized and counted. Funding sources, both private and public, are generally organized around a disease or disability. Appropriate classification of children becomes necessary when applying for funds and also when accounting for how the funds were spent [8]. Although there are individual benefits and agency accounting procedures which dictate that children need to be labeled, the negative aspects of labeling should not be overlooked. The stigmatizing effect, the decreased performance expectations, and the disproportionately large number of minority children labeled with special needs are aspects that must be considered both before and after classifying children [13]. The classification and identification of special needs children become important for both the individual child and the agency that provides services to these children or that conducts research with these children.

Under Pub. L. 94–142, programming needs are governed by a written individualized educa-

tion program (IEP). The IEP is required for children who have been identified and labeled through the assessment process and who have been approved as being eligible to receive special education or related services. The IEP is similar to other forms of treatment planning in which strengths and needs are identified in regard to the child's current level of performance. Reasonable goals are established with objective criteria, enabling the examiner to judge whether the goals have been met. Under Pub. L. 94–142, assessment serves classification and identification purposes as well as programming purposes. The need to administer more than one evaluation instrument (stated in the law) when assessing the child for classification and placement is particularly useful when trying to meet identification and programming purposes. The norm-referenced test (which compares the child's performance with that of his or her peers) provides more information in regard to the purpose of identification and classification, while the criterion-referenced test (describes level of performance in relation to components needed to perform a task) provides information that is helpful for the purpose of programming [8].

TECHNICAL ADEQUACY AND SOURCES OF ERROR

The quality of the individual test in regard to psychometric properties, the purpose for which the test is to be used (referral question), and to whom the test will be given (age, disability) are all important factors to consider when selecting the appropriate evaluation tool. It is the responsibility of the examiner to be informed about the technical adequacy, the purpose, and the population for which the test was designed. Chapter 3 provides extensive information for the reader concerning reliability and validity measures for both norm-referenced and criterion-referenced tests, and an explanation of standard error of measurement. Basic considerations and expectations for the normative data from a norm-referenced test include the following:

1. Sufficient number in the normative sample to be representative of the population
2. Sufficient representation of the population (usually based on a U.S. census) on age, sex, socioeconomic status, geographic region, race, intelligence level
3. Data updated periodically to reflect the changes in the population over time
4. Inclusion of a representative sample of the population for which the test was designed [8]

Frequently, however, evaluation instruments do not measure up to these basic expectations for the normative sample. The Standards for Education and Psychological Tests [3], published by the American Psychological Association, describes additional expectations and guidelines for what information should be included in a test (e.g., a test's rationale, development, technical characteristics, administration and interpretation procedures).

Even if an evaluation tool is judged to be technically adequate, it can still yield misleading information if administered under inappropriate conditions. Therefore, standardized procedures should be strictly adhered to. According to Anastasi [6], *standardization* implies a uniformity of procedures in administering and scoring the test. Following the specific directions for administering the test, using the correct test materials (which should be in good condition), and adhering strictly to the established time limits are all part of the standardized procedure. The proper testing conditions are also part of the standardized procedure. A table and chair (if needed) that appropriately fit the child and a well-lighted place free from distraction and interruptions are generally considered to be part of a standard testing environment [8]. Sometimes it is impossible to follow the outlined standardized procedures; for example, a child with physical limitations may be unable to provide the needed motor or verbal response. Ap-

propriate assessment of this type of child is explored in Chapter 4. Examples of other common situations involving nonstandardized procedures include a poor testing environment (e.g., the school cafeteria or storeroom) and assessment of the very distractible child who needs a sticker reinforcement to complete the test with reliable and valid information. Deviations occurring in standardized procedures should be carefully explained in the test report. Taylor [13] reported on several studies that researched the effects of reinforcement on test-taking ability. The presence of a reinforcer and the type of reinforcer (tangible versus social, culturally appropriate social reinforcement versus culturally inappropriate) generally increased performance levels.

In addition to potential errors in the administration of a standardized test, difficulties in scoring unique, atypical, or ambiguous answers as well as a lack of training in the standardized procedure for administration, scoring, and proper interpretation of test findings can also influence test reliability and validity.

Additional potential sources of error affecting test results relate to both the child and the examiner. The increased stress and anxiety in a test situation and the lack of motivation on the part of the child may be potential sources of error. Therefore, the examiner should spend time initially in the test situation to be supportive and nonthreatening and to establish rapport; this procedure may help to minimize anxiety and achieve a best effort performance from the child. In addition, taking time to discuss test results with the teacher or parent to determine if the performance is "typical" for the child can help to validate results. For example, human figure drawings can vary substantially due to factors such as stress, fatigue, motivation, attention, and rapport. Therefore, obtaining confirmation of the child's "typical" performance from outside sources can be helpful. The practice effect from repeated test administration can also influence test results and is in part the reason why psychological reevaluations are administered only every 3 years in the public schools.

Examiner bias, although not necessarily conscious, can also have an influence on test outcomes. Depending on what has been heard in interviews or read in the child's records, the examiner may be more lenient or conservative when scoring test results. Although at times difficult, the examiner must use the information obtained about a child in a responsible manner and make a conscious effort to avoid bias [13].

LEGAL ISSUES

The one law that has had the most impact on pediatric assessment is the Education for All Handicapped Children Act (Pub. L. 94–142). Although state regulations and guidelines seem to change frequently, the general impact of Pub. L. 94–142 on special education, evaluation, and programming has been far-reaching and positive. The law [7] outlines six principles that pertain to all handicapped children in need of special education. They are as follows:

1. Zero reject. All handicapped children shall be provided with a free and appropriate public education. The exact age range for children varies from state to state.
2. Nondiscriminatory evaluation. The procedures used to identify a handicapped child and the nature and extent of services needed (special education and related services) for that child shall be free of discrimination. This principle covers both the classification and determination of programming needs.
3. Individualized Education Programs (IEPs). An overall plan for educational programming needs shall be developed and include several components such as current level of performance, annual goals, objectives, evaluation procedures, and documentation of the type and duration of the special services.
4. Least restrictive environment. To the maximum extent possible, handicapped children should be educated with nonhandicapped

children. However, mainstreaming should occur when the child's performance can be successful in that environment. The intent of the law is that education should work toward mainstreaming but that the type and severity of the disability may preclude education in a mainstreamed environment.
5. Due process. The persons making educational decisions shall be accountable and subject to a system of checks and balances.
6. Parental participation. Parents must be informed of decisions made about their children and are encouraged to participate in the decision-making process.

Each of the six principles indirectly affects and is in turn affected by the assessment process. However, the nondiscriminatory evaluation principle has the most impact on assessment and is reviewed in more detail below.

Nondiscriminatory Evaluation

Regulations implementing Pub. L. 94–142 state specific guidelines with regard to the nondiscriminatory evaluation principle. These guidelines are discussed below [7]:

1. "Tests and other evaluation materials:

   (a) Are provided and administered in the child's native language or other mode of communication, unless it is clearly not feasible to do so."

   The selection of an appropriate test must take into account the ability of the child to respond to test items. Therefore, motor free tests (Motor Free Visual Perception Test, Test of Visual Perceptual Skills, Pictorial Test of Intelligence [French]) are useful with a cerebral palsy population. Chapter 8 provides useful information regarding selection of a response mode and appropriate test for the child with physical limitations. Tests requiring minimal or no visual skills (Reynell-Zinken Scales: Developmental Scales for Young Visually Handicapped Children) are useful for the visually impaired and blind population, and tests requiring no auditory comprehension or spoken instructions (Hiskey-Nebraska Test of Learning Aptitude, Leiter International Performance Scale) are useful with the hard-of-hearing and deaf populations. Administering tests in sign language or in other languages may be needed to ensure optimal performance and a valid measure of skills. Unless a test in another language has been published in that language, caution must be exercised in regard to interpretation due to a lack of standardized administration procedures.

(b) "Have been validated for the specific purpose for which they are used."

Technical adequacy of a test is essential for a meaningful evaluation and interpretation of results.

(c) "Are administered by trained personnel in conformance with the instructions provided by their producer."

Proper training in the standardized administrative procedures and interpretation of test results, and knowledge of the areas of assessment are important for a valid assessment. Some tests (e.g., Southern California Sensory Integration Tests and the revised version Sensory Integration Praxis Tests) involve a certified training process, and other tests (e.g., Wechsler Intelligence Scale for Children—Revised [WISC-R], Stanford-Binet) can be administered only by a licensed psychologist.

2. "Tests and other evaluation materials include those tailored to assess specific areas

of educational need and not merely those which are designed to provide a single general intelligence quotient."

Intelligence testing alone is no longer acceptable for classifying and determining educational needs. Additional performance tests related to specific educational ability and disability are included.

3. "Tests are selected and administered so as best to ensure that when a test is administered to a child with impaired sensory, manual, or speaking skills, the test results accurately reflect the child's aptitude or achievement level or whatever other factors the test purports to measure, rather than reflecting the child's impaired sensory, manual, or speaking skills (except where those skills are the factors which the test purports to measure)."

This guideline refers to obtaining a valid measure of a child's skill level and not a measure that reflects the child's handicap. Motor free tests should be used to measure the intelligence of children with very poor motor coordination.

4. "No single procedure is used as the sole criterion for determining an appropriate educational program for a child."

At least two measures of performance are needed to determine the appropriate educational program. Most court cases have involved the use of a single intelligence test for school placement [13].

5. "The evaluation is made by a multidisciplinary team or group of persons, including at least one teacher or other specialist with knowledge in the area of suspected disability."

A team approach, which includes educators and related service personnel (physical therapist, occupational therapist, speech therapist, adapted physical educator) depending on the area of suspected disability, becomes necessary in making placement and program decisions based on a comprehensive evaluation.

6. "The child is assessed in all areas related to the suspected disability, including, where appropriate, health, vision, hearing, social and emotional status, general intelligence, academic performance, communicative status, and motor abilities."

This guideline reinforces the need for the multidisciplinary approach to assessment. In addition to specific guidelines, the Federal Register [7] also indicates that testing shall not be racially or culturally discriminatory.

Other enactments that have resulted in federal laws regarding assessment include the Rehabilitation Act of 1974 (Pub. L. 93–112) as amended by (1) the Rehabilitation Act Amendments of 1974 (Pub. L. 93–576) and (2) the Education Amendments of 1974 (Pub. L. 93–380). Section (Sec.) 504 of Pub. L. 93–112 was the first federal civil rights law for handicapped persons and was originally restricted to the employment of handicapped persons. Sec. IIIa of Pub. L. 93–516 amended the original public law and extended the civil rights of handicapped persons into educational settings [8]. Pub. L. 93–380 provided the basic framework for Pub. L. 94–142 and contained the Family Educational Rights and Privacy Act (Title V, Sec. 513 and 514), which is often referred to as the *Buckley Amendment* [8]. Under this act, parents have access to their children's school records. If parents do not agree with statements in their child's record, they can challenge the records and request that school officials amend the statements of concern. The schools must provide a hearing so that records can be challenged by parents or students. At age 18 and for all students attending postsecondary educational facilities, the rights to records transfer from the parents to the student. In addition, schools must obtain parental consent to release any school records to other agencies, and schools must inform parents of their right of access to school records. Failure to comply with these guidelines can result in loss of federal funding for the school [8, 11].

Sattler [11] states (primarily in relation to psychological reports) that there have been both positive and negative results from the Privacy Act. On the positive side, a closer relationship between parents and schools has developed, and there has been greater attention to the written evaluation reports in regard to labeling and conjectural and speculative statements. On the negative side, there has been an increase in paperwork, watered down reports, and concern about lawsuits.

ETHICAL ISSUES

Evaluators usually maintain membership in their professional organization. These professional organizations have developed and accepted codes of ethics which provide guidelines for professional behavior [1, 2, 4, 5]. These guidelines address several areas of behavior, including areas of clinical competence, evaluation techniques, and report writing.

Professional competence is an essential condition of ethical practice. A task force under the American Occupational Therapy Association has outlined eight basic competencies in assessment in a paper, "Hierarchy of Competencies Relating to the Use of Standardized Instruments and Evaluation Techniques by Occupational Therapists." These competencies are listed below.*

1. Recognizes the importance of using standardized, reliable, and valid instruments whenever such are appropriate

*Reprinted with permission of The American Occupational Therapy Association, Inc., Copyright (1984), *The American Journal of Occupational Therapy* 1984, p. 804.

2. Distinguishes between subjective and objective data, and uses each accordingly
3. Distinguishes the critical differences between standardized and nonstandardized instruments
4. Recognizes the need to use standardized instruments according to the instructions given in the test administration manual
5. Recognizes that using standardized instruments in an unstandardized (or adapted) manner may result in an invalid assessment
6. Recognizes that specialized training may be necessary to administer certain instruments correctly and to interpret the data appropriately
7. Uses assessment data to document work with a client so as to provide a logical, continuous record of performance, therapeutic goals and media, and outcomes
8. Follows ethical practices in the use of assessments: recognition of copyright, protection of the security of tests, protection of the confidentiality of test results, use of assessments for which one's education and experience is sufficient [9].

These codes and guidelines indicate that all evaluators should recognize their individual competencies and incompetencies. In honoring the ethical responsibility of using only those instruments which they are personally qualified to use, a competent evaluator, when unfamiliar with a certain instrument, should refer a child to another practitioner who possesses the necessary expertise [8].

In regard to report writing, ethical codes state that the test results should be presented objectively and should not be misused by other professionals [1, 4]. In addition, "any reservations regarding the validity or reliability resulting from testing circumstances or inappropriateness of the test norms for the person tested" [1, 4] should be reported. Further responsibilities of the evaluator toward the individual being served include confidentiality in all areas and understandable explanations of the nature, the

purposes, and the results of assessment activities [1, 4].

REVIEW

The examiner plays a critical role in the assessment process, and with that role comes the responsibility of being competent. Knowledge of test mechanics and specific areas of disability are necessary background skills for effective assessment practices. Four considerations that have an impact on and must be integrated with the clinical practice of assessment were reviewed. These four areas are (1) purpose of an assessment, (2) technical adequacy, (3) legal issues, and (4) ethical issues.

The purpose of an assessment can be divided into (1) classification and identification and (2) programming for intervention and remediation. The classification of children becomes important for deciding who receives services, funding, accounting of funds, and doing research. The programming aspect of assessment is governed by Pub. L. 94–142 for school age children and is implemented through an IEP.

Technical adequacy of a test instrument includes psychometric characteristics, the purpose of and rationale for the test, and the population for which the test was designed (age, disability). Evaluation of psychometric characteristics is explored in depth in Chapter 3. Standardized procedures were also reviewed in this section; even though a test is technically adequate, it can yield misleading information if administered inappropriately. Additional potential sources of error can arise from the child in the form of test anxiety, practice effect, and atypical performance, and from the examiner in the form of examiner bias and scoring errors.

Pub. L. 94–142 provides specific guidelines in relation to providing nondiscriminatory evaluation. Specifically, the guidelines indicate that

1. Valid and appropriate tests are selected and administered by trained clinicians.

2. Specific areas of educational need are assessed.
3. Performance on tests reflects the child's achievement level and not his or her handicap.
4. At least two tests are administered.
5. More than one person is involved in the assessment.
6. All areas related to the suspected disability are evaluated.

Clinical competence is governed by professional codes of ethics. Competence in proper evaluation practices and in report writing is essential to the assessment process. As the clinician becomes more aware of the responsibility of the evaluator role, the highest of professional standards can be achieved, resulting in effective delivery of services for the child and his or her family.

REFERENCES

1. American Occupational Therapy Association. Principles of occupational therapy ethics. *Am. J. Occup. Ther.* 38 : 799, 1984.
2. American Physical Therapy Association Judicial Committee. *Code of Ethics and Guide for Professional Conduct.* Alexandria, Va.: American Physical Therapy Association, 1984.
3. American Psychological Association, American Educational Research Association, and National Council on Measurement in Education. *Standards for Educational and Psychological Tests.* Washington, D.C.: American Psychological Association, 1974.
4. American Psychological Association. Ethical principles for psychologists. *Am. Psychol.* 36 : 633, 1981.
5. American Speech-Language-Hearing Association. Code of Ethics of the American Speech-Language-Hearing Association. 1983–1984 Directory. Washington, D.C.: American Speech-Language-Hearing Association, 1983.
6. Anastasi, A. *Psychological Testing* (5th ed.). New York: Macmillan, 1982.
7. Federal Register. Education of Handicapped Children. Regulations Implementing Education for All Handicapped Children Act of 1975. August 23, 1977. Pp. 42474–42518.
8. Helton, G. B., Workman, E. A., and Matuszek, P. A. *Psychoeducational Assessment Integrating Concepts and Techniques.* New York: Grune & Stratton, 1982.
9. Maurer, P., et al. Hierarchy of competencies relating to the use of standardized instruments and evaluation techniques by occupational therapists. *Am. J. Occup. Ther.* 38 : 803, 1984.
10. Rules Governing Programs and Services for Children with Special Needs. Raleigh, N.C.: State Department of Public Instruction, Division for Exceptional Children, 1984.
11. Sattler, J. M. *Assessment of Children's Intelligence and Special Abilities* (2nd ed.). Boston: Allyn & Bacon, 1982.
12. Shea, V. Overview of the Assessment Process. In C. S. Newmark (ed.), *Major Psychological Assessment Instruments.* Boston: Allyn & Bacon, 1985.
13. Taylor, R. L. *Assessment of Exceptional Students: Educational and Psychological Procedures.* Englewood Cliffs, N.J.: Prentice-Hall, 1984.

Selection of Evaluation Instruments 3

Joan C. Rogers

The evaluator, in addition to understanding the assessment process and knowing the responsibilities involved in this process, must carefully select evaluation instruments. Informed selection requires knowledge of the psychometric properties of the test in order to determine (1) the usefulness of a particular test in a particular situation and (2) the correct interpretation of the test results.

One therapist plans to screen preschool children for learning disabilities. Another seeks to evaluate a third grader's motor skills, and a third needs to diagnose the speech problems of a child with cerebral palsy. Standardized evaluation instruments can be used by all three therapists to assist them in making these assessment decisions. A *standardized* instrument has a fixed content and is administered and scored according to explicit procedures. In selecting an instrument from those that are available, the therapist seeks to choose a ''good'' test, since the use of an instrument of poor quality increases the likelihood of making an erroneous decision. A ''good'' evaluation instrument is one that provides information relevant to the decision to be made, yields results that are consistent, and is easy to administer and interpret. In other words, it is valid, reliable, and practical.

This chapter is designed to assist therapists in selecting evaluation instruments. It begins by discussing the importance of clearly specifying the behavior domain that is to be evaluated and the objectives of the evaluation. Norm-referenced and criterion-referenced instruments are then distinguished to aid the therapist in deciding the kind of interpretative data that is wanted. Subse-

quently, the qualities of validity and reliability, which constitute the primary criteria for instrument selection, are applied to norm-referenced and criterion-referenced instruments. The chapter concludes with a discussion of practical considerations, such as ease of test administration and interpretation, which also influence instrument selection.

EVALUATION OF TESTING INSTRUMENTS

Content

An instrument is useful to the therapist to the extent that it yields information that facilitates clinical decision making. If a therapist suspects that a child's learning difficulties stem from visual-perceptual problems, the child should be given a test that measures aspects of visual-perceptual functioning believed to be important for learning. Prior to beginning a review of evaluation instruments, the therapist must have a well-formulated idea of the behavior domain he or she wishes to measure. If one is interested in a comprehensive evaluation of visual-perceptual skills, a test that is restricted to visual figure-ground perception will not serve this purpose no matter how well constructed the test is.

Objectives

In addition to knowing the content of the evaluation, the objectives of the evaluation also need to be outlined. An instrument that is capable of distinguishing (screening) children who have visual-perceptual problems from those who do

19

not may be of little value in describing (diagnosing) the nature of the visual-perceptual deficit. If an instrument is to be used to chart a child's progress during intervention or to recommend placement in school or a special residential environment, evidence of the instrument's capability to serve these objectives must be sought. A good understanding of what is to be measured and why is a prerequisite for reviewing tests to ascertain their suitability for the use intended.

Psychometric Properties

After identifying the behavior domain that is to be evaluated and the objective of the evaluation, the therapist must decide whether to use a norm-referenced or a criterion-referenced instrument.

Norm-referenced tests compare a child's performance with that of the child's peers. A child's performance is regarded as high or low, depending on how his or her score falls in relation to those of the peer reference group. A peer reference group is any group to which the child's performance may be appropriately compared. For example, a child's musical talents might be compared with the performance of peers of the same age or of child prodigies. Norm-referenced tests are constructed in a manner that encourages a wide distribution of scores, and thus enables the examiner to discriminate those children who perform better from those who perform less well. Test items that elicit correct responses from the majority of children are likely to be eliminated, since such items furnish little discriminative information.

Criterion-referenced tests describe a child's level of performance. These tests consist of items that reflect the components needed to complete a task or perform a skill. The child's performance is described according to what he or she can and cannot do. In other words, a child's performance is compared with a standard, such as accomplishment of 80 or 90 percent of the test items, rather than with the performance of the peer group. Unlike norm-referenced tests, it is possible for many children to obtain perfect or near perfect scores on criterion-referenced tests.

In selecting an evaluation instrument, the therapist must decide if a measure that compares the child's performance with that of other children (norm-referenced test) is desired or if a measure that compares the child's performance with task or skill objectives (criterion-referenced test) is preferred. The former type of measure gives an indication of the child's relative position within a group, while the latter gives an indication of mastery level. The development of criterion-referenced measures is relatively recent, which in part accounts for the reason that the majority of tests used by therapists are norm-referenced. Since the determination of validity and reliability differs for norm-referenced and criterion-referenced tests, the type of evidence needed to judge the technical adequacy of a test depends on the type of evaluation instrument.

NORM-REFERENCED INSTRUMENTS

Validity

The essential concern in selecting an evaluation instrument is that the test gives a true measure of the behavior domain that is being evaluated (Table 3-1). If one is seeking to evaluate visual-perceptual problems, one would prefer a test that did not confuse the measurement of visual-perceptual abilities with other abilities, such as reading or fine motor skills. In other words, one would desire a test that measured *only* visual-perceptual abilities and that did this well. One would want a valid test.

Validity refers to the extent to which a test measures what it says it measures. Although we commonly speak of the validity of a test, validity really refers to the results yielded by a test. Test results are not valid or invalid. Rather, they are more or less valid depending on the use to which they are put. A test may have high validity for one purpose and low validity for another.

Table 3-1. Summary of validity and reliability indicators for norm-referenced and criterion-referenced evaluation instruments

I. Norm-referenced evaluation instrument (compares child's performance with that of other children)
   A. Validity (refers to the meaning of test results)
      1. Content (the extent that test items reflect an accurate or adequate sampling of the behavior domain)
      2. Criterion-related (concurrent and predictive use of test results to estimate performance on behavior other than that measured in the test itself)
      3. Construct (appraisal of the underlying structure [theory] of the behavior or trait measured)
   B. Reliability (refers to the consistency of test results)
      1. Test-retest (stability of test results over time)
      2. Equivalent forms (consistency of test results with different item samples)
      3. Equivalent forms plus time interval (stability over time and consistency of test results with different items)
      4. Internal consistency (item homogeneity)
      5. Examiner (agreement among test scorers)
      6. Standard error of measurement (error in an individual score)
II. Criterion-referenced evaluation instrument (compares child's performance with an absolute performance standard)
   A. Validity
      1. Descriptive (evaluation of clarity of test specifications)
      2. Functional (use of criterion-referenced tests for other than descriptive purposes)
      3. Domain selection (defensibility of the domains selected to represent a task or skill)
   B. Reliability
      1. Decision consistency (consistency of the decision made regarding skill mastery)
      2. Norm-referenced reliability estimates (applicable if an appropriate spread of scores is achieved)

For example, a test of visual-perceptual abilities may have a high degree of validity for diagnosing visual-perceptual problems, moderate validity for predicting reading ability, and low validity for forecasting prosocial behaviors. Thus, validity is not a general characteristic of an instrument. Rather, it is specific to the objectives of testing.

The validity of a test score is not self-evident and cannot be assumed. Validity must be established. Evidence of validity should be given in the test manual. The three basic types of validity are *content validity, criterion-related validity,* and *construct validity.* Each type is concerned with a different kind of data interpretation. In determining the usefulness of an evaluation instrument, the therapist must be careful to ascertain that the evidence of validity covers the specific use that is to be made of the test results.

Content Validity

Content validity is of critical importance when the therapist is interested in describing a child's performance in a particular area of behavior. *Content validity* refers to the extent to which the behaviors measured by an evaluation instrument reflect an accurate and adequate sampling of the behavior domain and thus enable valid inferences to be made.

In assessing a child's manual dexterity, for example, it would not be feasible to test every possible way in which the hand is used. Instead, a sample of hand skills is taken to construct the test of manual dexterity. The child's performance on the test is used to draw a conclusion about his or her manual dexterity. The performance demonstrated on the sample is used to generalize about the child's overall manual dexterity. For the conclusion about the child's manual dexterity to be valid, the test items must be representative of the behavior domain associated with manual dexterity. Thus, in evaluating the content validity of a test, the focal question is: How well do the items comprising the evaluation instrument represent the domain of behavior that the instrument is supposed to measure?

Evidence of content validity is obtained from the test author's discussion of the test's development and rationale. The discussion should provide an indication of how the behavior domain measured by the test was conceptualized, how the limits or parameters of the domain were set, and how the sample of test items was drawn. This information is easier to document if the entity being measured is concrete, such as self-feeding, rather than abstract, such as adaptive behavior. To support the content validity of a test, one would expect to find task analyses, test plans and outlines, and the testimony of experts in the field in the test manual.

As a potential test user, the therapist has to decide how well the content of the test measures the behavior domain he or she seeks to assess in a particular child or group of children. For example, a test manual may indicate that manual dexterity is defined as skill in manipulating small objects and that the test tasks involve objects for which one would normally use pincer or lateral prehension patterns. The therapist would have to decide if this definition of manual dexterity and the way in which it is to be tested met his or her need for information. Since the test excludes actions regarded as developmentally significant, such as gross grasp, it may be inappropriate for assessment of a particular child or group of children.

If the therapist agrees with the conceptualization of manual dexterity, he or she proceeds to ascertain how adequately the author has translated the definition into a testable form. The manual and test items are examined in detail to determine if the comprehensiveness of the coverage and the relative emphasis given to various behaviors or tasks is appropriate. In making this judgment, the therapist relies on the expert opinion provided by the test author, his or her own experience, and knowledge gleaned from the literature. If the agreement between test specifications and knowledgeable opinion is high, the test would be regarded as having high content validity. If the correspondence is low, content validity would be regarded as low.

In essence, the determination of content validity involves a judgment of the extent to which concept definition is adequate and is ef-

fectively operationalized in the test design, and the extent to which the test as designed meets the needs of the test user. To the extent that the therapist's need for information is met, the evaluation instrument is valid for use with the child.

Criterion-Related Validity

If the therapist is interested in using a test score to estimate a child's current or future performance on a measure other than the evaluation instrument, evidence of criterion-related validity is sought. For example, the therapist may wish to use manual ability at age 15 to indicate current potential for success in typewriting, or to predict the potential for success in an assembly line job at age 20. The estimation of present status from a test score requires *concurrent validity,* while the prediction of future performance requires *predictive validity.*

Both concurrent and predictive validity are types of criterion-related validity and involve the comparison of test data with behavior that is external to the test itself. The behavior external to the test is called the *criterion behavior.* Concurrent and predictive validity differ only in the time period between measurement on the test and measurement of the criterion behavior. In concurrent validity, the two measures are taken at the same time, while in predictive validity, measurement of the criterion behavior takes place after the appropriate lapse of time. To use data on manual ability collected at age 15 to predict performance on the assembly line at age 20, one would have to wait 5 years to collect the criterion measure. On the other hand, to establish the utility of manual dexterity for judging present typewriting skills, the tests of manual and typewriting skills could be given at the same time. A test that has concurrent validity is not necessarily valid for predictive purposes. Similarly, a test that has predictive validity is not necessarily valid for making generalizations about current abilities.

The establishment of criterion-related validity involves a comparison of the status obtained on the test with the status obtained on the criterion. For example, the test of manual ability might be given to a group of students with mental retardation at age 15. The test allows us to rank these students from those having the most skill to those having the least. Five years later these same individuals are rated on their level of performance on the assembly line. Scores on the manual dexterity test are then compared with the ratings of on-the-job performance. The validity of the manual dexterity test as a predictor of assembly line performance is indicated by the extent to which the students are ranked similarly by both the test and the job performance index. The degree of similarity between how the students are ranked on the test of manual dexterity and the ratings of their on-the-job performance is expressed by the *validity coefficient.*

The validity coefficient is a correlation coefficient. *Correlation* is the statistical technique for determining the degree of relationship between two measures. The correlation coefficient is designated by the symbol r. Theoretically, the relationship between a test and a criterion can be anywhere from $+1.00$ to -1.00. An $r = +1.00$ indicates that the position of each individual relative to other group members on the test and on the criterion was identical, with individuals scoring high on the test also scoring high on the criterion and those scoring low on the test also scoring low on the criterion. An $r = -1.00$ means that there is a perfect inverse relationship between test and criterion rankings, with persons scoring high on the test scoring low on the criterion and vice versa. An $r = .00$ is interpreted as no linear or simple relationship between the test and the criterion.

Ideally, one would like to have a perfect relationship between the test and the criterion behavior. However, differences typically occur between the two sets of scores, and validity coefficients generally range between .40 and .80. This finding raises the question of how high the validity coefficient should be to be useful, a question to which there is no simple answer. Obviously, one would like the validity coeffi-

cient to be as high as possible, since the higher the validity coefficient, the more accurate the prediction. One method of judging the adequacy of a validity coefficient is to compare it with other validity coefficients involving the same criterion behavior and other methods of predicting or estimating that performance. Even if a validity coefficient is low, if the test is the best available indicator, it can provide useful information. Validity coefficients are high or low only in relation to each other.

In the clinical situation, tests are generally used to make decisions about individual children rather than groups of children, as might be the case in a classroom setting. For individual decisions, validity coefficients of .70 or above are desirable. Validity coefficients below .70 should be viewed cautiously, since the relationship between the test and the criterion is weak. For this reason, evidence about the child's performance should be obtained.

In interpreting validity coefficients, several factors must be taken into consideration besides the magnitude of the coefficient itself. An awareness of the range of performance within the group used to calculate the coefficient is critical. The more restricted the group's performance abilities, the lower the resulting validity coefficient because it is harder to differentiate individuals whose performance is highly similar than it is to differentiate those who performance is very diverse.

A major problem in the establishment of criterion-related validity is that of coming up with an acceptable criterion and a feasible method of measuring it. For example, the ingredients of job success, independent living, or personal adjustment are not easily identified or measured. The criterion acts as a standard against which success is gauged and clinical judgments are made. In critiquing criterion-related validity, the criterion standard must be scrutinized as cautiously as the test. If that standard is found to be lacking or if it has been carelessly measured, the value of that evaluation instrument is questionable.

When selecting a test for predictive purposes, the therapist bases the decision on how much new information the test provides, in addition to how well it relates to the criterion. For example, suppose a therapist was debating about using a test of manual ability and a test of visual perception to predict future job performance on small assembly line tasks. If these two tests correlated highly with each other, and both had been shown to correlate well with future job performance, they would yield essentially the same information, and little would be gained by using both tests. On the other hand, if the correlation between the two tests was low, it would be advantageous to use both tests to assist in decision making, since each would be contributing different information regarding future job performance.

Construct Validity

A *construct* is an idea that is abstract (e.g., numerical reasoning ability) rather than concrete (e.g., the ability to do addition). Intelligence, manual ability, spatial visualization, and tactile defensiveness are examples of constructs. Constructs are described by certain measurable behaviors that tend to occur together. Once the behaviors that infer the presence of a certain construct have been identified, individuals can be ranked based on the extent to which they exhibit those behaviors. Although constructs cannot be directly observed, some agreement exists about how they operate in human actions. We expect a tactually defensive child to demonstrate discomfort or avoidance of touch, especially if the touch is unexpected. Children who are not tactually defensive do not exhibit these behaviors. Underlying the construct of tactile defensiveness is a theory that explains how the construct operates or is overtly manifested.

The establishment of construct validity is essentially a process of theory validation. The theory allows one to predict test scores, if the test is a valid indicator of the construct. If the test scores are as predicted, the validity of the test as a measure of the construct is supported. If the test scores differ from the predicted scores, the validity of the test, as well as perhaps the underlying theory, is suspect.

Evidence of construct validity is needed when the therapist seeks to interpret test scores in terms of constructs. Construct validity emerges from the accumulation of evidence from multiple methods.

One method of establishing construct validity is to compare the scores of groups that are known to differ or are theorized as performing differently. Theories often predict that scores will vary because of age, sex, training, or pathology. For example, the hypothesis that children of drug addicts exhibit more tactile defensive behavior than normal children might be tested.

If the theory suggests that the behaviors comprising the construct will be altered as a consequence of some intervention, test scores obtained before and after treatment can be compared. If the theory predicts that sensory integrative therapy reduces tactile defensiveness, and the test scores are as theorized, the test can be regarded as valid.

A third method emerges from studying the relationships between scores obtained from the same individuals on different tests. A theory may lead us to expect that our construct is related to some things but not others. For example, we would expect one test of tactile defensiveness to be highly related to another test of tactile defensiveness because they are presumably both measures of the same construct. On the other hand, we might expect a low correlation between tests of tactile defensiveness and eye color because they are measuring different things and we have little reason to expect an association.

Factor analysis is another common method of establishing construct validation. If the items comprising a test or subtest are all measuring the same construct, we would expect them to be highly related. *Factor analysis* is a complicated statistical procedure that identifies the overlap and underlying structure of a set of test items. Suppose that the results of a 20-item tactile defensiveness scale from 500 children were subjected to factor analysis. We would expect all 20 items to load heavily on one factor. If, instead, two factors emerged, each with 10 items, we would be more inclined to rethink our test, since this finding suggests that the test is tapping two dimensions of the construct of tactile defensiveness as defined in the instrument. Results of the factor analysis would lead us to revise our original idea about the structure of tactile defensiveness. Factor analysis thus yields a more insightful description of constructs.

It is apparent that the supporting evidence of a test's construct validity entails logical as well as empirical procedures. The process of establishing construct validity is a cumulative and unending one. The more complex the construct, the more difficult it is to establish the construct validity of the instrument devised to measure it.

Reliability

For an instrument to be useful, it must be reliable as well as valid. Whereas validity pertains to the meaning of what is being measured, *reliability* refers to the consistency or reproducibility of results (see Table 3-1). An evaluation instrument that grades a child's motor performance as retarded one day and superior the next is of limited value. A reliable test yields the same results over and over again, provided the child's behavior or traits have not actually changed.

Ideally, the test results should be "absolutely consistent." For example, if we were to repeat an evaluation after several hours or the next day, we would like to obtain the same scores. Consistency of results enables us to have confidence in them.

Although perfect consistency is desirable, it is rarely attainable. Many factors other than the characteristics being measured influence test scores. Let us assume that the computer game Pac Man provides a measure of eye-hand coordination. The first time Mike plays he achieves a score of 650. On the next trial, his score falls to 590. Many factors could account for the inconsistency of his score. During the first time, he may have been more motivated to play or less tired than during the second. Or, the first maze may have been easier than the second. The higher score may have reflected more "luck" than the lower score. Depending on which score was used as the "true" measure of Mike's eye-hand coordination, his relative position within his peer group would probably change. Hence, our judgment of his eye-hand coordination skill would change. The reliability of a measuring device gives an indication of how accurately a finding would be reproduced if the child were tested again. Alternatively, reliability may be viewed as an indicator of the amount of error in a score.

Like validity, reliability refers to the scores obtained from measurement, not the measuring instrument per se. Reliability can be expressed in two ways—the *reliability coefficient* and the *standard error of measurement*. The reliability coefficient provides a useful means of comparing one test with another, while the standard error of measurement is useful for interpreting individual scores.

Reliability as a Correlation Coefficient

Unlike the determination of validity, in which a test is correlated with an external performance criterion, in the determination of reliability, the test is correlated with itself. Several approaches may be used to compute reliability coefficients. Each approach looks at score reliability differently. Scores may be reliable over different time intervals or different samples of test items. Reliability, like validity, is not a general property of test scores but is always specific to some purpose. Thus, in selecting an evaluation instrument, the therapist must be careful to obtain an estimate of reliability that meets the intended purposes of testing. The three major approaches to evaluating the reliability of norm-referenced measures that are commonly used are test-retest, equivalent forms, and internal consistency. Reliability can also be estimated in terms of examiner agreement.

The reliability coefficient is a correlation coefficient, and therefore is interpreted in much the same way as the validity coefficient. If a test manual reports a reliability coefficient of + .93, one could conclude that the test was reliable. The correlation coefficient approaches 1.00 and suggests that the set of scores on each of the two measures was highly similar.

When a test is being used to make an important clinical decision regarding a child, a reliability coefficient of .90 or above is needed. For screening tests, a reliability coefficient of .80 or above is acceptable.

Test-Retest Reliability

Test-retest reliability is obtained by administering a test to a group of children and subsequently readministering the same test to the same children. Scores on the two tests are correlated, and the resulting correlation coefficient provides an estimate of the stability of the test results over the time interval. Test-retest reliability provides an estimate of how confidently one can generalize from a score obtained by a child to a score that would be obtained if the test were given at another time.

The time between the first and second testing may vary. Consequently, there are as many test-retest reliabilities as there are time intervals between testing. In selecting an evaluation instrument, the therapist must note whether the reported test-retest reliabilities were calculated in a manner that matches the aims of testing. If the therapist's interest is in knowing how accurately a score characterizes a child at a specific point in time, a procedure for determining reliability in which the two measures are carried out

one right after the other is appropriate. Such a procedure takes into account variation or score error that is due to the measuring process. With such a short time span, it is safe to assume that the characteristic being measured has remained the same.

If the therapist plans to use test results to make a long-range prediction, a longer interval between testing and retesting is needed. If the test score will be used to predict behavior 2 or 3 years into the future, the therapist needs assurance that the score will remain stable over this interval, or the long-range prediction will be inaccurate. A procedure for determining reliability that separates the two testings by a considerable time interval takes into account score variation due to fluctuation of the individual's performance as well as variation due to the measuring process. In interpreting test-retest reliability coefficients, the interval between test administrations must be considered. We can expect the estimate of reliability to be higher the shorter the time interval, because there is less chance that a true change has occurred in the characteristic measured.

The interpretation of a test-retest reliability coefficient is often difficult. When retaking a test, children are not presented with the same task as they were the first time because they have already reacted to the test items. Particularly if the interval between testings is short, a child may respond to test items the second time the same way as the first time simply because previous responses were remembered. Alternatively, a child may have learned something from the first testing that causes him or her to respond differently the second time. A child tested only one time would not be so influenced.

Equivalent Forms

Tests are comprised of items that have been chosen to represent a behavior domain. Some variation in test scores arises out of the selection of some items as opposed to other items.

Concern about score variation due to the sampling of test items is taken into account in the equivalent forms method of calculating reliability. If the therapist is interested in using a test score to generalize about a child's performance to the domain of behaviors represented by the test, the equivalent forms method of estimating reliability is appropriate. Other terms for the equivalent forms method are *parallel* forms and *alternate* forms.

In the equivalent forms method, two forms of a test are administered to the same children and the results are correlated. The two forms of the test are constructed according to the same specifications; that is, the items, although different, cover the same area of behavior and require responses that are equally difficult. Since the two tests are designed to evaluate the same behavior, they should be highly correlated. The equivalent forms method of estimating reliability enables the therapist to determine how confidently a child's score can be generalized to what would have been received if the test were comprised of different items.

The equivalent forms of a test can be given one right after the other, or they can be separated by a longer time interval. If the two testings follow each other immediately, only score variation due to the specificity of items is considered. This procedure is appropriate when the stability of behavior over time is not a concern.

If the two testings are separated by a longer time interval, score error from the three main sources of error—error arising from the measurement process, from changes within the individual over time, and from item sampling—is taken into account. While fluctuations due to day-to-day changes in the child and changes in the measurement process are taken into account by the test-retest method, variation due to item sampling is not. Incorporating a time interval into the equivalent forms method constitutes the most precise test of reliability. Thus, reliability coefficients calculated by this method are likely to be lower than those calculated by other methods. The rigorousness of the test must be taken into account in interpreting these coefficients. If the purpose of testing is to make long-range predictions, a coefficient that takes into account all sources of error is desirable.

Internal Consistency

To estimate reliability using the test-retest and equivalent forms methods, two tests must be administered. Since it is often not feasible to administer two tests, a method of estimating reliability from a single testing has been devised. In this method, two scores are derived from a single testing by dividing the test into two presumably equal halves for the purpose of scoring. For example, the odd-numbered test items may be regarded as one test, and the even-numbered items as another. The odd-numbered items may then be correlated with the even-numbered items. A high reliability coefficient indicates that the test is measuring something consistently from beginning to end. Split-half reliability furnishes an indication of the internal consistency of the measuring device, that is to say, of the homogeneity of the item content.

The correlation coefficient obtained by correlating odd- and even-numbered items is actually based on two half tests, and fails to portray accurately the full length test. Test reliability is somewhat dependent on the length of the test. A longer test gives us a larger sampling of the behavior domain than a shorter test, and therefore is generally more reliable. A reliability coefficient computed on the basis of two half-length tests tends to underestimate reliability.

The Spearman-Brown Prophecy Formula is used to correct for the reduction in test length and provides an estimate of the reliability of the whole test. Coefficient alpha can also be used to estimate internal consistency; this coefficient takes into account all possible ways in which a test can be divided into two parts. If the test items are scored dichotomously (i.e., true or false), the Kuder-Richardson formulas can be used. Kuder-Richardson Formula 21 assumes that all test items are of equal difficulty; Formula 20 does not make this assumption.

When using a split-half reliability coefficient it must be remembered that both scores reflect the child's performance at one point in time. Daily variation of the individual is not taken into account. It should also be noted that split-half reliability is *not* applicable for timed tests, since it spuriously inflates the estimate.

Examiner Reliability

Examiner reliability constitutes a fourth index of reliability. It refers to the extent to which test results vary because of factors introduced into the testing situation by persons doing the evaluation or scoring. In paper and pencil tests, the examiner's influence is usually negligible, although it may be an issue if an examiner gives more directions or allows more time than the instructions indicate. For other kinds of tests, such as personality tests or perceptual-motor tests, the examiner's influence on the test results may be considerable. The more objective the test, the greater the reliability. When objectivity of the examining or scoring process is of concern, examiner reliability should be reported in the test manual. In this case, the reliability coefficient reflects the extent of agreement between examiners.

Factors Influencing Reliability

As has been noted, the size of the reliability coefficient is influenced by test length, speed, the interval between testings, and the calculation method employed. When interpreting reliability coefficients, it is also critical to take group characteristics into account. The reliability coefficient tells us how consistently a test ranks each child relative to other children. Obviously, it is easier to rank individuals if the range of ability in the group is large rather than small. Less shifts will occur in the rank of the manual abilities of 2, 3, and 4 year olds than of 2 year

olds alone. For this reason, reliability coefficients calculated using heterogeneous groups will be higher than those using homogeneous groups, and the former should be scrutinized more rigorously.

Standard Error of Measurement

The reliability of an instrument can be gauged by the standard error of measurement as well as by the reliability coefficient. The reliability coefficient is useful for comparing tests, while the standard error of measurement is the appropriate statistic for evaluating the amount of error in an individual score.

Suppose that Mike played Pac Man 100 times, resulting in 100 scores. If his scores were tallied and graphed, they would tend to approximate the bell-shaped normal curve. The average of the resulting frequency distribution can be thought of as Mike's "true score." The standard deviation of this distribution provides a description of the variation of Mike's score on repeated measurement. The deviation of these scores around the "true score" is called the *standard error of measurement* and gives a measure of intraindividual variability.

Obviously, in testing, there is only one score per test, rather than multiple scores, for each child. Thus, the standard error of measurement is projected from group data. The standard error of measurement provides an indication of reasonable limits of a child's score. For example, if a child obtained a score of 70 on a test, we would want to know how accurately this score reflected his or her "true score." If the standard error of measurement for this test were 6, we could expect the child to score between 64 and 76 (70 ± 6) about 68 percent of the time. This estimate is based on the characteristics of the normal curve, since 68 percent of all cases in a normal distribution fall within + 1 and − 1 standard deviation from the mean. There remains a 16 percent chance that the true score is less than 64 and a 16 percent chance that it is greater than 76. If we were unwilling to accept this possibility of error, a more rigorous confidence level could be established. For example, we could be about 95 percent certain that the child's true score was between 58 and 82, or 2 standard errors of measurement. This estimate is also based on the normal curve and the knowledge that about 95 percent of the cases in a normal distribution fall between +2 and −2 standard deviations from the mean. The standard error of measurement should be included in the test manual.

The relationship between the reliability coefficient of a test and its standard error of measurement is such that as the reliability coefficient increases (indicating greater consistency of results), the standard error of measurement decreases (indicating less score error). Unlike the reliability coefficient, which varies with the range of ability that is present in a group, the standard error of measurement is independent of the group's ability range.

CRITERION-REFERENCED INSTRUMENTS

Validity

Content validation constitutes the principal concern for criterion-referenced tests (see Table 3-1). Descriptive clarity of the behavior domain being measured is critical. Although the process of establishing the content validity of criterion-referenced tests is essentially the same as that for norm-referenced tests, the former is generally done more conscientiously and explicitly. For criterion-referenced tests, content validity is sometimes called *descriptive validity.*

Descriptive validity is established by ascertaining (1) the adequacy of the test specifications for generating homogeneous test items to measure the desired behavior domain and (2) the homogeneity of the test items generated. Homogeneity is a marker of clarity. To evaluate the clarity of the test specifications, experts in the behavior domain to be measured may devise items according to the rules set forth in the test specifications. The homogeneity of the items generated may then be judged by an independent group of experts or may be evaluated empirically by administering the test items to an appropriate group of learners and calculating the intercorrelations between the items. Having ascertained that the test specifications are clear, the test items themselves are more carefully scrutinized. Each of the test items is rated as congruent or incongruent with the test specifications by multiple independent experts. An average congruency percentage is calculated from these ratings. Congruency percentages of 90 or higher are viewed as acceptable.

In criterion-referenced testing, the counterpart to criterion-related validity of norm-referenced tests is *functional validity.* Functional validity involves the use of criterion-referenced tests for purposes other than descriptive purposes; for example, the use of a test to make decisions regarding an impaired child's readiness for mainstreaming into a regular classroom. Functional validity has limited applicability, since criterion-referenced tests are almost always used for descriptive purposes only. However, if tests are used to generalize beyond the behaviors tested, functional validity may be ascertained by the same procedures used to establish criterion-related validity.

Domain-selection validation is the third type of validity of concern for criterion-referenced measures and is similar to construct validation of norm-referenced tests. Domain-selection validity involves the defensibility of the domain or domains selected to represent a task or skill. Generalizability is the critical issue. Since tasks or skills are often comprised of several behavior domains, test developers have several options to consider when formulating the test. The domain that best generalizes to performance of the other domains comprising the task or skill should be selected.

One method of establishing domain-selection validity is to provide a careful description of the qualifications of the individuals who selected the behavior domain and the procedures used for selection. Their credentials lend believability to the test. In addition, each of the domains comprising the task or skill can be taught until mastered to a group of children, and the influence of this mastery on the other domains can be systematically assessed.

Reliability

The procedures developed to determine the reliability of norm-referenced instruments require a spread of scores, that is, a wide range of variation among the subjects tested. For this reason, these procedures are often inappropriate for gauging the reliability of criterion-referenced instruments, where test mastery is highly probable. Correlational analyses yield spurious results when response variation is restricted. When the spread of scores is markedly reduced, it is suggested that reliability be determined according to the consistency of the decision made regarding skill mastery.

Criterion-referenced tests yield data that are used to judge whether a child has mastered or not mastered the competencies required for some task or skill. The determination of reliability rests on the consistency of the categorization of the child as master or nonmaster. Reliability is expressed as the percentage of children whose scores resulted in the same categorization on repeated measurement. The index of reliability is called the *percentage of decision consistency.*

The standard for delineating mastery or nonmastery might be the median performance level or a performance level (such as 70 or 80 percent of the items) that has been empirically or clinically determined as the minimum required for test mastery. If the median is used as the performance standard, the phi coefficient can be used to calculate reliability. This coefficient is a nonparametric statistic that is appropriate to use when response variation is limited.

The percentage of decision consistency can also be used as an indicator of reliability if more than two options are under consideration. For example, if children are being classified as masters, level I remedial, and level II remedial, the proportion of identical decisions would be calculated for each category.

Equivalent forms are important for criterion-referenced tests, since examinees may retake different versions of a test to demonstrate mastery. Items for the different forms may be randomly selected from a large item pool. Equivalency can be calculated using the correlation coefficient, nonparametric statistical tests, or the percentage-of-decision-consistency approach depending on the decision to be made and the kind of data available.

Usability

In addition to validity and reliability, a number of practical considerations must be taken into account in selecting an evaluation instrument. The potential user of an instrument must consider the ease with which the instrument can be administered, scored, and interpreted. The therapist needs to ascertain how much skill is required to manage the evaluation and whether special training is needed. These issues relate to an instrument's usability or practicality. The easier a test is to give, score, and interpret, the more practical it is to use.

ADMINISTRATION OF TESTS

An evaluation instrument is easy to administer if the instructions are simple, clear, and comprehensive. After reviewing the directions, it should be clear what the test administrator is to do, and what the child taking the test is to do. The ease with which the test can be administered is increased if the testing procedures do not require a high degree of skill to carry out and can be readily learned. The need for special training reduces the usability of the test.

The test administrator's task is complicated if the test includes many subtests that either have separate instructions or are timed. The need to time multiple subtests requires considerable concentration, particularly if the subtests are short and close timing (i.e., to a fraction of a second) is needed. Standardized tests are designed to be given according to the specifications in the test manual. If these specifications are vague and the testing procedures are unclear or if errors are made in test administration, the validity and reliability of the evaluation results are adversely influenced.

Since the time available for evaluation is usually limited, an evaluation instrument's usability is generally increased the shorter it is. Thus, a shorter test is usually preferable to a longer one, as long as adequate reliability and validity are maintained.

Scoring of Tests

A test is easy to score if the directions indicate clearly how the score is to be computed. The directions should inform the test user about the management of test items that were missed (i.e., not completed), responses that were wrong, and the calculation of subscores and the total score. Ease of scoring is facilitated if scoring decisions are automatic, that is, they follow directly from the scoring instructions and require little or no judgment on the part of the test scorer.

Interpretation of Test Scores

A test is easy to interpret to the extent that the raw score can be readily translated into usable data. Raw scores in and of themselves are rather meaningless. A child's score of 70 on a spelling test is difficult to interpret unless it can be compared with some standard. For example, spelling 70 of 80 words correctly would reflect greater ability than spelling 70 of 100 words, assuming that the words were at the same level of difficulty. In this case, a perfect test score provides the standard against which performance is judged. The percentage of correct answers is a suitable score for criterion-referenced tests.

In norm-referenced testing, a child's performance is compared with the performance of other children rather than with an absolute standard. This comparison is accomplished by interpreting raw scores in reference to percentile, standard score, age norms, or grade norms. Each of these norms indicates that relative status of a child within the norm group. For the interpretation to be meaningful, the norm group must be an appropriate group from which to view the child's performance. Thus, it is important for the characteristics of the norm group to be specified in the test manual.

One way of interpreting a child's raw score is to ascertain, by using the raw score, where a child's performance falls within a particular reference group. This is commonly accomplished by converting the raw score to a percentile or standard score, which enables the score to be interpreted in terms of the bell-shaped normal curve.

A *percentile* indicates the percentage of cases falling below a particular score. For example, a child's score of 70, that falls at the eightieth percentile, indicates that 80 percent of the cases in the reference group received a score lower than 70. To guard against attaching unwarranted precision to a test score, percentile bands, rather than percentiles, can be used. For example, a raw score of 70 may be interpreted as reflecting performance from the seventy-fifth to the eighty-fifth percentile. The percentile bands are often constructed to represent standard deviation units from the mean.

Although percentiles are easily understood, they have a major drawback stemming from the inequality of percentile units. The difference between the ninetieth and ninety-fifth percentile is greater than the difference between the fiftieth and fifty-fifth percentile. Since standard scores have a uniform meaning over the range of values, they have an advantage over percentiles.

Standard scores are expressed in terms of standard deviations above or below the mean of the reference group. Common standard scores are *z* scores, *T* scores, and stanines. A *z* score represents a raw score expressed in terms of a mean of 0 and a standard deviation of 1. Since *z* scores can result in negative numbers and fractions, *T* scores are often preferable. *T* scores express a raw score in terms of a mean of 50 and a standard deviation of 10. *Stanines* are standard scores having a mean equal to 5 and a standard deviation of about 2. The stanine scale is confined to the numbers 1 through 9; that is, stanines divide the normal distribution into nine parts.

Most intelligence tests are now interpreted in terms of standard deviation units rather than ratio intelligence quotients (ratio of mental age to chronological age). Typically, deviation intelligence quotients have a mean of 100 and a standard deviation of 15 or 16.

Percentiles and standard scores use the bell-shaped normal curve as a reference point for score interpretation. A scoring system based on the normal curve assumes that the behavior or trait being measured is normally distributed in the population. If this is not the case, the raw scores can be "normalized" or "pushed" into a distribution that more closely approximates the normal probability distribution. These scores are referred to as *normalized standard scores*. There is a direct relationship between percentiles and standard scores, if the raw scores are normally distributed or have been normalized.

Raw scores can be used to determine which group a child belongs to rather than where a child falls in a particular group. This is accomplished through age norms and grade norms. A child's raw score is compared with the average score obtained by successive age or grade groups to identify the group which matches his or her performance.

Pediatric instruments often use age and grade norms. Age norms are appropriate for characteristics that improve with age. They are problematic in the sense that growth from 1 year to the next lacks a uniform meaning. The growth between ages 1 and 2 is not the same as between ages 11 and 12. A year's growth in figure-ground perception is not comparable to a year's growth in gross motor skills. Age norms on various characteristics are also not comparable. As individuals mature, many characteristics stabilize or change only minimally from year to year. Thus, age norms usually plateau or level off.

Grade norms pose many of the same problems as age norms. The equality of grade units is suspect, and there is little assurance that the amount of growth from grade to grade is uniform. Grade norms are most useful for academic performance at the elementary school level in areas where instruction is continuous from grade to grade. The interpretation of grade norms must be approached with caution. For example, if a third grader obtains a score indicative of a fifth grade reading level, this does not mean that fifth grade reading skills have been mastered. Rather, the grade probably reflects superior performance on third grade work. Grade norms reflect the average score obtained at each grade level, and thus by reading third grade material well, a student may achieve a score equal to that of the average fifth grader.

Percentiles, standard scores, age scores, and grade placement scores are derived scores. They are derived from raw scores and enable us to attach meaning to the raw scores. Tables giving raw scores and the value of their corresponding derived score are contained in the test manual. Generally, several such norm tables are displayed to give the norms calculated on different samples of children. The normative samples should be described in terms of pertinent characteristics, such as sex, socioeconomic status, intelligence, and geographical area, so that the potential test user can judge the sample's adequacy for serving as a peer reference group.

REVIEW

Evaluation instruments can be classified as norm-referenced or criterion-referenced. *Norm-referenced instruments* are designed to compare a child's performance with that of other children, while *criterion-referenced instru-*

ments compare a child's performance with an absolute performance standard.

Validity is the major concern in test selection and involves the extent to which the evaluation instrument measures what it says it measures. There are three types of validity, and test users should seek evidence in the test manual of the type of validity that is required for the intended use of the test. Content validity refers to the extent to which the test items reflect an accurate and adequate sampling of the behavior domain of interest. Criterion-related validity implies the use of test results to estimate performance on a behavior (the criterion) other than that measured in the test itself. Construct validity involves an appraisal of the underlying structure of the behavior measured by the instrument. When these concepts of validity are applied to criterion-referenced instruments, the terms content validity, criterion-related validity, and construct validity are sometimes replaced with descriptive validity, functional validity, and domain-selection validity, respectively.

Reliability is a precondition for validity and refers to the consistency of test results. When comparing one instrument with another, the correlation coefficient is the appropriate statistic, while the standard error of measurement is used to interpret individual scores. Reliability coefficients can be calculated in various ways to give an estimate of stability (test-retest method), or equivalence (equivalent forms method), stability and equivalence (equivalent forms adminis-

tered after an appropriate time lapse), and internal consistency (split-half and other methods). Examiner reliability suggests the degree of agreement among test scorers. Like validity, reliability is always purpose-specific, and one evaluates the reliability coefficient in terms of the purpose for testing. The reliability of criterion-referenced instruments is generally determined by the percent of decision consistency, since the norm-referenced techniques have limited utility when test score range is restricted. Table 3-1 summarizes the important features of the scientific properties of tests.

While the technical adequacy of evaluation instruments is of primary importance, practicality also plays a role in test selection. One's capability for administering, scoring, and interpreting the test can influence the reliability and validity of the test results.

REFERENCES

1. Anastasi, A. *Psychological Testing.* London: Macmillan, 1968.
2. Lyman, H. B. *Test Scores and What They Mean.* Englewood Cliffs, N.J.: Prentice-Hall, 1971.
3. Mehrens, W. A., and Lehmann, I. J. *Measurement and Evaluation in Education and Psychology.* New York: Holt, Rinehart, and Winston, 1984.
4. Popham, J. *Criterion-Referenced Measurement.* Englewood Cliffs, N.J.: Prentice-Hall, 1978.
5. Thorndike, R. L. *Applied Psychometrics.* Boston: Houghton Mifflin, 1982.
6. Thorndike, R. L., and Hagen, E. P. *Measurement and Evaluation in Psychology and Education.* New York: Wiley, 1977.

Use of Standardized Tests with the Physically Handicapped

4

Bonnie J. Hacker
Patricia B. Porter

The importance of assessment has been stressed throughout this text. Screening, program placement, program evaluation, and measurement of student progress are dependent on appropriate nonbiased evaluation [20]. Results of the majority of tests reviewed in this text rely on the child's ability to execute a verbal and/or motor response to stimuli items. Often neither of these responses is available to the severely physically handicapped child. Duncan et al. [7] report that the "market literally abounds with standardized tests . . . [but] few attempts have been made to create instruments for use with a physically handicapped population."

Significant strides have been made toward more appropriate assessment of subcultural and sensory-impaired children [16, 17]. Nonverbal physically handicapped children, however, continue to be placed in remedial programs without benefit of testing [21] or on the basis of subjective, teacher-adapted testing [11].

Vicker [21] suggested a solution to the difficulty of inappropriate assessment of the severely handicapped, nonverbal child when she pointed directly to the remediation of the communication deficit as the key. She wrote that the verbal expressive problems of the child with severe neuromuscular difficulty can be successfully circumvented via use of another expressive mode. Following evaluation of 12 severely handicapped, institutionalized children with cerebral palsy, Baumann, Hanker, and Schian [1] reported that "objective findings as to the psychic [psychological or cognitive] capabilities of the disabled person *cannot* be obtained until the communication possibilities have been ex-

ploited." Baumann et al., in this same review, proposed three alternatives to the inappropriate assessment of nonverbal, physically handicapped individuals:

1. Design and standardization of new test instruments not based on motor performance or speech capabilities.
2. Administration of our present standardized tests with adaptation and interpretation being the responsibility of the individual examiner.
3. Use of an augmentative communication aide to allow the child a consistent response potential to the items administered from currently used standardized tests.

Duncan et al. [7] addressed the difficulty in testing severely physically handicapped, nonverbal children. They suggested that design of a single standardized test (see 1 above) may be a "meaningless task due to the variability in motor involvement, vocal abilities, experiential background and motivational history" of the population [7]. Various approaches to the modification of standardized tests are briefly described in the Duncan et al. paper. The areas they list are (1) methods of presentation, (2) content, and (3) response mode.

Modification in means of presentation and style of response can be made in many tests in order to allow the physically handicapped child to demonstrate his or her understanding and knowledge. Modification of test content would serve to render the standardization meaningless. Very careful consideration must be given to selecting a functional motor response to be used in testing. Positioning, motor capabilities of various body parts, consistency and specificity of response, fatigue, and motivation are all extremely important factors in the selection process.

The practical systematic strategies for accurate assessment of nonverbal physically handicapped persons are discussed in this chapter, as well as standardized tests currently in use that can be easily adapted for administration.

POSITIONING FOR TESTING

Before testing a child or selecting a response indicator, the child must be adequately positioned. The purposes of appropriately positioning the child are to provide (1) good visual contact with test materials, (2) postural foundation for potentially controlled voluntary movements, and (3) a comfortable position that will be minimally fatiguing.

Positioning is best accomplished with the assistance of an occupational or physical therapist. Most commonly, the child will be positioned in a wheelchair that has been specifically adapted to that child's motoric needs. Less severely handicapped children may be able to use a straight-back wooden chair with minimal support such as a seat belt. General guidelines for seating include hips well back in chair and feet supported, providing 90 degrees flexion at hips, knees, and ankles. Children may also be able to use various pieces of adapted equipment such as a corner chair or bolster chair. One alternative to sitting is the use of a prone stander, which can be successful even for many severely handicapped children because of the trunk stabilization offered.

In addition to positioning the child in a chair, consideration must also be given to the child's relationship to the testing table and/or test materials. If the child is able to point directly to materials, a surface will be needed and can be either a tray attached to the wheelchair or a freestanding table, preferably with a semicircle cutout. Table height should be at least at the child's waist level and often slightly higher. The child should be positioned close to the table because its surface provides additional support and stability. For children relying on visual scanning and eye gaze, an easel or vertically attached Plexiglas should be placed at a comfortable distance from the child (usually 24–36 in.) depending on the child's visual acuity and size of pictures being presented (Fig. 4-1).

DETERMINING METHOD OF INDICATION

When severe motor impairment precludes verbal responses, alternate methods of indication must be identified in order to adequately assess a child's knowledge. The response mode chosen must be accurate, reliable, reasonably efficient, and under voluntary control. Unfortunately, in the face of severe neurological disorders, the movements demonstrated are frequently poorly controlled and unreliable, making selection of the best method of indication a difficult task. Training in a response must be approached with caution as the desired response may not be within the child's neuromotor repertoire. Secondly, it is important to select a response that

Fig. 4-1. Visual scanning system.

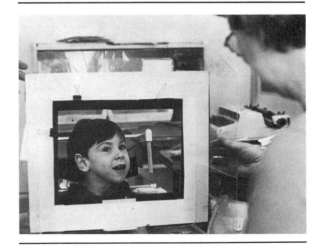

the child can reliably use for a 30- to 60-minute testing period. Due to the amount of effort many children must exert to accomplish a motor act, the method of indication selected for testing may not be the child's highest level of response. For example, a child may be able to touch four discrete areas on a tray using one or both hands, but the response requires so much effort that little concentration remains to devote to the test questions. In this case, an eye gaze system may be a better choice.

The most efficient system of testing would be to use a method of direct indication if this is within the child's motoric means. The best option is use of a hand or finger to point to choices. After the child is adequately positioned, present a board divided into grids on the child's tray or table. Using simple pictures or colors, ask the child to show or point to "_____." Start with a board the size of the test being used and divided in the same way (usually four quadrants). Several trials will be needed and the child's response may need to be shaped. The child's response must be clear enough for the examiner to accurately read it 100 percent of the time. If the child's responses are not clear, but some voluntary upper extremity control is demonstrated, at least three options can be explored: (1) the size of the quadrants can be enlarged; (2) the grids can be rearranged (e.g., the choices can be placed in a horizontal line); or (3) an assistive device such as a T-bar pointer can sometimes be used.

Some children can head point with an assistive device, either a head pointer or an optical pointer to indicate choices. Usually this approach is best if a child is already experienced in using such a device. Headsticks must be custom designed and fitted, and both devices require a significant training period.

If the child is unable to use hand or head pointing, visual indication is an option that has proved successful in testing many severely motorically handicapped children. A sheet of Plexiglas, approximately 24 by 30 in. with a central space cutout, is often used. The board is positioned vertically directly in front of the child, at a distance of about 2 feet. The child indicates the choice by gazing at the appropriate picture or symbol. The examiner can read the child's choice by looking at the child's eye movements. The examiner should sit at eye level, across from the child. Directions to the child and recognition of eye gaze choice can be conducted by the examiner through the cutout area in the center of the Plexiglas. Usually the four corners of the board are the easiest to clearly read. In assessing the child's ability to eye gaze, ask him or her to look to each corner as you point to it. If the child can do this successfully, he or she must then be taught to scan the four corners, return gaze to center, look at the chosen answer for 2 or 3 seconds, and then return to center. This method makes it easy to determine the child's choice during testing.

If these methods of direct selection prove unsuccessful or too tiring, a scanning system can be used if the child has a yes/no response. In general, it is preferable to have two discrete motor responses, such as raising hand for "yes" and shaking head for "no." Very motorically handicapped children may have to rely on eye gaze to the side to indicate "yes" and a nonresponse to indicate "no." After the "yes"/"no" system is established, the examiner can then scan the choices for the child, pointing to each one, while asking "Is it this one?" or a similar phrase. This type of scanning is usually more efficient for testing purposes than an electronic system.

ADAPTING TEST MATERIALS

Psychological, Language, and Educational Tests

Children with severe physical handicaps frequently are unable to effectively interact with standardized psychological tests or language or education tests, because the presentation format requires relatively good eye-hand coordination. Even tests designed for the physically handicapped may be beyond the motor capabilities of some individuals. Attempts to interpret a child's poorly directed movements as indication of a particular test choice may result in either under- or overestimating a child's abilities. These difficulties may be alleviated to some extent by adapting the test materials. A list of tests suitable for adaptation is found in Table 4-1.

Evaluation of the child's motor skills, positioning, and best method of indication by an occupational therapist and/or physical therapist should occur before proceeding with the testing of severely physically handicapped children. The therapist can then consult with the examiner regarding test presentation to facilitate reliable assessment.

The tests most suitable for adaptation have multiple picture displays, such as the *Pictorial Test of Intelligence* [10] or the *Peabody Picture Vocabulary Test-Revised* [8]. If the child is able to use one or both arms to indicate a choice, but movements are poorly controlled, cutting the test cards apart and placing the pictures widely spaced on the laptray or table may make it easier for the child to indicate a choice. Sometimes the placement of pictures should be modified either by placing the four pictures in a symmetrical arrangement with one in each corner or by placing them in a straight horizontal line. If the child points with only one hand, the pictures may need to be placed more to one side, keeping in mind the child's pointing range. It may be useful to divide the tray into quadrants using colored tape so that the child's indication can be more easily determined.

For children who must rely on eye gaze, the cut apart test can be easily affixed to a sheet of clear Plexiglas placed vertically between the examiner and the child. The pictures are usually placed in the four corners with clothespins, tape, or removable adhesive with the center of the board being reserved as a neutral place to make eye contact with the examiner. To successfully test the child using this method, the child must first have demonstrated reliable eye pointing. The use of at least two examiners fa-

cilitates test administration. One examiner sits behind the Plexiglas, presents the question, and records the response, while the other examiner places and removes the pictures. (The second person can be an aide or parent, if given a brief orientation.) Techniques such as the use of two boards (while the child is responding to pictures on one board, the next question can be prepared on a second board) or a flip chart can speed presentation.

Tests of Motor Skills

Tests of motor skills are often of little value and sometimes quite inappropriate to use with the severely motorically impaired child. Children with little control of motoric movements, balance, or posture will score extremely low on developmental tests of movement; however, this score yields little specific information about the child's problems or approaches for intervention. Similarly, such tools offer little help for measuring subtle changes in quality of movement.

Currently available measures of motor development should therefore be approached with caution in assessing the severely motorically impaired child. Evaluations must be accompanied by clinical descriptions of quality and patterns of movements with clear identification of the limitations of any standardized tools used.

REVIEW

While standardized tests can be of value in the assessment of physically handicapped nonverbal children, careful consideration must be given to selection of the test instrument, modification of it, and interpretation of test results. In many instances, use of standardized test instruments can provide an *estimate* of the child's level of functioning. In reporting test results, examiners should be careful to specifically note modifications made in the test instrument or procedures and the mode of response used by the child. It is inappropriate to assign the child a specific age or developmental level based on

Table 4-1. Tests that can be modified for use with physically handicapped children

Test	Age range	Comments
GENERAL INTELLIGENCE TESTS		
Peabody Picture Vocabulary Test-Revised (PPVT-R)	2½–18 yr	Measure of receptive vocabulary; requires selection of a choice from a set of four picture arrays; adapted pointing or eye gaze can be used
Pictorial Test of Intelligence Scale (French)	2 yr–adult	Good nonverbal measure of learning aptitude; only a pointing response is needed
Leiter International Performance Scale	2 yr–adult	No verbal response is required; pointing and some object manipulation is required
Columbia Mental Maturity Scale	3 yr 6 mo–9 yr	Requires principally a pointing response
Hiskey-Nebraska Scale of Learning Abilities	3 yr–adolescence	Requires no speech
LANGUAGE TESTS		
Sequenced Inventory of Communication Development (SICD)	4 mo–4 yr	Results based on child's performance and parental report; many items require no verbal or complex motor response; omission of some motor and speech items is possible in final scoring
Test for Auditory Comprehension of Language (TACL)	3–6 yr	Child is required to respond to examiner's verbal stimuli by pointing to one of three line drawings
Boehm Test of Basic Concepts	Kindergarten–grade 2	Multiple choice format; child is asked to select the picture that illustrates the concept being tested
Test of Language Development-Primary (TOLD-P)	4 yr–8 yr 11 mo	Several subtests require only pointing response
EDUCATION TESTS		
Peabody Individual Achievement Test (PIAT)	5–18 yr	Pointing response is required
Key Math Diagnostic Arithmetic Test	Preschool–grade 6	Requires ability to indicate a response
Detroit Tests of Learning Aptitude	6 yr–17 yr 11 mo	Several subtests require only a pointing response
SENSORIMOTOR TESTS		
Motor-Free Visual Perception Test	4–8 yr	Pointing response usually used; easily adapted to other response mode
Test of Visual-Perceptual Skills (Non-Motor)	4 yr–12 yr 11 mo	Pointing response used

norms established on a population not representative of this child's handicapping condition. Furthermore, deviation from the standard method of presentation may violate the standards under which the test was developed, rendering standardized data inapplicable. Results of testing adapted in this manner yield primarily descriptive rather than normative information.

More precise assessments of severely physically handicapped children will require the development of test instruments specifically geared to their needs, abilities, and life experiences. Such efforts have already been made in the field of visual impairment through a standardized adaptation of the Stanford-Binet specifically designed for partially sighted and blind children [10]. Clinical adaptations as described in this chapter offer some insight into a child's ability, but fail to take into account the very different environmental reality for a child unable to negotiate in or manipulate the environment. The physically limited child may have an exceptional understanding of medical and therapy terms or experiences, yet lack information about the community or have difficulty understanding spatial or action concepts. Tests specifically designed with content appropriate to the life focus of nonverbal physically handicapped children and standardized on this population must be developed. Until then, appropriate modifications of currently used tests, selection of a child's best response mode, and careful interpretation of test results must suffice.

REFERENCES

1. Baumann, U., Hanker, B., and Schian, M. M. Carba Linguaduc: *Application of Electronic Systems for the Physically Disabled.* Liebefeld-Bere, Germany: Carba A.G., 1977.
2. Boehm, A. E. *Boehm Test of Basic Concepts.* New York: The Psychological Corporation, 1971.
3. Bugemeister, B. B., Blum, L. A., and Lorge, I. *The Columbia Mental Maturity Test.* New York: Psychological Corporation, 1972.
4. Carrow, E. *Test for Auditory Comprehension of Language.* Austin, Texas: Educational Concepts, 1973.
5. Connolly, A. J., Nachtman, W., and Pritchett, E. M. *Key Math Diagnostic Arithmetic Test.* Circle Pines, Minn.: American Guidance Service, 1976.
6. Davis, J. *Perkins-Binet Tests of Intelligence for the Blind.* Watertown, Mass.: Perkins School for the Blind, 1980.
7. Duncan, D., et al. Nondiscriminatory assessment of severely physically handicapped individuals. *J. Assoc. Sev. Handicapped* 6 : 17, 1981.
8. Dunn, L. *The Peabody Picture Vocabulary Test-Revised.* Circle Pines, Minn.: American Guidance Service, 1981.
9. Dunn, L., and Markwardt, F. *Peabody Individual Achievement Test.* Circle Pines, Minn.: American Guidance Service, 1970.
10. French, J. *Pictorial Test of Intelligence.* Boston: Houghton Mifflin, 1964.
11. Hammel, D. *Detroit Tests of Learning Aptitude-2.* Austin, Tex.: PRO-ED, Inc., 1985.
12. Harris-Vanderheiden, D. Field Evaluation of the Auto-Comm. In G. Vanderheiden and K. Grilley (eds.), *Nonvocal Communication Techniques and Aids for the Severely Physically Handicapped.* Baltimore: University Park Press, 1975.
13. Hedrick, D., Prather, E. M., and Toben, A. R. *Sequenced Inventory of Communication Development.* Seattle: University of Washington Press, 1975.
14. Hiskey, M. *Hiskey-Nebraska Test of Learning Aptitude.* Lincoln, Nebr.: Union College Press, 1966.
15. Leiter, R. *Leiter International Performance Scale.* Chicago: Stoelting, 1959.
16. Mercer, J. *Labeling and the Mentally Retarded.* Berkeley, Calif.: University of California Press, 1973. (HV 3006 C 3M4)
17. Meyers, C. E., Sundstrom, P. E., and Yoshida, R. K. The school psychologist and assessment in special education. *School Psychol. Monogr.* 2 : 1, 1979.
18. Newcomer, P., and Hammill, D. *The Test of Language Development.* Austin, Tex.: PRO-ED, Inc. 1977.
19. Raven, J. *The Coloured Progressive Matrices.* Dumfries, Scotland: Grieve, 1963.
20. Salvia, J., and Ysseldyke, J. E. *Assessment in Special and Remedial Education.* Boston: Houghton Mifflin, 1978.
21. Vicker, B. (ed.). *Nonoral Communication Systems Project.* Iowa City: Campus Stores Publishers, The University of Iowa, 1974.

Test Reviews

Part II of *A Therapist's Guide to Pediatric Assessment* provides an in-depth evaluation of standardized tools in four areas: developmental and screening tests, sensorimotor tests, language tests, and psychological and cognitive tests.

All tests have been reviewed using the outline in Appendix B. Reviews are divided into five major sections, each with a concluding summary and references. The first section, *Descriptive Information,* includes preliminary information such as title, author, and publisher, type of client, and who can give the test. This section is useful for scanning a number of tests to find one that is appropriate for a particular child. The *Historical Perspective,* which follows, provides test development information. A review of pertinent literature is also found, which often includes studies providing further psychometric information (i.e., correlative or predictive validity). The third section, *Content and Test Administration,* gives detailed information regarding specific procedures. A description of scoring procedures and complexity is also included. *Psychometric Properties* are discussed in the fourth section, providing the examiner with a wealth of information regarding the confidence with which a particular test may be used. In Part I, Chapter 3, "Selection of Evaluation Instruments," provides the foundation for discussion of the terminology and concepts inherent in the standardization, reliability, and validity of published tests. The fifth section, *Guidelines for Use in a Clinical Setting,* offers practical information based on the reviewer's experience, for using a particular test, in-

cluding how it relates to other tests, the value of clinical observations, and use with different populations. For tests that can suitably be used with the physically handicapped, more detailed information can be found in Part I, Chapter 4, "Use of Standardized Tests with the Physically Handicapped."

The tests selected for review in Part II are the ones more commonly used by pediatric evaluators. However, the selections are also influenced by the regional bias of the authors. Developmental tests for the infant and toddler (from birth through 3 years) are one group of tests excluded from this book. Rather, the book focuses on the preschool and school-aged child. The impact of Pub. L 94–142 has provided increased impetus for the use of well-standardized evaluation tools with this population. Another group of tests that are excluded pertain to educational and special education assessment tools. Several published books have reviewed this group of tests [3–5, 7]. In addition, reference books such as *Tests in Print* [2] and *The Mental Measurement Yearbook Series* [1] provide an extensive listing of published tests and include brief critical reviews. A newly published book in the psychology field provides a very extensive review of 10 commonly used evaluation tools for children and adults, including the Halstead-Reitan Neuropsychological Test Battery [6], which is mentioned in the summary for Chapter 6.

Often tests provide in-depth evaluation of specific areas of function. In assessment, it is important to remember that a dysfunction or delay in one area can impede development in other areas. For example, the clumsy and poorly coordinated child may develop low self-esteem and poor social skills with peers secondary to lack of motor skills mastery. The visually handicapped child whose environmental experiences are severely limited may demonstrate secondary developmental delays in cognitive and social-emotional skills. Comprehensive assessment must be designed to evaluate the potential interaction of strengths and weaknesses in one area affecting skills development, positive or negative, in another area. Therefore, therapists are strongly encouraged to consider the concepts of team evaluation and ecological assessment discussed in Part I, Chapter 1, "The Assessment Process." With responsible assessment by skilled and knowledgable therapists, the lives of children with special needs can be enhanced.

REFERENCES

1. Buros, O. K. *The Ninth Mental Measurements Yearbook.* Highland Park, N.J.: Gryphon Press, 1985.
2. Buros, O. K. *Tests in Print,* Vol. 1. Hillsdale, N.J.: L. Erlbaum, 1984.
3. Compton, C. *A Guide to Seventy-five Tests for Special Education.* Belmont, Calif.: Fearon Education of Pittman Learning, 1984.
4. Donahue, L., et al. *A Guide to Special Education Tests.* Annapolis, Md.: Anne Arundel County Public Schools, 1982.
5. Mulliken, R. K., and Buckley, J. J. *Assessment of Multihandicapped and Developmentally Disabled Children.* Rockville, Md.: Aspen Systems, 1983.
6. Newmark, C. S. (ed.). *Major Psychological Assessment Instruments.* Newton, Mass.: Allyn & Bacon, 1985.
7. Salvia, J., and Ysseldyke, J. *Assessment in Special and Remedial Education.* Boston, Mass.: Houghton-Mifflin, 1981.

Developmental and Screening Tests

Shelley Stowers
Cathee J. Huber

A *developmental test,* for the purposes of this chapter, is defined as a nondiagnostic test from which information about more than two discrete aspects of development can be obtained. The test usually includes a survey of skills in several areas important to the progression of normal growth and development. Areas frequently tested include gross and fine motor skills, adaptive behavior skills, social skills, and language skills. Developmental testing provides a means for practitioners to assess the degree of maturation that a child has achieved in reaching a variety of developmental milestones relative to the degree of maturation expected for the child's chronological age.

Developmental tests typically fall into one of two categories: screening tests and assessment tests. *Screening tests* are intended to identify the presence, or possible presence, of deviations from normal growth and development as early as possible. Screening tests should never be thought of as diagnostic. *Assessment tests* are intended to document a pattern of strengths and weaknesses across the several developmental areas. They result in a description of functional age levels rather than in specific scores. Assessment test results are useful for designing intervention programs. The pattern of the child's strengths and weaknesses cues the practitioner as to which functional levels the child has already achieved, and what the next appropriate step is. Some assessment tests are so detailed that they can actually be used as the step-by-step intervention plan as well as the assessment instrument. Detailed assessment tests grew out of

a need expressed by preschool and developmental day-care program personnel for help in designing educational plans appropriate to the variety of individuals being served.

Tests in this chapter were selected for their appropriateness in surveying a variety of developmental skills, and on their applicability to a variety of settings. Some tests have as their purpose identification of developmental progress in medical settings, while others recognize that educational settings are appropriate places to document child development. Some were selected as examples of tests to be used only for screening or assessment, while others are examples of tests that can also be used to design specific programs of intervention. Some instruments were selected because of their focus on development of children with special sensory problems such as blindness; most, however, can be used for children with a variety of disabilities. All of the tests are focused on the early identification of problems or potential problems so that children can be placed in appropriate treatment settings (medical or educational) at the youngest age possible. All of the tests are available commercially.

Several instruments in this chapter are limited in presence or sophistication of standardization, reliability, and/or validity data. Their strengths are in areas such as potential for individual programming or assessing children with special sensory problems (blindness). Limitations in standardization and validation should not be ignored, but also should not preclude use of any test. Rather, professionals selecting such tests must accept responsibility for recognizing the weaknesses and taking them into account when deciding on their appropriateness.

The instruments reviewed in this chapter are divided into four general categories: tests designed specifically for screening, tests to be completed by parent report, tests that require a combination of parent report and examiner observation of the child, and tests for examining the development of visually impaired children. The following instruments are included:

Screening Tests
    Denver Developmental Screening Test
    Meeting Street School Screening Test
    Miller Assessment for Preschoolers
Tests Requring Parent Report
    Developmental Profile II (Alpern-Boll)
    Vineland Adaptive Behavior Scales
Tests Requiring Parent Report and Examiner
        Observation
    Gesell Preschool Test
    Learning Accomplishment Profile-
        Diagnostic
    Learning Accomplishment Profile-Revised
    Vulpé Assessment Battery
Tests for Visually Impaired Children
    Reynell-Zinkin Developmental Scales for
        Young Visually Handicapped Children
    A Social Maturity Scale for Blind Preschool
        Children

Screening Tests

DENVER DEVELOPMENTAL SCREENING TEST

Descriptive Information

Test Identification

The title of this test is the Denver Developmental Screening Test (DDST). It was first published in 1967 and has been revised several times (1970, 1973, 1975). The most recent editions include a *Manual/Workbook for Nursing and Medical Personnel* (1973), and a *Reference Manual* (1975). W. K. Frankenburg, M.D., and J. B. Dodds, Ph.D., are the authors of the original DDST; W. K. Frankenburg, M.D., J. B. Dodds, Ph.D., and A. W. Fandal are authors of the 1970 and 1973 editions; and the authors of the 1975 edition are W. K. Frankenburg, M.D., J. B. Dodds, Ph.D., A. W. Fandal, E. Kazuk, M.A., and M. Cohrs. Frankenburg and Dodds were with the Departments of Pediatrics and Psychiatry, respectively, in the Clinical Psychology Division, University of Colorado School of Medicine, Denver at the time the DDST was developed. DDM Inc. P.O. Box 20037, Denver, Colorado 80220 publishes the test. Approximate prices for the various items pertaining to the DDST are listed below:

Item	*Price*
DDST Complete Package (Test Kit, 1 pad of forms, 1 manual/workbook)	$37.00–$41.00
DDST Test Kit	$19.00–$21.00
DDST Test Forms-Original (100/pad)	$10.00–$11.00
	$11.00–$13.00 in Spanish
DDST Test Forms-Revised (100/pad)	$10.00–$11.00
DDST Manual/Workbook (English only)	$15.00–$17.00
DDST Reference Manual	$10.50–$12.00
	$11.00–$13.00 in Spanish

Item	Price
DDST Training Film or Videotape for Nurses	
Film	
Rental	$100.00–$110.00
Videotape	
Rental	$ 90.00–$100.00
Purchase	$300.00–$350.00
DDST Training Film or Videotape for Paraprofessionals	
Film	
Rental	$100.00–$110.00
Videotape	
Rental	$ 90.00–$100.00
Purchase	$300.00–$350.00
Introduction to the DDST for Professionals	
Videotape	
Rental	$ 60.00–$70.00
Purchase	$200.00–$250.00

10% Shipping and handling will be added to all orders.

Age and Type of Client

The DDST can be used with any child between birth and 6 years of age.

Purpose

The DDST is designed to help health providers detect early indications of developmental deviations in young children. There are currently two approaches to using the DDST. Item administration is exactly the same using either approach. The difference is in whether the original DDST (Fig. 5-1) or revised DDST-R (see Figs. 5-3, 5-4) score sheet is used and whether the long or abbreviated testing procedure is used [13].

Time Required to Administer and Score Test

The original version of the DDST takes approximately 15–30 minutes to administer (Fig. 5-2), while the revised version takes approximately 5–7 minutes. Scoring either version takes only a few minutes.

Evaluator

The authors of the DDST state that most interested adults (professional or nonprofessional) can be taught to administer the DDST with only a few hours of training and supervision. It has been pointed out by other authors that examiners must be prepared to make some subjective observations in addition to the standardized objective observations. Because of the use of subjective observations, it has been argued that examiners should have some understanding of child development in order to make judgments about events that may be affecting test performance such as relationship to tester and attention span [6, 15].

Historical Perspective Of Test Construction

Development and Source of Test Items

The 105 items comprising the DDST were selected from 12 preschool intelligence tests and

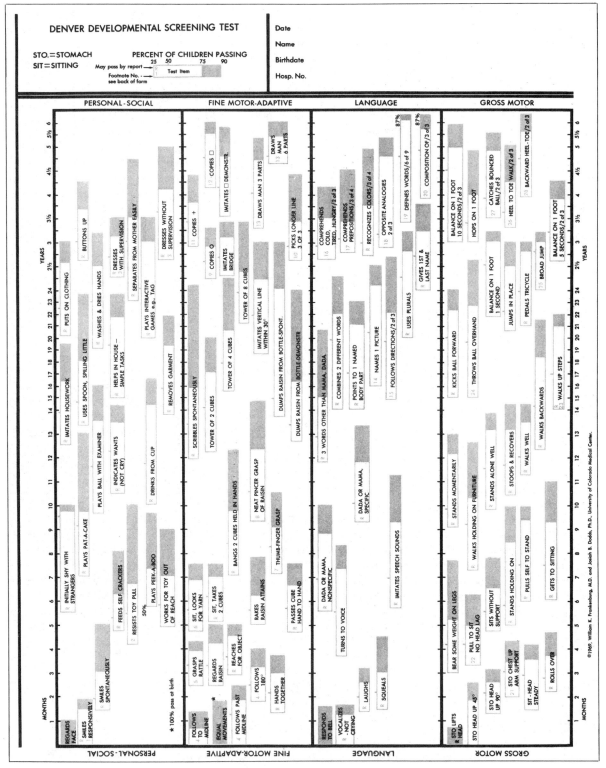

Fig. 5-1. Original scoring form for the Denver Developmental Screening Test. (Reproduced by permission.)

		DATE
		NAME
DIRECTIONS		BIRTHDATE
		HOSP. NO.

1. Try to get child to smile by smiling, talking or waving to him. Do not touch him.
2. When child is playing with toy, pull it away from him. Pass if he resists.
3. Child does not have to be able to tie shoes or button in the back.
4. Move yarn slowly in an arc from one side to the other, about 6" above child's face.
    Pass if eyes follow 90° to midline. (Past midline; 180°)
5. Pass if child grasps rattle when it is touched to the backs or tips of fingers.
6. Pass if child continues to look where yarn disappeared or tries to see where it went. Yarn
    should be dropped quickly from sight from tester's hand without arm movement.
7. Pass if child picks up raisin with any part of thumb and a finger.
8. Pass if child picks up raisin with the ends of thumb and index finger using an over hand
    approach.

9. Pass any en-
    closed form.
    Fail continuous
    round motions.
10. Which line is longer?
    (Not bigger.) Turn
    paper upside down and
    repeat. (3/3 or 5/6)
11. Pass any
    crossing
    lines.
12. Have child copy
    first. If failed,
    demonstrate

When giving items 9, 11 and 12, do not name the forms. Do not demonstrate 9 and 11.

13. When scoring, each pair (2 arms, 2 legs, etc.) counts as one part.
14. Point to picture and have child name it. (No credit is given for sounds only.)

15. Tell child to: Give block to Mommie; put block on table; put block on floor. Pass 2 of 3.
    (Do not help child by pointing, moving head or eyes.)
16. Ask child: What do you do when you are cold? ..hungry? ..tired? Pass 2 of 3.
17. Tell child to: Put block on table; under table; in front of chair, behind chair.
    Pass 3 of 4. (Do not help child by pointing, moving head or eyes.)
18. Ask child: If fire is hot, ice is ?; Mother is a woman, Dad is a ?; a horse is big, a
    mouse is ?. Pass 2 of 3.
19. Ask child: What is a ball? ..lake? ..desk? ..house? ..banana? ..curtain? ..ceiling?
    ..hedge? ..pavement? Pass if defined in terms of use, shape, what it is made of or general
    category (such as banana is fruit, not just yellow). Pass 6 of 9.
20. Ask child: What is a spoon made of? ..a shoe made of? ..a door made of? (No other objects
    may be substituted.) Pass 3 of 3.
21. When placed on stomach, child lifts chest off table with support of forearms and/or hands.
22. When child is on back, grasp his hands and pull him to sitting. Pass if head does not hang back.
23. Child may use wall or rail only, not person. May not crawl.
24. Child must throw ball overhand 3 feet to within arm's reach of tester.
25. Child must perform standing broad jump over width of test sheet. (8-1/2 inches)
26. Tell child to walk forward,   heel within 1 inch of toe.
    Tester may demonstrate. Child must walk 4 consecutive steps, 2 out of 3 trials.
27. Bounce ball to child who should stand 3 feet away from tester. Child must catch ball with
    hands, not arms, 2 out of 3 trials.
28. Tell child to walk backward,   toe within 1 inch of heel.
    Tester may demonstrate. Child must walk 4 consecutive steps, 2 out of 3 trials.

DATE AND BEHAVIORAL OBSERVATIONS (how child feels at time of test, relation to tester, attention
span, verbal behavior, self-confidence, etc,):

Fig. 5-2. Directions for Denver Developmental Screening Test. (Reproduced by permission.)

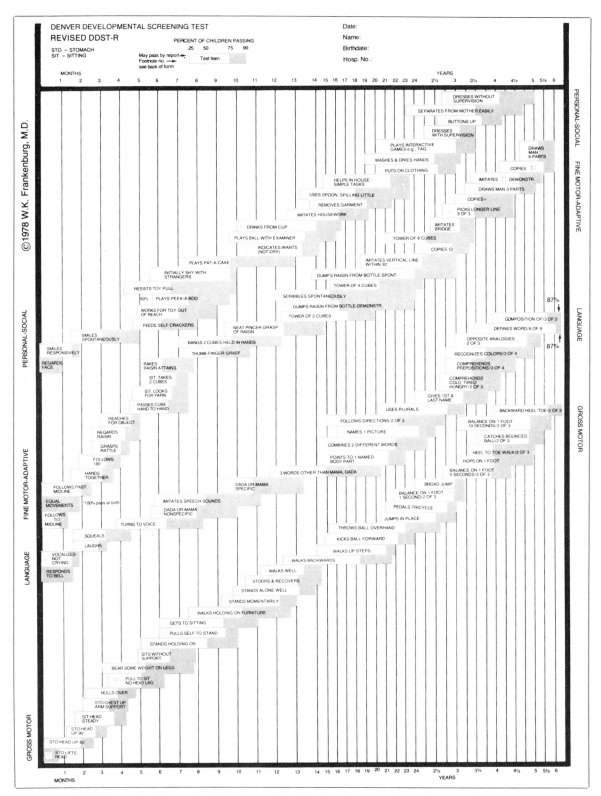

Fig. 5-3. *Revised scoring form for the Denver Developmental Screening Test (DDST-R). Items on the revised form are identical to those on the original scoring form and are arranged on the revised form to approximate a growth chart, providing a more "dynamic profile" of progression and development. (Reproduced by permission.)*

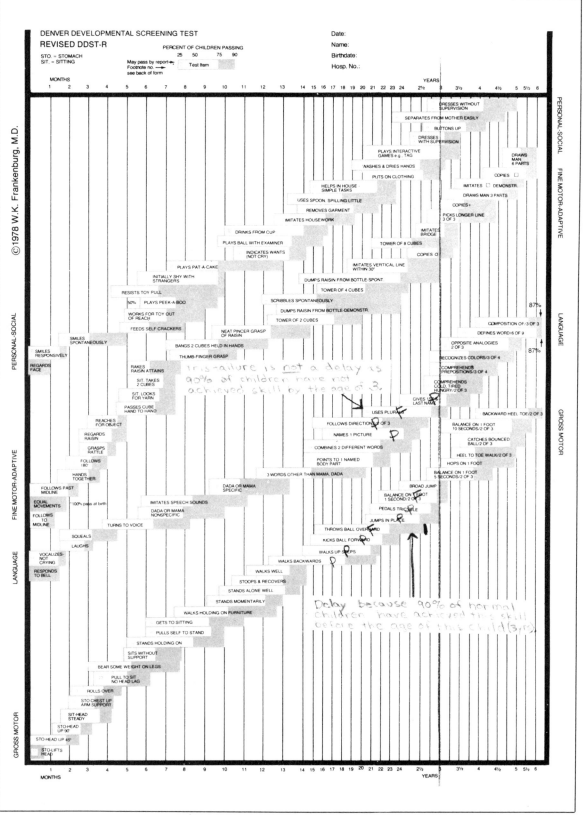

Fig. 5-4. Sample scored DDST-R demonstrating scoring of failed item versus delay.

developmental instruments. Inclusion in the final version required that each item be easy to administer, easy to score without ambiguity, and have a relatively short distribution (brief span of time between age at which some children begin to do a task and age by which most of the standardization sample had accomplished the task).

Review of Literature in Terms of Test Use

The DDST is widely used by a variety of professionals. It can also be used by a variety of non-professionals since there is no need to have special training in psychology or testing in order to qualify as a test user. The test format is particularly useful since the rate of development can be charted on one form over a 6-year period, and since relatively few items must be administered during any one testing session. Its adaptability is further enhanced since some items can be responded to by parent report, thus allowing the tester to make constructive use of time while the child adjusts to the testing situation. Finally, the format promotes giving anticipatory guidance to parents regarding upcoming expectations for their child's developmental progress.

This screening test has been used routinely in many settings where child health and developmental surveillance is carried out. Pediatricians' offices, health department well-child clinics, and preschool programs are common sites where it is frequently administered. The DDST is one of several observational screening tests that have been recommended for use in the Early and Periodic Screening, Diagnosis and Treatment (EPSDT) Program sponsored by Medicaid.

Some attempt has been made to predict school-related problems from early DDST scores. Camp et al. followed 65 children from low socioeconomic environments in Denver, Colorado, who were evaluated during their preschool years (ages 4–6 years) with the DDST and the Stanford-Binet Intelligence Test [5]. These 65 children were at least of third-grade age when studied for presence of school-related problems, and all had

been administered additional IQ tests after school entrance. School problems were defined as (1) repeating a grade, (2) enrollment in a program for educationally handicapped children, (3) enrollment in a program for educable or trainable mentally retarded children, (4) third grade achievement test scores more than 1½ years below grade level, or failing grades, (5) presence of significant behavior problems interfering with school performance as indicated by teacher checklist scores, and (6) referral for evaluation of hyperactivity or behavior or learning problems as indicated by health center records. From these data, the 65 children in the study were divided into three groups: (1) educational retardation and individual intelligence quotient (IQ) test scores below 80, (2) learning problems in school in combination with adequate intelligence (IQ 80 and above), and (3) normal (IQ above 80 and no learning or behavior problems in school). It was found that 88 percent of the children with abnormal DDSTs, 66 percent of those with questionable DDSTs, and 32 percent of the children with normal DDSTs had school problems. The authors concluded that the relationship between classification on the DDST and later school status is highly significant, and that children with either abnormal or questionable results should be referred for further testing when the purpose of the DDST is to identify children with potential learning problems. (*Note:* When the purpose of screening with this test is to achieve the best separation between children who are potentially mentally retarded and those who are not, other data suggest that questionable scores should be grouped with normals [11]).

The DDST has been widely used on various populations throughout the United States and in other countries. Sandler et al. emphasize that caution must be exercised when applying published normative data to dissimilar groups [17]. They studied one hundred four 4 to 6 year olds living in a lower-class, urban neighborhood. Many of these children were found to have delayed language acquisition, to seem to have little interest in doing the "right thing" rather than what they wanted to do, and to be suspicious of the examiner. Sandler et al. suggest that performance on a test such as the DDST is of little value without accompanying information regarding family background, cultural behavioral expectations, and normal adaptive responses to living experiences encountered. It is of note that several studies have been conducted in attempts to derive norms for specific populations [1, 3, 19, 20].

Theoretical Constructs and Implications for Intervention

The DDST is based on theories underlying normal growth and development. It is also based on theories on which the 12 developmental tests from which items were selected are based (i.e., Bayley Scales of Infant Development; Cattell Infant Intelligence Scale; Gesell Developmental Schedules; Griffith Developmental Scale; Hetzer-Wolf Baby Scales from the Vienna Test; Merrill-Palmer Scale of Mental Tests; Revised Yale Developmental Schedules; Stanford-Binet Intelligence Scale; Vineland Social Maturity Scale; Lincoln-Oseretsky Motor Development Scale; Communication Evaluation Chart; and the California Developmental Charts) [7]. The DDST was constructed because of concern of the authors that developmental delays were not being discovered until the children suffering from them entered school and objective testing was done for the first time. Children were not being seen routinely after infancy in pediatric settings where developmental testing could occur; or if they were, their pediatricians were frequently not doing objective testing. If testing was done, it was more often from nonstandardized developmental scales devised by the pediatricians themselves (consisting of items taken from various standard psychological tests).

This screening test has a number of implications for intervention. Of objective, standardized developmental screening tests used in places where young children gather (e.g., health departments, pediatricians' offices, preschools),

the DDST is probably the best known and the most widely used. Use of this test has led to increased opportunity for early detection and intervention for more children and to increased opportunity to give anticipatory guidance to more parents. It has occasionally been used as an outcome measure in research studies [16], and it is possible to determine a mental age on the DDST, although this is not recommended since the test was not designed for that purpose [11].

Some concern has been expressed regarding the possibility of cultural bias by the DDST. O'Pray points out that varying experiences and family background may influence children's behaviors (verbal responsiveness, relationship to tester, attention span, and self-confidence) as well as specific knowledge such as the word definitions required as part of DDST performance [15]. Sandler et al. agree that knowledge of environmental conditions (including living conditions and significant interpersonal relationships) is necessary before deficiencies in functioning can be interpreted [17]. Fleming states, "The test is not entirely sensitive to antecedent events, historical background including socioeconomic background, or to individual variations" [6]. She concludes, however, that if it is used as a screening tool (as designed) and not an assessment tool, it is capable of serving its purpose as a valid and reliable instrument for alerting examiners to possible problems.

Content and Test Administration

Content

The four areas tested by the DDST include personal-social (awareness of and response to people and things in the environment), fine-motor adaptive (eye-hand coordination activities, visual- and audioperceptual activities), language (receptive and expressive), and gross motor (large-muscle coordination activities). Age levels proceed at 1-month increments to 24 months, and at 3-month increments from 24 months to 6 years. Most test items span intervals of several months.

Test items for the DDST come in a bag shaped like a shaving kit and include the following:

Red wool pompom
Rattle with narrow handle
Small bell
Tennis ball
Small clear glass bottle with ⅝-in. opening
Pencil
Ten 1-in. square wooden blocks
Small box of raisins

The kit also comes with a small card on which a summary of how to interpret DDST results is printed. The only thing necessary for test administration that is not included in the kit is drawing paper for the older children.

Score sheets for the DDST are currently available in two formats. Each contains exactly the same items and the same number of items. The age range of each item is exactly the same. The most familiar format is arranged in four horizontal sectors, with items in each sector spanning the appropriate chronological age (see Figs. 5-1, 5-2). Chronological ages from birth to 6 years are listed across the top and bottom of the form. An age line is drawn to connect the child's current chronological age at the top with that at the bottom. Items intersected or touched by the age line are indicative of the items that must be administered at any testing session.

In 1981, a second DDST score sheet format was designed in order to ". . . provide a more dynamic profile of a child's developmental growth" [13]. This format resembles a normal growth curve. The four sectors are still discrete, but items at the lowest age levels in each sector begin at the bottom left side and progress upward to the right with increasing chronological age. This revised form is referred to as the *DDST-R* (see Fig. 5-3). The age line, defining which items need to be administered, is drawn in the same manner as on

the original form. Helpful footnotes referring to administration of selected items are found on the back of both forms.

Setting and Equipment

Administration of the DDST requires a relatively quiet room with enough space for a child to perform gross motor activities. Since comfort is a prerequisite for best performance, furniture should include a child-sized table and chair, and adult-sized chairs for the parent or caretaker and screener. The only testing equipment required, other than that in the test kit, is drawing paper for older children.

Administration Procedures

The DDST must be administered to just one child at a time. It requires observation of the child's response to directions given by the screener. Some items can be credited through report of a parent or caretaker who knows the child well. If a child is particularly shy, the parent or caretaker may administer the test items, but only after careful instruction by the screener.

Two versions of the test manual are available: the *Manual/Workbook for Nursing and Paramedical Personnel* [9] and the *Reference Manual* [12]. (*Note:* Either test format can be used with either manual.) The *Manual/Workbook* contains information about standardization and validation of the test, as well as practice questions with worksheets and answers. The *Reference Manual* is similar to the *Manual/Workbook* but does not contain the sample questions and worksheets. Both manuals contain clear, concise directions for administration of each test item.

Once familiarity with the DDST is gained, it is not a complex procedure to administer. Inaccurate information will result, however, if time is not taken to gain adequate rapport with the child, or if the items are not correctly administered. This point cannot be emphasized too strongly; if accurate information is to result from use of the DDST, it *must* be administered according to standardized directions included in the manual.

Scoring

Very precise, clear instructions are available for scoring the DDST. Instructions for scoring each test item are given in the manual immediately following the instructions for its administration.

There are two acceptable methods of scoring the DDST, one most appropriately used with each of the two versions of the test form. The original format requires that each item touched or intersected by the age line be scored as pass (P), fail (F), refused (R), or N.O. (no opportunity for the experience, i.e., no exposure to use of materials required in test item, such as a tricycle). In each sector it is necessary to test forward from the age line until the child has failed three items, and backward until at least three items have been passed. When the test is administered and scored in this manner, it is referred to as the *full DDST*.

The DDST-R is an abbreviated version. On the form the screener identifies and administers the three items immediately to the left of the age line in each sector for a total of 12 items. If any of these three items in any sector is failed (indicating a delay) or refused (indicating a potential delay), a full DDST must be given.

The DDST can be interpreted as being normal, abnormal, questionable, or untestable. The category into which each individual test result falls depends on the number of items indicating presence of a delay. A *delay* is defined as any item falling completely to the left of the age line that was failed. A failed item intersected by the age line is not considered a delay (see Fig. 5-4). The total number of delays determines whether a test result is normal, abnormal, questionable, or untestable. The procedure for determining presence of each category is clearly outlined in the test manual.

Whenever the results of a child's DDST are ab-

normal, questionable, or untestable, plans for rescreening in 2 to 3 weeks should be made. The rescreening appointment should be at a time during the day when the child would not be expected to be tired or hungry. If rescreening results are still abnormal, questionable, or untestable, and if the performance is reported to be a typical one, the child should be referred to a person qualified to do developmental testing.

Psychometric Properties

Standardization

Both the *Reference Manual* and the *Manual/Workbook* contain the specific instructions necessary for administering items on the DDST in a standard fashion. Equally specific instructions are included for talking with parents, preparing the test form, and interpreting results. In addition, other materials are available to aid in learning the correct method to administer the test. These materials include a training film (or videotape) for paraprofessionals and a videotaped introduction to the DDST for professionals who will be involved in supervising the administration of the DDST (including rationale for developmental screening, rationale for development of the DDST, and demonstration of proper DDST administration).

The same standardization data were used as the basis for both the DDST and DDST-R. Standardization took place in the 1960s on 1036 children (543 male, 493 females), in Denver, Colorado, who were considered normal. They ranged in age from 2 weeks to 6 years 4 months, and were divided into 25 age groupings, with from 34 to 47 children in each group. The sample in the standardization study reflected socioethnic and occupational characteristics of the Denver population according to the 1960 census.

Normative data were obtained through calculations of the percent of children in each age group passing each test item. A smoothed percent-passing curve was computed for each item, and a point on the curve was determined to represent the chronological age at which 25, 50, 75, and 90 percent of the children passed the test item.

Reliability

Test-retest reliability (stability over time) has been reported for the DDST as a whole [15]. One hundred and eighty-six children were tested 1 week apart by each of two examiners. These examiners achieved 97 percent agreement on classification of the same sample of children. Test-retest reliability has also been reported for individual test items [12]. Twenty children ranging in age from 2 months to 5½ years were tested by the same examiner at an interval of 1 week. Stability between test items over this short interval was 95.8 percent.

Interobserver reliability (consistency) has also been reported for both individual test items and for the DDST as a whole. Several children from the standardization study took part in determination of interobserver reliability of individual test items [12]. Four examiners each tested a group consisting of children of varying ages. The average percentage of agreement on items passed or failed was 90 percent.

Consistency for classification by the DDST as a whole was reported in a study done in Cardiff, Wales [2]. Ninety-six babies approximately 1 year of age were examined by two of six designated screeners. Percentages of children on whom there was exact agreement between two examiners were as follows: personal and social sector, 79 percent; fine motor–adaptive sector, 83 percent; language sector, 83 percent; gross motor sector, 95 percent; whole test, 96 percent.

A study to determine reliability between the DDST and DDST-R has also been reported. The purpose of the study was to determine the amount of agreement between " . . . the scoring of individual items and the total test when items were scored independently and simultaneously by two research assistants (who alternated examination and observation responsibilities)'' [13]. Two hundred children representing six age groups (birth–6 months = 50; 7–12 months = 15; 13–18 months = 15; 19–24 months = 15; 25 months–4 years = 55; 5–6 years = 50) were evaluated. Subjects were selected from several settings (Head Start, day care, inpatient pediatric units, health departments, private pediatric offices, local swim classes) in an effort to include children manifesting both normal and abnormal results. Three teams, each consisting of two reliable examiners, administered the tests. Results indicated a mean of 97 percent agreement between examiners on scoring of individual test items. Agreement between the DDST and DDST-R was determined for both the full version (22–25 items) and the short version (12 items). Agreement on classification by the two forms on the full test was 100 percent, and on the abbreviated test was 98 percent.

Validity

The DDST was validated most recently using the Bayley Scales of Infant Development or the Stanford-Binet Intelligence Test (depending on age of child) as the criterion test [12]. Validation apparently took place after one screening test administration, even though rescreening is recommended for children scoring questionable, abnormal, or untestable results on the DDST. A total of 1,292 children were screened with the DDST. All those receiving abnormal results (N = 20) or questionable results (N = 54), and 172 of those receiving normal results, were given either the Bayley or Stanford-Binet [10]. Depending on how the data are grouped, screening test validity (percentage of agreement between classification of same group of children by screening and by diagnostic measure) ranges from 96 to 75 percent; sensitivity (ability of screening test to identify abnormal as abnormal) ranges from 92 to 100 percent; and specificity (ability of screening test to identify normal as normal) ranges from 97 to 74 percent [18].

Frankenburg refers to *copositivity* (probability that screening test results will be positive when reference test results are positive) and *conegativ-*

ity (probability that screening test results will be negative when reference test results are negative) instead of sensitivity and specificity [8, 12]. They are similar measures and are calculated in the same way. Sensitivity and specificity are considered comparisons between the screening or reference test in question and the "true diagnosis" [11]. Copositivity and conegativity may be more appropriately used when comparing a screening test with a reference test.

When results of a second test are used for validation of the screening test, the indices of agreement derived from the 2 × 2 table are not identical with sensitivity and specificity, because these two qualities can be determined only in reference to the true diagnosis [4].

Decisions to use one set of terms or the other seems to be related, in part, to how diagnostically sound the test against which screening test results are to be compared is considered to be.

Guidelines for Use in a Clinical Setting

Since the DDST includes both parent report and child performance items, and since it examines several basic areas of development across a relatively wide age range, it can be appropriately used for any child with a chronological age between 0 months and 6 years. Performance on the DDST can indicate strengths and weaknesses in individual abilities and, therefore, is useful in deciding what kind of referral to make.

It is important to remember that the DDST is a screening test, and the results should never be interpreted as diagnostic. It provides a good, quickly administered look at general development and may be used to determine relative strengths and weaknesses as a basis for further referral and testing.

It is possible to make some valuable clinical observations on the basis of the DDST. Clinicians should be aware that the test fails to require observations of bilateral activities in some instances where that may be of importance (e.g., balancing on one foot, stacking and other activities using the hands). In addition, children doing

poorly in the language sector or in following directions should have their ears checked immediately rather than waiting 2 to 3 weeks for rescreening. Since the DDST is a general screening test, some of the more discrete steps in the various developmental areas are not observed. Close follow-up may be required for children who are not accomplishing items in any sector toward the end of the range of time generally considered to be within normal limits.

Review

The DDST is a test of general development covering the critical periods for development of social, fine motor, gross motor, and language skills. It can be used by a variety of professionals to identify developmental delays or to provide anticipatory guidance. The combined interview observation format is helpful for encouraging performance by shy children and for obtaining some information about children who cannot or will not perform.

Standardization data are available, but are limited to the Denver, Colorado, area. Unless local norms have been established, caution should be exercised when using the DDST on groups of children from rural or urban areas that may differ substantially from the Denver population. While the number of children in the overall standardization sample was adequate, the number in the various age groups was small.

Screening test validation data, based on positive correlations between the DDST and the Bayley Scales of Infant Development or the Stanford-Binet, do exist for the DDST. It should be noted that wide variations in interpretation of these data result depending on how the "questionable" category is used. Since the DDST is one of the few screening tests for which such data exist, it is the responsibility of the screener to be familiar with the test's strengths and weaknesses as supported by these data.

The DDST has been used for a variety of purposes including general developmental surveillance, preschool screening, EPSDT (Early

Periodic Screening, Diagnosis and Treatment) evaluation, prediction of school-related problems, and restandardization to additional population groups. Limitations of the DDST include limited sensitivity to antecedent events, to historical background including socioeconomic status, and to individual variation including prematurity [6, 14, 15].

In a recent study, the effect of prematurity on DDST performance was evaluated [14]. Although the basic validity of the policy for testing prematures set forth by Frankenburg, Dodds, and Fandal [9] is upheld, the Niparko study suggested:

1. Prematurity may be an influential factor on DDST performance that is *not* efficiently compensated for simply by adjustment of age (validity of scores may be increased by consideration of the nonadjusted score or, more important, by the amount of discrepancy between adjusted and nonadjusted scores).
2. Adjustment of age is not necessary after a chronological age of 6 months for children born after 34 weeks gestation.
3. Normal children resulting from pregnancies of less than 34 weeks tend to perform normally for chronological age sometime after 6 months chronological age, but the point at which this occurs could not be definitely determined.
4. "Very" premature infants were not shown statistically to achieve a normal performance according to their chronological age within the first year.
5. DDST results were uniformly inferior at 5 and 8 months. This may be the result of a greater number of items requiring recently acquired skills at these ages.

The DDST remains one of the most widely used developmental screening tools in the world. When a practitioner takes professional responsibility for knowledge of its strengths and weaknesses, it is a very useful screening instrument.

In general, screening and rescreening guidelines offered in the test manual are adequate. Practitioners should be alert to two exceptions:

1. Motor activities are tested unilaterally. Children with weaknesses involving an upper or lower extremity are likely to use the stronger side, and the weakness may be missed by the screener.
2. When language delays are found, immediate action should be taken to determine whether or not a hearing loss is present. Hearing loss may be due to an ear infection, which should be treated immediately and not left alone until rescreening can be accomplished.

REFERENCES

1. Barnes, K., and Stark, A. The Denver Developmental Screening Test: A normative study. *Am. J. Public Health* 65 : 363, 1975.
2. Bryant, G., et al. A preliminary study of the use of the Denver Developmental Screening Test in a health department. *Dev. Med. Child Neurol.* 15 : 33, 1973.
3. Bryant, G., et al. Standardization of the Denver Developmental Screening Test for Cardiff children. *Dev. Med. Child Neurol.* 21 : 353, 1979.
4. Buck, A., and Gart, J. Comparison of a screening test and a reference test in epidemiologic studies. *Am. J. Epidemiol.* 83 : 586, 1966.
5. Camp, B., et al. Preschool developmental testing in prediction of school problems. *Clin. Pediatr.* 16 : 257, 1977.
6. Fleming, J. An evaluation of the use of the Denver Developmental Screening Test. *Nurs. Res.* 30 : 126, 1980.
7. Frankenburg, W. K., and Dodds, J. B. The Denver Developmental Screening Test. *J. Pediatr.* 71 : 181, 1967.
8. Frankenburg, W. K. Criteria in Screening Test Selection. In W. K. Frankenburg and B. W. Camp (eds.), *Pediatric Screening Tests.* Springfield, Ill.: Thomas, 1975.
9. Frankenburg, W. K., Dodds, J. B., and Fandal, A. *Denver Developmental Screening Test: Manual* (Revised 1970 Edition). Denver: University of Colorado Medical Center, 1970.
9a. Frankenburg, W. K., Dodds, J. B., and Fandal, A.

Denver Developmental Screening Test: Manual/ Workbook for Nursing and Paramedical Personnel. Denver: University of Colorado Medical Center, 1973.

10. Frankenburg, W. K., Goldstein, A. D., and Camp, B. W. The revised Denver Developmental Screening Test: Its accuracy as a screening instrument. *J. Pediatr.* 79 : 988, 1971.

11. Frankenburg, W. K., Camp, B. W., and Van Natta, P. A. Validity of the Denver Developmental Screening Test. *Child Dev.* 42 : 475, 1971.

12. Frankenburg, W. K., et al. *Denver Developmental Screening Test: Reference Manual* (Revised 1975 Edition). Denver: University of Colorado Medical Center, 1975.

13. Frankenburg, W. K., et al. The newly abbreviated and revised Denver Developmental Screening Test. *J. Pediatr.* 99 : 995, 1981.

14. Niparko, N. The effect of prematurity on performance on the Denver Developmental Screening Test. *Phys. Occup. Ther. Pediatr.* 2 : 29, 1982.

15. O'Pray, M. Developmental screening tools: Using them effectively. *Matern. Child Nurs. J.* 5 : 126, 1980.

16. Robischon, P. Pica Practice and Other Hand-Mouth Behavior and Children's Developmental Level. In F. S. Downs and M. A. Newman (eds.), *A Source Book of Nursing Research.* Philadelphia: Davis, 1977.

17. Sandler, L., et al. Responses of urban preschool children to a developmental screening test. *J. Pediatr.* 77 : 775, 1970.

18. Stangler, S., et al. *Screening Growth and Development of Preschool Children: A Guide for Test Selection.* New York: McGraw-Hill, 1980.

19. Ulda, R. Standardization of the Denver Developmental Screening Test on Tokyo children. *Dev. Med. Child Neurol.* 20 : 647, 1978.

20. Ulda, R. Child development in Okinowa compared with Tokyo and Denver, and the implications for developmental screening. *Dev. Med. Child Neurol.* 20 : 657, 1978.

MEETING STREET SCHOOL SCREENING TEST

Descriptive Information

Test Identification

The title of this test is *Early Identification of Children with Learning Disabilities: The Meeting Street School Screening Test* (MSSST), 1969. Its authors are Peter K. Hainsworth and Marian L. Siqueland; both were working as psychologists at the time the MSSST was published.

The Easter Seal Society of Rhode Island, Inc., Meeting Street School (667 Waterman Ave., East Providence, Rhode Island 02914) publishes this test at a cost of $12–$15 for the manual, $5–$6 (for 50) or $9–$10 (for 100) test forms (four pages including child's work sheet and examiner's score sheet). Shipping and handling charges are paid on all *prepaid* orders.

Age and Type of Client

The MSSST is designed to be used with children of kindergarten and first grade age (5 years 0 months to 7 years 5 months) who do not have requisite language and visual-perceptual-motor control to absorb the symbolic information included in the traditional curriculum.

Purpose

The purpose of this test is to identify young children who exhibit psychoneurological skills frequently felt by teachers to be inefficient in those with learning disabilities. A child with learning disabilities is defined as one with ". . . adequate mental ability, sensory processes, and emotional stability, who has specific deficits in perceptual, integrative, or expressive processes which severely impair learning efficiency" [2]. More specifically, the MSSST is intended to aid in determination of a child's effectiveness in processing information through gross motor, visual-perceptual-motor, and language modalities. Concentration is placed on skills felt to be typically inefficient in children with learning disabilities, including ability to attend, organize, and carry through with specific tasks. The MSSST can be used as either a screening or a diagnostic test. It results in a profile of specific skills and in a rating of behavioral manifestations that can expose characteristics of children with learning disabilities.

Time Required to Administer and Score Test

Usually 15 to 20 minutes is needed to administer the MSSST once the examiner is thoroughly familiar with it. Scoring is simply a matter of summing numbers to obtain raw scores and then converting the raw scores to scaled scores.

Evaluation

This test can be used by any professional with interest and experience in working with young children, particularly in the educational, psychological, and medically related fields. No individual professions are specifically identified as being most appropriate. Professionals can use the test for either screening or diagnostic purposes, and must take responsibility for using it correctly in either instance.

The MSSST can also be used by nonprofessionals who have been well trained. Ability to make the test meaningful enough to the child to allow best performance is defined by the authors as a prerequisite ability. Nonprofessionals should not use the test unless they have received technical training and are under supervision by a professional. Interpretation of test results remains the responsibility of the professional.

Historical Perspective
Of Test Construction

Development and Source of Test Items

The MSSST was developed following concern about the large number of 7- to 14-year-old children who, because of difficulty learning in school accompanied by various degrees of behavioral and emotional disturbances, were referred to the Meeting Street School for evaluation of suspected learning difficulties. The items developed are based on experiences of the school's professional staff in evaluating children with neurological dysfunction, and were chosen to ". . . tap the common gross motor, visual-perceptual-motor, and language deficits and quirks manifested by the learning disability child" [2]. The test items

were taken from assessment procedures designed to assess neurological, psychological, physical, occupational, and language skills in children with cerebral palsy and related disorders [1]. The test contains 15 groups of items with varying numbers of individual tasks within each group.

Review of the Literature in Terms of Test Use

The MSSST can be used as part of a program for early identification of learning disabilities, either as a screening measure or as an adjunct to a diagnostic evaluation. As a screening test it is expected to identify children who have poor information processing skills. As part of a diagnostic evaluation it can be expected to add an additional dimension to the "traditional" evaluation by identification of information processing skills. The authors envisioned its use as part of an overall program for early identification in school systems; this program might include the following steps:

1. Establish need and encourage staff participation in a way that will demonstrate the constructive educational plans that can result from such participation.
2. Incorporate efficient use of all available sources of information, perhaps through implementation of the "progressive screening process":
   a. Administer "gross indices" (teacher observation, group tests of IQ or readiness).
   b. Investigate the suspect children with a more complex procedure (such as the MSSST).
   c. Refer the children who do poorly on the MSSST to appropriate sources for more in-depth evaluation (e.g., diagnostic testing, ongoing educational evaluation).
3. Follow up the early identification program in a way that will enhance its meaningfulness for both children (through placement in intervention programs) and personnel (e.g., through participation in curriculum change, increase in understanding of development

and in understanding of children with learning disabilities).

If the MSSST is used early in a child's school career, it may provide preliminary identification of those at risk for learning disability. If used later in the year, it may be combined with teacher observation and group testing results, leading to further isolation of the problem and appropriate intervention. Results of the MSSST could be used by a variety of professionals. Some, such as medical or nursing professionals, may use the results primarily as a basis for referral. Others, such as teachers or occupational therapists, may use the results to provide input for individualized plans.

Theoretical Constructs and Implications for Intervention

The theoretical framework within which development of the MSSST took place is called the Information Processing Model (an adaptation of the Psycholinguistic Model on which the Illinois Test of Psycholinguistic Abilities is based) [3, 4]. Specific components of this model are included in Table 5-1. It is felt that children with learning disabilities characteristically have trouble either in one or more of the five processes through which information flows (i.e., orientation, intake, integration, output, and feedback) or across one or more of the three major modalities through which education usually takes place (visual-perceptual-motor, language, or body awareness and control). In addition, they may have trouble with behavioral organization (do not orient, integrate, or feedback properly). There is a complex relationship between information processing skills and intelligence, but the authors feel that, compared with intelligence tests, the MSSST measures different aspects of performance. For this reason, use of the MSSST as an adjunct to a diagnostic test battery, particularly in school system evaluation settings where time may not allow extensive testing of information processing skills for all children, may be desirable.

It is felt that the information processing model has the following implications for understanding children with learning disabilities as part of the basis for intervention:

1. It can aid in understanding the way in which information flows through any one of the three major modalities, and provides a unified basis for evaluating different aspects of performance within that modality.

Table 5-1. An information processing model

	Visual-perceptual-motor	Language	Body awareness and control
Orientation		Focus of attention	
		Selection of appropriate cues from background	
Intake		Discrimination of form, space, and time cues	
	Visual	Auditory	Kinesthetic
		Retention of pattern and sequence of incoming information	
Integration		Set selection	
		Association to previous learning	
		Retrieval of relevant information	
		Selection of appropriate sequences for outgoing information	
Output		Execution of precise and controlled movement patterns	
	Eye-hand	Articulation	Body control
Feedback		Immediate response monitoring	
		Relevance of response to overall goals	

Source: Adapted from S. Kirk and J. McCarthy. The Illinois Test of Psycholinguistic Abilities—An approach to differential diagnosis. *Am. J. Ment. Defic.* 66 : 399, 1961.

2. It provides a way of accounting for the interrelationships between modalities and processes rather than concentrating diagnostic and treatment efforts on just one.

3. It recognizes that most information processing skills are general and not specific to any one modality; therefore, problems may arise in several areas.

4. Many of the behavior problems associated with learning disabilities can be understood in terms of breakdowns of the same processes of orientation, integration, and feedback that are significant to information processing skills.

The MSSST encourages observation of children in various situations such as the classroom, in screening or diagnostic settings, and with peers. Both the products of performance (actual skill level) and the process or behavioral organization by which performance is achieved (child's ability to organize, attend, comprehend, formulate, and act on information) can be analyzed.

Content and Test Administration

Content

The MSSST contains three subtests: Motor Patterning, Visual-Perceptual-Motor, and Language. Each subtest consists of five separate skills, and each skill is broken down into between three and eleven segments. Table 5-2 indicates the skills within each subtest and the purpose of each. There is no separate kit containing test items. All materials, except for a pencil, are contained in the test manual. Materials in the manual consist of nine test administration cards with stimulus materials printed on them.

The Meeting Street School Test Record Form is a two-page form (printed on both sides and attached at the top). The first page consists of the examiner's score sheet (Fig. 5-4). It includes a behavior rating scale and a grid on which to chart a profile of scores, and the test items. The second page consists of a work sheet for the child and provides space for making required drawings and for matching forms, letters, and words.

Setting and Equipment

A setting that is quiet and free from distraction is required for administration of the MSSST. It is helpful if the test area contains at least 5 to 6 feet of open space for demonstration of motor skills (skipping requires the most space), but these skills can be demonstrated in a hallway if absolutely necessary. The testing area should contain a table and chair of appropriate size for the child being tested and a chair for the examiner. No equipment other than the manual, score sheet, and a pencil is required.

Administration Procedure

The MSSST must be administered to one child at a time. It is not appropriate for group administration. The test requires observation of various responses to directions given by the examiner. No items can be credited by report of parent, teacher, or other individual. In most instances, the testing situation should include only the child and the examiner, although no specifications that a third person not be in the room are stated. When screening a group of children in school, it is suggested that the teacher prepare the children by presenting the testing as a "special opportunity," and then choose a confident child to go with the examiner first. This is to help less confident children follow the eager example.

Standardized directions are included for each test item. Material to be quoted directly to the child is underlined, and items to be demonstrated are indicated. Additional clarifying instructions for the examiner regarding numbers of trials and methods of encouragement are also included. The directions for imitation of hand patterns are illustrated. Directions are, in general, clearly stated in a detailed fashion.

Even though directions are generally clear and detailed, administration of the MSSST is complex. Many aspects of the test require varying

Table 5-2. Meeting Street School Screening Test subtests

Subtest	Skill and skill purpose
Motor Patterning	1. Gait patterns: measure motor output through learned skill patterns
	2. Clap hands: sample ability to imitate unfamiliar body movement patterns
	3. Hand patterns: sample ability to imitate unfamiliar movement patterns
	4. Follow directions I: assess verbal understanding (integration) of body space (uncomplicated motor output)
	5. Touch fingers: assess fine finger coordination in rapid, sequential movements
Visual-Perceptual-Motor	1. Block tapping: assess integrative memory for place (spatial) sequences
	2. Visual matching: sample visual-perceptual discrimination of form in differing spatial orientations
	3. Visual memory: sample short-term memory for geometric and letter forms
	4. Copy forms: assess ability to coordinate eye and hand in reproduction of geometric and letter forms (shape, orientation, spacing)
	5. Follow directions II: sample understanding of spatial and directional concepts when drawing on paper
Language	1. Repeat words: assess ability to listen to and repeat unknown and familiar speech sound sequences in correct form, order, and rhythm
	2. Repeat sentences: assess ability to listen and repeat complex language in correct length and grammatical form
	3. Counting: assess ability to sequence numbers in automatically learned and in interrupted sequences
	4. Tell a story: assess ability to formulate and express thoughts about an abstract picture in a meaningful way
	5. Language sequencing: assess ability to sequence time concepts and to understand order and meaning of time units

Source: Adapted from P. Hainsworth and M. Siqueland. *Early Identification of Children with Learning Disabilities: The Meeting Street School Screening Test.* Providence, Rhode Island: Meeting Street School, 1969.

kinds of directions, some of which the examiner must demonstrate. To provide a fair test administration, the examiner *must* be thoroughly familiar with the instructions to be given. The importance of gaining good rapport with the child, as well as attention the examiner must pay to properly orienting the child to each task, is emphasized in the manual.

Scoring

Directions for scoring the MSSST are succinctly stated and very easy to follow. A special appendix with examples is included for scoring the section regarding copying of forms. There are no specific instructions for scoring the Behavior Rating Scale. Subjective judgment, placed on a continuum (see Fig. 5-4), is required.

While scoring is not particularly difficult, the procedure for accomplishing it is somewhat complex. Varying numbers of points can be given for quality of performance of most items. The examiner must be well versed both in how to give the instructions and in the variations to watch for in order to score appropriately. The test can become confusing to both child and examiner when there has been inadequate preparation. Once the correct number of points has been given for each item, they are simply totaled to yield subtest raw scores and an overall MSSST total raw score. Scoring the behavior rating scale is also complex, particularly because it calls for a degree of subjective judgment. Descriptions of behaviors that may be observed are included in the manual, guiding the examiner in what to look for but not necessarily in where to place the

MEETING STREET SCHOOL SCREENING TEST RECORD FORM

Name _____ Class _____ Examiner _____

	yr.	mo.	day
DE	___	___	___
DB	___	___	___
Age	___	___	

GRADE	MSSST Total	Cut-off	Risk for Learning Disability
K-1	Raw Score	Score	
___	___	___	HIGH ? LOW

PROFILE OF SCORES

	Raw Score	Scaled Score
Motor Patterning	___	___
Vis-Percept-Motor	___	___
Language	___	___
MSSST	___	___

MP	VPM	L	MSSST	IQ
19			80	138
16			70	128
13			60	118
10			50	108
7			40	98
4			30	88
1			20	78

BEHAVIOR RATING SCALE

TEST COOPERATION |L_____|
passive resistance, non-involved / cooperates / active resistance, manipulative

ATTENTION |L_____|
preoccupied or dreamy / attends / hyperactively inattentive

CONCENTRATION |L_____|
perseverative / concentrates / distractible

FEEDBACK |L_____|
lacks energy or willingness to check / monitors self / impulsively uncritical, inconsequential

MOTOR CONTROL |L_____|
clumsy / smooth, lithe

PENCIL SKILLS |L_____|
clumsy / dextrous

EYE CONTROL |L_____|
irregular movements / smooth tracking

SPEECH |L_____|
unintelligible / clearly intelligible

LANGUAGE |L_____|
agrammatical, impoverished / grammatical, rich

OVERALL EFFICIENCY |L_____|
inefficient / efficient

GAIT PATTERNS (5)

0 1	Hop-1: five times on both feet, stationary
0 1 2	Skip-2, Lame duck skipping-1
0 1 2	Dance-2, with counting steps-1

CLAP HANDS (6)

	0 1	Up-Down -- 1
S	0 1 2 3	Front-Front-Back - No. in 3 or second trial - 1
	0 1 2	Up-Up-Down-Back - No. in 2

HAND PATTERNS (6)

	0 1	Up-Down -- 1
S	0 1	Out-Cross-Out-In - 1
	0 1 2	Up-Down-Out-In - No. in 2
	0 1 2	Slant-Up-Down-In - No. in 2

FOLLOW DIRECTIONS I (6)

0	1	Put this pencil above your head and then behind you
0	1	Put this pencil between us and then nearer to you
0	½ 1	Take two steps forward and one step backward
0	1	Turn to your right
0	½ 1	Take three steps toward me and then turn and face away from me
0	½ 1	Turn right, take two steps backward and turn left.

Fig. 5-5. Meeting Street School Screening Test Record Form. (Reproduced by permission.)

TOUCH FINGERS (6)		
	0 1	Hands Separate - 1 both correct
S	0 1 2	Hands Together - 2 if under 7"
		1 if 7" plus
	0 1	Hands Together - 1 if under 7"
	0 1 2	Thumb to 2, 4, 3, 5 - 2 if under 7"
		1 if 7" plus

MOTOR PATTERNING TOTAL (29)

BLOCK TAPPING (6)		
0 1	.....	1 3 3
0 1	.....	5 4 2
0 1	.....	1 5 3
0 1	.....	5 1 4 3
0 1	.....	3 5 2 4 1
0 1	.....	3 2 4 3 1 4

VISUAL MATCHING (5)	
0 1	Row One - 1 for figure 2
0 1 2	Row Two - 1 each, figures 2 & 3
0 1 2	Row Three - 1 each, figures 2 & 4

VISUAL MEMORY (6)	
0 1	Backward N
0 1	Circle-Square
0 1	Diamond - Triangle
0 1	b
0 1	may
0 1	with them

COPY FORMS (8)

Circle 0 ½ 1
Square 0 ½ 1   Spacing 0 ½ 1
Diamond 0 ½ 1
Triangle 0 ½ 1   Spacing 0 ½ 1
May   0 1 2

FOLLOW DIRECTIONS II (5)	
0 1	Draw a ball behind the car
0 1	Draw a line from the bottom of your paper to the car
0 1	Draw a line from the right hand side of your paper to the car
0 1	Draw an X in the upper left hand corner of your paper
0 1	Draw a ball in the bottom right hand corner of your paper, put an X inside it, and draw a square around them.

VISUAL - PERCEPTUAL - MOTOR TOTAL (30)

REPEAT WORDS (5½)	
0 ½	ah-man-ee
0 ½	laudy-tu-dum
0 ½	kaka-kada-kat
0 ½	tum titty um tum tum
0 ½	dia-do -ko-ki-nee -sis
0 ½	quack duck quack
0 ½	feminine
0 ½	above and below
0 ½	musicology
0 ½	transcontinental
0 ½	popocatepetal

REPEAT SENTENCES (5)

_____ Please pass the meat and peas (6)

_____ Joan and Jane had a chocolate sundae after the movie yesterday (11)

(0-6=0, 6-8=1, 9-11=2, 12-4=3, 15-6=4, 17=5)

COUNTING (7)		
	0 1	Counting Blocks - 1
S	0 1 2	Forward 1-10 - 2 if under 7"
		1 if 7" plus
	0 1 2 3	Backward 10-1 - 3 if under 7"
		2 if 7" plus
		1 if gets 5-1
	0 1	Count to 10 by 2's - 1

TELL A STORY (5)

_____

_____

_____

_____

0	for irrelevant detail or nothing
1	for naming two figures
2	for one figure in action
3	for two figures in action
4	for three figures interacting
5	for score of 4 plus imagination

LANGUAGE SEQUENCING (6)	
0 1	breakfast, lunch . . . (give answer if fails)
0 1	morning, afternoon . . . (give answer)
0 1	yesterday, today . . . .
0 1	fall, winter. . . . .
0 1	Sunday, Saturday, Friday . . .
0 1	week, day, hour . . . .

LANGUAGE TOTAL (28½)

MSSST TOTAL (87½)

Fig. 5-5 continued.

observation on the scale. It is likely that the Behavior Rating Scale will be most easily completed by those with considerable experience in working with children.

Raw scores from each subtest (Motor Patterning, Visual-Perceptual-Motor, and Language), and from the total MSSST, are converted to scaled scores using tables (organized by chronological age) in the manual. The four resulting scaled scores can then be plotted on the Profile of Scores located on the front of the record sheet. When the MSSST is used as a screening tool, *raw scores* are used to determine which children have insufficient information processing skills to meet curriculum demands of the kindergarten or first grade. Cutoff points at or below which a child may be considered "at risk" for learning disabilities are 39 for kindergarteners and 55 for first grade. These points essentially distinguish those children falling below the mean ("low achievers") from those falling above the mean ("high achievers"). The authors point out that when the test is used prior to school entrance or early in the year, these cutoff points may be slightly low. If use of raw scores produces "questionable" results according to those deciding how to classify the children, scaled scores can be used. If one or more scaled scores on the three subtests is 1 standard deviation from the mean or if the total MSSST scaled score is 43 or below, *and* the MSSST raw score is within 5 points of the cutoff, the child is considered "suspicious" for learning disability.

When the test is used as part of a diagnostic evaluation, results are interpreted by using the scaled scores, the Behavior Rating Scale, and clinical observation. Scaled scores range from 1 to 19 (mean of 10) for each of the four subtests and from 20 to 80 (mean of 50) for the total test score. Scaled scores are available for five age groups, arranged in 6-month increments, from 5 years to 7 years 5 months. Scores falling at or near the mean show average performance for chronological age. Indications of 1, 2, and 3 standard deviations above and below the mean are also included on the Profile of Scores. Although it is not made particularly clear on the score profile grid on the score sheet, means, standard deviations (1, 2, and 3 SD) above and below the mean, and percentiles of performance can be gleaned after plotting scaled scores; Fig. 5-6 is an adapted version of this profile grid.

The IQ scores indicated to the right of the scoring profile grid were obtained by the standardization sample of 500 children. Using the Science Research Associates Primary Mental Abilities group IQ test, this group obtained a mean IQ of 108 with a standard deviation of 10.

No suggestions are given for situations in which rescreening would be considered advisable. Emphasis is placed on the responsibility of the examiner to provide a comfortable environment, to establish good rapport, and to be sure that directions are clearly given.

It is implied in the manual that the MSSST is most likely to be used within school systems, either for identifying children at risk for learning disabilities or for adding additional dimensions to more traditional school evaluations. School systems must work out for themselves an acceptable way of gathering and using such results. Suggestions for ways in which this might be done are included in the manual. If the MSSST were to be used in other screening settings, it would be assumed that the screening cutoff scores would be used as the basis for referral.

Psychometric Properties

Standardization

Specific, step-by-step instructions for administering the MSSST are included in the test manual. Items for which it is permissible to repeat administration or rearrange order are indicated. The test administrator should establish rapport and orient the child appropriately; only then will it be possible to administer the item as described.

According to the test manual, the MSSST was standardized on 500 children in kindergarten and first grade. They were selected from a small geographical area (primarily East Providence,

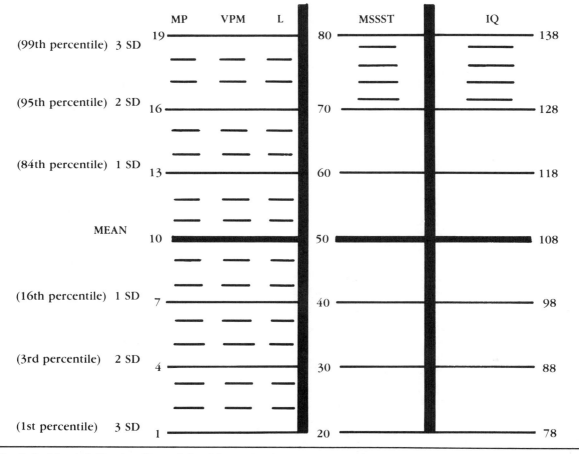

	Raw	Scaled
Motor Patterning (MP)	————	————
Visual-Perceptual-Motor (VPM)	————	————
Language (L)	————	————
MSSST	————	————

Profile of Scores

Fig. 5-6. Adapted Meeting Street School Screening Test (MSSST) Profile Grid.

Rhode Island) that supposedly was representative of population characteristics of the United States according to 1966 U.S. census figures for fathers' occupations. One hundred children in each of five 6-month age ranges were tested. Boys and girls are reported to have been equally distributed across each age range and socioeconomic level. The standardization sample was drawn from the regular school population ". . . in one geographical area that does not include hard core deprived groups" [2]. No further definitive information is given about the standardization sample, including how it was selected. This limited sample size in relation to race, socioeconomic status, and geographic area is a weakness of the test. According to the manual, more extensive standardization was planned, however.

Based on MSSST scores of the 100 children at each of five 6-month age ranges, five normative tables were constructed. No further information regarding construction of these tables is included in the manual.

Reliability

Test-retest reliability (stability over time) has been reported for the *total* MSSST score. Children (number unspecified) were retested 2 to 4 weeks apart. Correlation coefficients are reported to "cluster" at .85. Correlation coefficients for the individual subtests are said to range from .75 to .85. The authors state that, provided test performance by a child is "reasonable," these scores are stable enough to be used for comparison between children. They also report that ". . . test-retest coefficients of the 15 individual items are not high enough to justify a pattern analysis of the functions tapped by these items" [2].

Correlation coefficients for interobserver reliability are reported to be "consistently above .95" for the three subtest scores and total MSSST score. Two raters are reported to have scored the same child at the same time. There is no further information regarding how many children were so rated. The authors report the results of an unpublished master's thesis in which similar results were obtained by both an experienced and an inexperienced examiner [2].

Validity

The authors state that the MSSST has ". . . strong face and clinical validity since the items come from the experience of Meeting Street School's professional diagnostic team in evaluation of those children failing in school because of neurological dysfunction" [2].

The reported relationships between the MSSST and two tests used to diagnose language and visual-motor-perceptual skills (i.e., the Illinois Test of Psycholinguistic Abilities [ITPA] and Frostig Developmental Tests of Visual Perception) appear to be the evidence available concerning concurrent validity. These results were part of an unpublished master's thesis [2]. Subjects for this study were 40 kindergarten boys selected from a group of 120 who had IQs above 90 and who had been given the MSSST. They were divided into two groups: high risk (lowest MSSST scores) and control. No indication is given regarding the range of MSSST scores. Table 5-3 illustrates the resulting correlations. It is concluded that the above data indicate that children who are identified as suspicious or high risk on the MSSST do indeed have language and visual-perceptual-motor difficulties as measured by these two well-accepted tests, and that the MSSST can be used with confidence as a short screening procedure for difficulties in these areas [2].

Predictive validity is reported as correlations between the MSSST and school readiness and school achievement scores. Specific readiness and achievement tests used are not identified.

The authors point out that IQ scores are not the only, or even the most efficient, predictors of school success. They suggest combining IQ and MSSST scores as a more efficient predictor, even though this score still cannot account for the influence of factors such as motivation, socialization, cultural expectation, prolonged illness, and lack of adequate educational experience. From the normative sample, 220 kindergarten

Table 5-3. Correlations between Meeting Street School Screening Test and two diagnostic tests

Tests and test scores	MSSST	Correlation
ITPA Composite Score (5 subtests)	Total	.77
ITPA Composite Score	Language Subtest	.71
ITPA Composite Score	Motor Patterning Subtest	.62
ITPA Composite Score	Visual-Perceptual-Motor Subtest	.42
Frostig (all five subtests)	Total	.57
Frostig	Visual-Perceptual-Motor Subtest	.54
Frostig	Language Subtest	.55

Source: Adapted from P. Hainsworth and M. Siqueland. *Early Identification of Children with Learning Disabilities: The Meeting Street School Screening Test.* Providence, Rhode Island: Meeting Street School, 1969.

and 274 first grade children were followed for 1 *or* 2 years (number of each in each time period is not identified). Table 5-4 demonstrates the resulting correlations. Combining MSSST and IQ scores was found to be more predictive of school achievement than either score alone, even though it was recognized that overlapping skills were tested. No indication is given regarding the specific IQ test used.

The authors followed 163 randomly selected children (67 kindergartners, 96 first graders) from the standardization sample for 2 years. At the end of that time (end of first grade and end of second grade), the children were all given standard achievement tests. Performance on the achievement tests was designated as being above or below the median. Table 5-5 demonstrates a method for fitting the data into a fourfold classification table and also demonstrates screening test validity, sensitivity, and specificity [5]. There are no absolute guidelines above or below which sensitivity or specificity are routinely considered acceptable or nonacceptable. In general, the higher the percentage, the better. Sensitivity and specificity can be manipulated by changing the cutoff point. If the cutoff point is changed to increase sensitivity, specificity will be lowered and more overreferrals will result. It is essential that those doing screening and those receiving referrals agree on an acceptable level of sensitivity and be willing to manage the effects of lowered specificity.

There are no data in the manual regarding vali-

dation with a criterion test for the purpose of measuring skills thought to be involved in learning disabilities. The authors state clearly that sole reliance should not be placed on scores of the MSSST or of any other test. They provide multiple illustrations of ways in which the MSSST can be used in combination with achievement and IQ test results to determine those most likely to be at risk for learning disabilities.

Guidelines for Use in a Clinical Setting

The MSSST is one of the few tests classified as a screening test that purports to identify children at risk for learning disabilities. Therefore, it is potentially widely useful in any program with early identification of learning disabilities as its purpose. It is most likely that some preselection process such as those suggested by the authors (e.g., brief medical and developmental history, brief general screening procedures, observation in group setting, teacher ratings) will make this a more practical test to use. Some evaluators may prefer to not use a test with only a 51 percent sensitivity if they feel other measures or combinations of measures give better data. (Note: The test was not validated using a criterion test that measures skills thought to be involved in learning problems; rather it was validated using "standard achievement tests.") The authors claim the best use of the MSSST is in combination with other tests and observations.

The MSSST is viewed by its authors as contrib-

*Table 5-4. Correlations between Meeting Street School
Screening Test (MSSST) scores and achievement scores 1 or 2 years later*

Subjects	Readiness scores at end of kindergarten	Achievement scores at end of first grade
Kindergarten children given MSSST	$r = .66$	$r = .63$
First grade children given MSSST	$r = .53$	$r = .46$

Source: Adapted from P. Hainsworth and M. Siqueland. *Early Identification of Children with Learning Disabilities: The Meeting Street School Screening Test.* Providence, Rhode Island: Meeting Street School, 1969.

*Table 5-5. Comparison between Meeting Street School Screening
Test (MSSST) performance and "Standard Achievement Tests"* [a, b, c]

Classification by MSSST	Abnormal (below median)	Normal (above median)	Totals
Referrals (below cutoff point)	Correct referrals, $n = 43$	Overreferrals, $n = 11$	54
Nonreferrals (above cutoff point)	Underreferrals, $n = 41$	Correct nonreferrals, $n = 68$	109
Totals	84	79	163

[a]Screening test validity (percentage of agreement between classification of same group of children by both screening and diagnostic measure):

$$\frac{43 + 68}{163} \times 100 = 68\%.$$

[b]Sensitivity (ability of screening test to identify abnormal as abnormal):

$$\frac{43}{43 + 41} \times 100 = 51\%.$$

[c]Specificity (ability of screening test to identify normal as normal):

$$\frac{68}{68 + 11} \times 100 = 86\%.$$

Sources: Adapted from P. Hainsworth and M. Siqueland. *Early Identification of Children with Learning Disabilities: The Meeting Street School Screening Test.* Providence, Rhode Island: Meeting Street School, 1969; and from S. Stangler, C. Huber, and D. Routh. *Screening Growth and Development of Preschool Children: A Guide for Test Selection.* New York: McGraw-Hill, 1980.

uting information that is different from that of most other tests. Considerable discussion is included in the manual as to how the MSSST can be used (1) to confirm teacher suspicion of a child who is at risk for learning problems, (2) to augment information supplied by IQ testing (particularly for children who have normal and above IQs but are still performing poorly), and (3) even to supplement diagnostic measures intended to identify learning disabilities (such as the Frostig and the Bender-Gestalt) since these tests vary in their comprehensiveness.

Review

The MSSST is designed to identify young children of kindergarten and first grade age who may be at risk for developing learning disabilities. It is based on an information processing model and specifically tests in the areas of motor patterning, visual-perceptual-motor skills, and language skills. Although there are drawbacks to the test, it does represent an important effort to meet a critical need of school-aged children.

The organization of the MSSST manual is difficult to follow. It is filled with interesting and valuable material, but it is difficult to know where in the manual to find this information. Directions for actual test administration are clear but complex and, with practice, can be easily replicated. It is not recommended that an untrained examiner administer this test, however, since thorough familiarity is required before test administration can be done smoothly and correctly.

The authors point out, correctly, that since learning disabilities usually represent combinations of problems, devising a test to detect them is particularly difficult. This also makes it difficult to validate such a test. The MSSST was validated as a diagnostic measure by correlating scores with several diagnostic tests measuring aspects of skills critical to diagnosis of learning disabilities including the ITPA, Frostig, a group IQ test, readiness measures, and achievement measures. It was validated as a screening measure by correlating scores with "standard achievement tests." Neither set of validation data is particularly complete, and test users are cautioned to take this into consideration when choosing to use the MSSST.

The MSSST was standardized on a group of children from one geographic area. Very little specific information about this group is given in the manual. Although the group was said to be representative of the United States population as a whole at that time (according to use of 1966 U.S. census figures for fathers' occupations), additional normative data would increase the value of the test.

REFERENCES

1. Denhoff, E., et al. Developmental and predictive characteristics of items from the Meeting Street School Screening Test. *Dev. Med. Child Neurol.* 10 : 220, 1968.
2. Hainsworth, P., and Siqueland, M. *Early Identification of Children with Learning Disabilities: The Meeting Street School Screening Test.* Providence, R.I.: Meeting Street School, 1969.
3. Kirk, S., and McCarthy, J. The Illinois Test of Psycholinguistic Abilities—An approach to differential diagnosis. *Am. J. Ment. Defic.* 66 : 399, 1961.
4. Osgood, C. E. *Contemporary Approaches to Cognition.* Cambridge, Mass.: Harvard University Press, 1957.
5. Stangler, S., Huber, C., and Routh, D. *Screening Growth and Development of Preschool Children: A Guide for Test Selection.* New York: McGraw-Hill, 1980.

MILLER ASSESSMENT FOR PRESCHOOLERS

Descriptive Information

Test Identification

The title of this test is *Miller Assessment for Preschoolers* (MAP), 1982. Its author is Lucy Jane Miller, Ph,D., O.T.R. The Foundation for Knowledge in Development (1855 West Union Ave., Suite B-8, Englewood, Colorado 80110) publishes the test at a cost of $225–$275 for the MAP Test Kit and $7–$10 for a packet of score sheets. Miller is an occupational therapist with pediatric experience who is now providing training in use, administration, and interpretation of the MAP through the Foundation for Knowledge in Development.

Age and Type of Client

The MAP was designed to screen normal children from 2 years 9 months to 5 years 8 months of age for identification of mild to moderate developmental delays.

Purpose

The MAP was designed as a screening instrument to identify children who demonstrate mild to moderate developmental delays and who may be in need of further evaluation. An extended version of the MAP includes Supplemental Scores and Observations and was designed to provide the professional with more clinical information for the purpose of "defining a child's strengths and weakness and an indication of possible avenues of remediation" [6].

Time Required to Administer and Score Test

Administration time for an experienced examiner is 20 to 30 minutes. Scoring time of the screening version is stated to be less than 2 minutes; the extended version requires more time.

Evaluator

The MAP can be administered by a variety of professionals or nonprofessionals. The author suggests that professionals administering and interpreting the MAP Supplemental Scores and Observations should attend an accredited MAP Seminar.

Historical Perspective Of Test Construction

Development and Source of Test Items

In 1971, Lucy Miller was frustrated by the lack of standardized screening tools for preschool and kindergarten children. Her goal was to develop a test sensitive enough to detect children "at risk for future school-related problems, such as learning disabilities" [6].

An extensive review of normal and abnormal child development literature and preschool standardized and nonstandardized tests provided Miller with over 800 items for field testing. Each item was field tested and revised or discarded based on the data analysis. Items were discarded if they (1) lacked solid statistical support, (2) required too much time for administration and scoring, and (3) required extensive equipment.

Five editions of the MAP have been field tested, with approximately 4000 children participating. The final version of the MAP contains 27 core items.

Review of Literature in Terms of Test Use

No studies other than standardization, validity, and reliability have been published regarding this screening tool. No literature reviewing the use of the MAP is available.

Theoretical Constructs and Implication for Intervention

An extensive review of normal preschool child development and a review of factors associated with school-related difficulties provide the basis for item selection on the MAP. In the manual the author provides a short review of the literature for each content area. It appears that the sensory and motor areas are derived from sensory integration and neurodevelopmental theories of evaluation as well as developmental theories. The theoretical constructs of the cognitive and combined areas are discussed and referenced in the manual.

Content and Administration

Content

The 27 core test items are divided into three ability areas: sensory and motor abilities, cognitive abilities, and combined abilities.

The sensory and motor abilities area contains two indices: the Foundation Index and the Coordination Index. The Foundation Index evaluates sensory awareness and basic motor tasks that are theoretically linked to the ability to perform complex tasks. Items in this index can be found in the general neurological examination, sensory integrative examination, and the neurodevelopmental examination. Specific areas listed are position and movement sense, touch, and basic movement components such as flexion, extension, and rotation. Core test items are stereognosis (The Feely Game), finger localization (The Finger Game), hand-to-nose coordination (The Mr. Thumbuddy Game), Romberg's sign (swaying of the body or falling when the eyes are closed while standing with the feet close together) (The Statue Game), stepping (The Marching Game), supine flexion (The Make-A-Ball Game), and kneel stand (The Stand-Up Game).

The Coordination Index contains items involving gross, fine, and oral motor activities. Core test items are tower (The Big Building Game), motor accuracy (The Draw-A-Cage

Game), tongue movements (The Funny Tongue Game), and articulation.

Core test items considered to be a combination of the Foundation and Coordination Indices are vertical writing (The Bunny Hop Game), walks line (The Walking Game), and rapid alternating movements (The Stamp Game).

The cognitive abilities area contains two indexes: Verbal Index and Nonverbal Index. The Verbal Index contains language activities involving memory, sequencing, comprehension, association, and verbal expression. Core test items are general information, follows directions, sentence repetition, and digit repetition.

The Nonverbal Index contains activities involving memory, sequencing, and mental manipulations that do not require verbal expression. Core test items are sequencing (The Put Away Game), block tapping (The Watching Game), object memory (The Remembering Game), puzzles (The Make-A-Picture Game), and figure ground (The Hide and Seek Game).

The combined abilities area contains one index—the Complex Task Index—which involves activities requiring a combination of sensory, motor, and cognitive abilities. Core test items are block designs (The Make-A-Building Game), Draw-A-Person, imitation of postures (The Simon Says Game), and maze (The Find Your Way Game).

A Behavior During Testing sheet is located on the back of the score sheet. The author states it was "designed to provide a framework for observing the subjective aspects of the child's behavior" [3]. The Behavior During Testing sheet contains three sections with nine items: Attention Section (activity level, concentration, ability to structure time/complete tasks, and need for reward/ability to delay gratification), Social Interaction Section (reaction to separation from caretaker, interaction with examiner, and verbal interaction), and Sensory Reactivity Section (reaction to movement and reaction to touch).

Supplemental Observations (approximately 70) are organized clinical observations that can provide the experienced clinician with more in-depth information. The areas included are quality of movement, draw-a-person interpretation, quality of speech and language, and the quality of visual and tactile responses. The author repeatedly states that the examiner's ability to evaluate a child's responses in this area is subjective and that the examiner should attend a certified MAP seminar to gain proficiency in these observations.

A Developmental History form is provided for children receiving a more in-depth assessment. Its purpose is to provide a framework for a detailed interview with the parents or caregiver.

The MAP Test Kit includes the examiner's manual, cue sheets, score sheets, record booklets, drawing booklets, scoring transparency, scoring and card notebook, and test materials. The examiner's manual is very complete, closely following the recommendations of the American Psychological Association and the American Educational Research Association's National Council on Measurement in Education Standards for Educational and Psychological Tests and Manuals. It includes information on the MAP's development; theoretical background; standardization, reliability, and validity data; description of administration, scoring, and interpretation; figures; tables; and a bibliography. Cue sheets are provided in the scoring notebook to allow the examiners to administer the test without the manual or the need to memorize administration procedures. The Item Score Sheet provides space for raw score documentation. On the back of this sheet is the Behavior During Testing Information. The Record Booklet includes the Summary Sheet, Family Information and Developmental History Sheet, the Supplemental Observation Sheet, and the Performances Indices Sheet. The Drawing Booklet is used by the child for Draw-A-Person, Vertical Writing, and Motor Accuracy items. The Scoring and Card Notebook holds the Cue Sheets, Scoring Sheets, test materials of figure-ground cards, puzzles, clown face, and scoring transparency. The test kit materials are contained in a sturdy carrying case that is well organized and maintains test materials in an accessible manner for the examiner. All needed test materials are available in the test kit. Since this test is standardized, substitution of materials by the examiner would make the normative data invalid. The author has done an exceptional job of including engaging materials for preschoolers and providing the examiner with well-organized equipment.

Setting and Equipment

Suggested environment for administration of the MAP is a well-lit room, at least 6 by 12 feet, with a child-sized table and chairs, a mat, and space to perform the gross motor items. All the equipment needed is provided in the MAP Test Kit.

Administration Procedures

The MAP is administered in a one-to-one situation. The presence of parents and other caregivers is acceptable only if absolutely necessary. The child must perform the activities; parental report is not acceptable. As this is a standardized test, the administration format must be followed to ensure valid results.

The manual provides specific administration instructions and verbal directions for each item. The author encourages the examiner to make the session "fun." In the administration section of the manual, each core item contains information on materials needed, procedure for administering the item and verbal directions, scoring instructions, supplemental observations, and age-specific information for core items that change according to the age of the child. The Cue Sheet makes it possible to administer items without the manual.

The examiner is instructed to calculate the child's chronological age and select the score sheet that matches the child's age. The score sheets are divided into six age groups (6-month intervals). It is important that the examiner use the correct score sheet because the only way to correct a mistake is to readminister the entire test using the appropriate sheet.

The examiner should be familiar with the test items and have organized the test materials and environment before administration. The author has provided very logical, straightforward directions, and all test materials are well organized; thus, the complexity of this test's administration has been kept moderately simple. The examiner must be careful to match the correct cue sheet with the correct score sheet and test materials to avoid confusion.

The scoring procedure of the MAP is clearly stated. Specific scoring directions are provided for each item in the manual. The examiner should be familiar with the color-coded scoring sheet prior to administration for ease in recording responses. All scores are converted into percentile ranks. Percentile scores are attainable for each item, each index, and/or a total test score.

The scoring procedure is fairly simple due to the color coding of the scoring sheet and charts. The green area on the scoring sheet indicates that the child is functioning in the 25 percent or higher rank and is felt to be within normal limits; the yellow area (suspect area) represents a 6 to 25 percent level and indicates that the child may need further evaluation. By adding a child's item responses in the red and yellow areas and converting that sum into a percentile ranking using Table 38 in the manual, a final percentile score is achieved.

It is possible to obtain supplemental percentile scores in each of the five indexes for examiners desiring more information regarding a child's strengths and weaknesses. A performance indices chart is provided for ease of scoring. A total percentile score for each index can be ascertained using Table 40 in the manual following the same procedure used to obtain the final percentile score.

The Behavior During Testing sheet and Supplemental Observation sheet do not receive a specific score, but guidelines are provided in the manual to assist in interpretation.

When using the MAP as a screening tool, the Final Percentile Score is color coded in the red-yellow-green format as previously described. The cutoff between normal and abnormal is left to the discretion of the examiner or school system. A predictive validity has been completed by the test developer, which involved 338 pre-schoolers who were initially tested in 1979–1980 and subsequently evaluated four years later. The highest predictive correlation was found to be IQ scores on the WISC-R. Predictive correlations were also found with (1) performance in math, reading, and language as measured by the Wood-cock-Johnson, (2) retention in a grade place-ment, (3) need for special services, and (4) report card grades [7]. Two other predictive validity studies, one follow-up after one year [4], and the other follow-up at 1¼ and 2½ years [2] found positive correlation with teacher rating and school performance. Since the test was designed to identify children at risk for school-related problems, it does not identify gifted children or children performing at the upper end of the scale.

If the examiner desires an indication of a child's strengths and weaknesses, the percentile score for each index can be computed. The same red-yellow-green format is used. Interpretation using these scores must be done cautiously as some in-dexes have only a few items. These scores can be useful in suggesting areas that require further evaluation.

The examiner can determine the amount of change in a child over time by using the raw score or percentile score of each item. The author sug-gests at least a 6-month interval between testings; this time interval can provide the examiner with information regarding treatment efficacy.

The Behavior During Testing and Supplemen-tal Observations do not affect the child's test scores. The information gained is subjective and very much dependent of the examiner's clinical experiences. Guidelines are provided to assist the examiner in interpretation of these areas.

The author continuously cautions the examin-er against overinterpretation of the MAP results.

She states that no medical diagnosis or specific neurological dysfunction can be ascertained from this test.

Referral Guidelines

Miller suggests the following referral resources for children performing poorly on the MAP in-dexes: Foundation Index, pediatricians and/or neurologists; Coordination Index, pediatricians, neurologists, occupational therapists, and/or physical therapists; Verbal Index, pediatricians, speech pathologists, and/or psychologists; Non-verbal Index, pediatricians, psychologists, and/or educational specialists; and Complex Task In-dex, pediatricians and/or psychologists.

Psychometric Properties

Standardization

The MAP manual contains specific instructions for each item regarding administration proce-dure, verbal directions, and scoring criteria. These instructions must be followed for valid results.

The final MAP screening was administered to 1200 normal children between 2 years 9 months and 5 years 8 months of age. A random, stratified research design was used involving the nine geo-graphic regions identified by the U.S. Census Bu-reau. The variables considered in the sample were age, geographic region, race, sex, size of community, and socioeconomic status. Six age groupings were delineated (age was the most im-portant variable in the data analysis). Sex and race differences were not analyzed. The manual contains many tables providing specific num-bers involved in the data collection.

The goals of the scoring system were (1) to be simple and quick, (2) to provide information comparing a child's performance with other children's performance, and (3) to identify chil-dren in need of further evaluation. Percentile rank scores were computed because they were felt to be simple to compute and easily understood. A raw score frequency distribution was obtained for each item in each age group. The red-yellow-green color-coded scoring format was established. The red area indicates the child's performance to be at or below the fifth percentile of the normative group, the yellow area indicates functioning between the sixth and twenty-fifth percentile, and the green area indicates functioning above the twenty-fifth percentile.

The green-yellow-red cutoff scoring criteria were somewhat arbitrarily decided. The data gathered from the normal sample was used. In a critique on the standardization of the MAP, De-Gangi [3] stated these cutoff criteria "should have been determined by comparing the performances of normal and delayed subjects."

Reliability

Test-retest reliability studies (stability over time) were conducted by three test administrators on 90 normal children. The two testing sessions were conducted 1 to 4 weeks apart by the same examiner. The total test reliability coefficient was 81 percent. The test-retest reliability coefficient for the five indexes were as follows: Foundation Index, 80 percent; Verbal Index, 80 percent; Nonverbal Index, 94 percent; Complex Tasks Index, 91 percent; and Coordination Index, 72 percent. Since the Coordination Index demonstrated the lowest stability, an analysis of each item was done to ascertain which items were unreliable. The three least stable items were the tower, cage, and vertical writing, ranging from 69.5 to 76.8 percent.

Interrater study was conducted with two test administrators and 40 normal children. One examiner administered and scored the tests; the other simultaneously scored the test. The correlation coefficient using the Pearson product-moment procedure was .978 for the total test. Correlations of the individual indexes ranged between .97 and .99, with the exception of the

Coordination Index, which was .84. An individual item analysis of this index found only the articulation item to have decreased interrater reliability.

Validity

Content validity was tested in the development of this tool with an extensive review of the literature of child development (Chap. 2 in the manual addresses the theoretical background used) and a review of approximately 113 preschool tests (listed in Appendixes AI–AV). Over 800 items were field-tested on approximately 4000 children. The final 27 items chosen were based on item difficulty (percentage of children passing each item at each age), item discrimination (point biserial correlation of each item), and correlation studies (relationship of items to subtest categories). A specification table providing information regarding items and behaviors assessed is available in the manual. A factor analysis regarding the interrelationships of test items found six factors being tested: verbal, nonverbal coordination, coordination, nonverbal, and two factors of foundation. Table 27 in the manual relates specifics of this factor analysis. A correlation analysis of each item and index revealed that test items contributed significantly to the total test (< 0.1 level) and that the contribution of each index was fairly equal (.647–.778).

Criterion-related validity was addressed by the administration of the MAP, the Wechsler Preschool and Primary Scale of Intelligence (WPPSI), the Southern California Sensory Integration Tests (SCSIT), and the Illinois Test of Psycholinguistic Abilities (ITPA) to 30 children. The results of these studies are discussed in Chapter 4 of the manual. Results must be interpreted cautiously due to the small sample size. Low correlations between the MAP and the WPPSI (.27) and between the MAP and the ITPA (.31) were demonstrated. Specific correlations and statistical analysis information is available in the manual for each test. The MAP and Denver Developmental Screening

Test (DDST) were administered to 90 children. It was found that, compared with the DDST, the MAP identifies 24 percent more children as delayed or high risk.

In order to evaluate construct validity, the MAP was administered to 90 children previously identified as having a functional delay (perceptual, behavioral, or language). Children with cerebral palsy, autism, or mental retardation were not included. The MAP identified 75 percent of the children in the "at risk" (red) or "suspect" (yellow) categories. When analyzing a breakdown of the numbers, it was found that the MAP identified 84 percent of the children between 3 years 8 months and 5 years 8 months of age but only 33 to 45 percent of the younger children. DeGangi [3] voiced concern that the "selection criteria were poorly defined for the delayed sample and did not include descriptions of the type and extent of the delay." She felt more descriptive information would provide the examiner with information "in determining which type of delays actually result in academic problems."

Predictive validity studies for a screening tool are essential. A predictive validity study of 338 of the preschoolers involved in the MAP standardization was completed in 1985 [2, 4, 8].

Guidelines for Use in a Clinical Setting

The MAP was designed as a preschool screening assessment to identify children who may be "at risk" for school-related problems. Guidelines and cautions are provided in the manual regarding the administration of this tool to children who are known to have a dysfunction, children functioning well below developmental expectations, children whose chronological age is outside the test's age range but who are functioning between 2½ and 5½ years of age, and children who do not speak English fluently.

The MAP provides a format and guidelines for collecting and interpreting clinical observations (supplemental observations) and behaviors observed during testing. The author recommends that the examiner using these observations attend a MAP Seminar for instruction. As with most clinical observations, the extent, specificity, and interpretation of the observations are dependent on the examiner's professional background and experience.

Review

The MAP is a standardized screening tool for children between the ages of 2 years 9 months and 5 years 8 months. Its purpose is to identify children at risk for school-related problems. The MAP is divided into three ability areas: sensory and motor, cognitive, and combined abilities. These areas are divided into five indexes: Foundation, Coordination, Verbal, Nonverbal, and Complex Tasks. Supplemental scores and supplemental observations can provide the more experienced examiner with additional information. A Behavior During Testing sheet and Developmental History format can also be used to gain more information.

The MAP was standardized on normal children using a random, stratified sampling procedure. "Fairly equal distributions were obtained for the six different age groups: for sex, region of the United States and for socioeconomic status, which were relatively close to U.S. Census Bureau figures" [3].

Good results were obtained from interrater and test-retest reliability studies [1, 3, 5, 6]. Validity studies were conducted with relatively good results although more studies are needed, using larger sample sizes. Initial reports of a predictive validity study appear promising [2, 4, 8].

The MAP has been described as "the best available screening test for identifying preschool children with moderate 'preacademic problems'" [6]; "an extremely promising instrument which should find wide use among clinical psychologists, school psychologists, and occupational therapists in assessing mild to moderate learning disabilities in preschool children" [6]; and "the MAP is a well-developed screening instrument that exhibits the qualities of good item discrimination, good test structure and content, good collection of data on normal subjects, and good interrater and test-retest reliability" [3].

REFERENCES

1. Barus, B. J. The Miller Assessment for Preschoolers (MAP: An introduction and review). *Am. J. Occup. Ther.* 37(5) : 333, 1983.
2. Cohn, S. Predictive Validity of the Miller Assessment for Preschoolers, dissertation. University of Denver, 1986.
3. DeGangi, G. A. A critique of the standardization of the Miller Assessment for Preschoolers. *Am. J. Occup. Ther.* 37(6) : 407, 1983.
4. Lemerand, P. Predictive Validity of the Miller Assessment for Preschoolers, dissertation. University of Michigan, 1985.
5. Linder, T. Review of the Miller Assessment for Preschoolers. In D. J. Keyser and R. C. Sweetland (eds.), *Test Critiques.* Kansas City, Mo.: Test Corp. of America, 1985. Pp. 443–454.
6. Michaels, W., and Deloria, D. Two Reviews of the Miller Assessment for Preschoolers. In J. Mitchell (ed.), *Ninth Mental Measurement Yearbook.* Lincoln, Nebr.: Buros Institute of Mental Measurement, 1985.
7. Miller, L. J. *The Miller Assessment for Preschoolers: Manual.* Littleton, Col.: The Foundation for Knowledge in Development, 1982.
8. Miller, L. J. Predictive Validity of the Miller Assessment for Preschoolers, dissertation. University of Denver, 1986.

Tests Requiring Parent Report

DEVELOPMENTAL PROFILE II

Descriptive Information

Test Identification

The title of this test is Developmental Profile II (Alpern-Boll), 1980–Psychological Development Publications; 1985, 1986–Western Psychological Services. The original edition, published in 1972, is entitled *Developmental Profile.* Gerald Alpern, Ph.D., and Thomas Boll, Ph.D., are the authors of the original edition. Alpern, Boll, and Marsha Shearer, M.A., authored the current edition. At the time the Developmental Profile was first written (1972), Dr. Alpern was Director of Research, Child Psychiatry Services, and Professor at Indiana University School of Medicine; in addition, he was Chief of Research, Marion County (Indiana) Association for Retarded Citizens. Dr. Boll was Associate Professor and Head of Psychology, Division of Child and Adolescent Psychiatry, University of Virginia Medical School, Charlottesville, Virginia. Revision author (1980) Marsha Shearer was Program Manager, Educational Services District 121, Seattle, Washington.

Western Psychological Services (12031 Wilshire Boulevard, Los Angeles, California 90025) publishes the test at a cost of $50–$55 for a test kit (manual and 25 test forms), $21–$24 for one test manual, $19.50–$21.50 each for two or more manuals, $22.50–$25.50 for one package of 25 forms, $19.90–$22.00 each for two-nine packages of 25 forms, and $18.75–$21.00 each for ten or more packages of 25 forms, plus 10 percent shipping and handling.

Age and Type of Client

The Alpern-Boll Developmental Profile II is designed to be used with any child between birth and 9½ years of age.

Purpose

The purpose of this test is to provide an inventory of skills (attainable by interview) designed to assess a child's development in five areas: motor, language, personal/self-help, social, and intellectual development. It results in functional age-level scores for each area tested and in an IQ equivalency score.

Time Required to Administer and Score Test

If all five scales comprising the Developmental Profile II are utilized, the test takes 20 to 40 minutes to administer.

Evaluator

The manual states that the Developmental Profile II was designed to be administered and scored by paraprofessionals "after brief training" (time unspecified). It is stressed that ultimate responsibility for use and interpretation rests with professionals who have training in psychological testing. Test users are expected to have knowledge of basic measurement principles, the limitations of test interpretation, and, in some cases, advanced training in evaluating children with handicapping conditions. Completion of a User Qualification form is required prior to purchase.

Development and Source of Test Items

The original Developmental Profile was designed in response to the need of an agency serving mentally retarded children. Children in the population served by this agency either had had no formal evaluation for several years or diagnostic tests that had been used were not providing useful information to their teachers.

Historical Perspective Of Test Construction

Items on the Developmental Profile were derived from (1) several scales of children's intellectual, physical, social, and language abilities, (2) normative data appearing in the developmental literature, and (3) the multidimensional concepts underlying the test. Administration of the total test results in a functional developmental age level.

Review of the Literature in Terms of Test Uses

The Developmental Profile II has been used as a standardized, functional assessment instrument to help meet the requirements of Pub. Law 94–142 (Education for All Handicapped Act). Specific uses of the test have included

1. Determination of eligibility for special education and/or related services

2. Planning tool for developing individualized educational programs (IEP) based on child's individual strengths and weaknesses
3. Measurement of individual progress through comparison of pretest (beginning of school year) scores with posttest (end of school year) scores
4. Program evaluation tool for comparing group scores

The Developmental Profile II has also been used as a general screening instrument to identify and document suspected developmental delay. It can be used in this way by professionals and nonprofessionals in any group interested in early identification and intervention for young children with potential developmental problems. For professionals with extensive experience in program planning, the Developmental Profile II provides information that can be used as the basis for intervention. The number of items/category/age range is too small, however, to allow for this use of results by inexperienced practitioners.

Theoretical Constructs and Implications for Intervention

The Developmental Profile II is based on theories from the literature of normal growth and development, and on the constructs underlying other (unidentified in manual) scales of intellectual, physical, social, and communicative abilities. The following four major goals guided construction of the Developmental Profile II:

1. Offering of an instrument that provides a multidimensional (in an attempt to provide a more accurate and functional view of individual children than is possible with tests measuring single-value depictions) view of child development
2. Providing an inventory with no significant bias as a function of race, sex, or social class (to minimize the possibility that it could be

used to discriminate against particular groups of children)

3. Providing a way to obtain a quick, inexpensive yet accurate description of development of individual children (but not at the expense of a high degree of reliability and validity)
4. Permitting administration, scoring, and interpretation by people without "specific expertise" in psychological testing (to expand use to a variety of settings where such assessment is needed but where such expertise might be unavailable)

The completed scales proved to have several implications for intervention. They were found to be useful in curriculum planning for individual children. Teachers were able to change their conceptualization of children because areas of strength, as well as deficit, were well-defined. Relatively accurate estimates of IQ were possible. Finally, teachers were able to evaluate the progress of children at the beginning and end of the school year, thus allowing evaluation of progress of individual children, classes of children, or groups of children with subsequent program revision.

Content and Test Administration

Content

The Developmental Profile II tests in the areas of physical, self-help, social, academic, and communication skills. The five scales contain a total of 186 items, with items arranged by age levels in each scale. Age levels proceed at 6-month intervals from birth to 3½ years, and by 1-year intervals thereafter (each yearly interval describes children within 6 months on either side of it). Most age levels within each scale contain three items. No equipment other than the test manual, scoring forms, and a pencil is necessary to administer the Developmental Profile II since it is an interview test.

The Developmental Profile II is scored in individual test booklets. Each of the five skill areas assessed (physical, self-help, social, academic, communication) is summarized and chronological age level equivalents determined (Fig. 5-7). Testing results in an overall profile, graphed on the first page of the test booklet, on which the age level equivalents for each skill area, the month deviant from true chronological age for each, and an IQ Equivalence Score can be recorded (Fig. 5-8).

Setting and Equipment

The Developmental Profile II can be administered in any setting that is conducive to an interview. The presence of two comfortable chairs, one for the interviewer and one for the interviewee, is required.

Administrative Procedures

The Developmental Profile II is an interview test. Questions may be answered by a parent or other person(s) who knows the child well. The purpose of the testing may dictate who the most appropriate person to be interviewed is (i.e., interview parent to gather information for program eligibility, teacher to measure child change, or even an older sibling for periodic developmental screening).

Administration and scoring directions are presented in detail in the test manual. The instructions are very clear and easily understood. The questions can be read exactly as printed in the manual or restated in language and style most comfortable for the situation. Instructions caution the interviewer not to change the *content* of the item if the wording is varied.

Administration of the Developmental Profile II is not complex. There are no items administered directly to the child. Items are easily presented and easily scored. Testing is begun at an age level where the child is likely to succeed, and a basal age (all items in two consecutive boxes on scoring form passed) obtained. Testing proceeds to higher age levels until a ceiling age (all items in two consecutive boxes on scoring form failed) is reached. It may not be possible to obtain ceiling if

SOCIAL DEVELOPMENTAL AGE SCALE (CONTINUED)

Item	Pass	Fail	Item	Pass	Fail
29. Does the child play table games such as checkers, Old Maid, Candy Land, or Lotto *with a friend of about the same age*? The child should be able to follow the rules, take turns, and there should be a "winner."	4	0	33. Does the child know that Santa Claus, the Easter Bunny, and the Good Fairy are not real? The child may get very excited about Christmas and even talk about Santa Claus, or the child may hide teeth under the pillow for the Good Fairy yet know that the Good Fairy is not real. Asking if Santa Claus is real is not sufficient to pass. The child must have come to *know* that these characters are not real.	6	0
PRIMARY ELEMENTARY II: **6–7 to 7–6 years (79–90 months)** **Basal Credit 90 months**					
30. Does the child have at least one real chore which is done at least weekly such as washing dishes, raking lawns, making a bed, taking out garbage cans, or some cleaning or dusting? The task should be done well and usually without urging more than two times.	6	0	**UPPER ELEMENTARY I:** **8–7 to 9–6 years (103–114 months)** **Basal Credit 114 months**		
31. Does the child know that voting is a way of deciding something? The child must understand that things are done in accordance with the way most of the people vote.	6	0	34. Is the child allowed to go outside the neighborhood alone? The distance should be comparable to at least four blocks.	4	0
PRIMARY ELEMENTARY III: **7–7 to 8–6 years (91–102 months)** **Basal Credit 102 months**			35. Does the child often prefer being somewhere away from home and family (at a playground or a friend's house) in order to be with his/her own friends?	4	0
32. Can the child work at home chores, for one-half hour, following a list on his/her own and do them acceptably without needing constant reminders?	6	0	36. Does the child, alone and without help, buy useful articles like gifts for others or family groceries? The child must know how much money is needed, choose appropriate items, *and* obtain correct change.	4	0

SOCIAL DEVELOPMENT SCORING SUMMARY

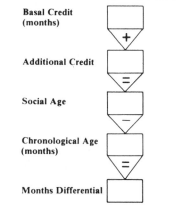

Basal Credit (months)

\+

Additional Credit

=

Social Age

−

Chronological Age (months)

=

Months Differential

Basal Credit is the oldest (highest) level in which all items are passed. Additional Credit refers to items passed beyond the basal.

10

Fig. 5-7. Example of portion of one subscale and subscale scoring summary for Developmental Profile II. (Copyright © 1984 by Western Psychological Services. Reprinted by permission of the publisher, Western Psychological Services, Los Angeles, California.)

Child's Name: _____ Testing Date: _____ Sex: M F
                                                       year   month

School: _____ Special Class: _____ Birthdate: _____ Grade: _____
                                                                 year   month

Examiner's Name: _____ Chronological Age: _____ (= _____ months)
                                                          year   month

Interviewee's Name: _____ Relationship to Child: _____

Months Differential Profile

	Physical	Self-Help	Social	Academic	Communication
	+48	+48	+48	+48	+48
	+44	+44	+44	+44	+44
	+40	+40	+40	+40	+40
	+36	+36	+36	+36	+36
	+32	+32	+32	+32	+32
	+28	+28	+28	+28	+28
	+24	+24	+24	+24	+24
Number of	+20	+20	+20	+20	+20
Months	+18	+18	+18	+18	+18
Advanced	+16	+16	+16	+16	+16
	+14	+14	+14	+14	+14
	+12	+12	+12	+12	+12
	+10	+10	+10	+10	+10
	+8	+8	+8	+8	+8
	+6	+6	+6	+6	+6
	+4	+4	+4	+4	+4
	+2	+2	+2	+2	+2
Chronological Age (months) [ ]	0	0	0	0	0
	−2	−2	−2	−2	−2
	−4	−4	−4	−4	−4
	−6	−6	−6	−6	−6
	−8	−8	−8	−8	−8
	−10	−10	−10	−10	−10
	−12	−12	−12	−12	−12
	−14	−14	−14	−14	−14
Number of	−16	−16	−16	−16	−16
Months	−18	−18	−18	−18	−18
Delayed	−20	−20	−20	−20	−20
	−24	−24	−24	−24	−24
	−28	−28	−28	−28	−28
	−32	−32	−32	−32	−32
	−36	−36	−36	−36	−36
	−40	−40	−40	−40	−40
	−44	−44	−44	−44	−44
	−48	−48	−48	−48	−48

Months Differential: _____ _____ _____ _____ _____

IQ Equivalence: _____	Physical Age	Self-Help Age	Social Age	Academic Age	Communication Age

Fig. 5-8. Scoring and profile form from the Developmental Profile II. (Copyright © 1984 by Western Psychological Services. Reprinted by permission of the publisher, Western Psychological Services, Los Angeles, California.)

a child's abilities are at the top of the scale. In this case, it must be noted that exact developmental age cannot be determined. The basal and ceiling methods are not appropriate for use with children with certain specific handicaps since they may not develop skills in the same sequence as other children. For these children, the authors suggest administering all items in the inventory in order to determine specific strengths and weaknesses.

Directions for scoring results of the Developmental Profile II are clearly stated and easily followed. Each test item is scored as pass or fail, depending on information given during the interview. If an informant is not sure of the answer, a "best guess" is acceptable. The passing or failing response is circled on the scoring form, directly opposite each item number. A failing response is always represented by a zero, while a passing response is always represented by a number (of months) other than zero (i.e., 2, 3, 4, or 6). Basal credit (highest or "oldest" box in which *all* items are passed) is determined for each of the five scales and recorded in years and months. Additional credit for each scale (sum of months credit, or "items passed" beyond basal level) is also recorded. Basal credit plus additional credit is then summed and becomes the total age score for each scale. This score can be entered onto the Profile Grid on the first page of the test booklet (see Fig. 5-8). This page provides a quick-glance summary of performance.

If a child is able to reach a double ceiling (all items failed in two consecutive boxes on scoring form) on the Academic Scale, an IQ Equivalency Score can be computed. This method is suitable for obtaining a descriptive label for administrative purposes, but should not be considered a substitute for full assessment of skills in the various developmental areas representing intellectual abilities. The IQ Equivalency Score is computed by dividing the score (in months) on the academic scale by the child's chronological age (in months) and multiplying by 100.

Administration of the Developmental Profile II results in determination of six "ages" for each child; the chronological age and five develop-

mental ages. In addition, the IQ Equivalency Score may be computed. Interpretation involves comparing the chronological and developmental ages in a variety of ways:

1. Determination of advanced or delayed skills in each area can be made using the Profile Sheet (see Fig. 5-8), which provides a graphic representation of the child's general development.
2. Determination of whether a lag between chronological age and developmental age is significant can be made. This determination is primarily dependent on the child's current chronological age and outcome age on the scale on which the lag is occurring.
3. Determination of relative developmental strengths and weaknesses based on the relationship of findings between the scale in question and on the other four scales.

Guidelines for referral are provided in the Developmental Profile II manual. The guidelines exist in the form of separate tables, for each of the five scales, in which any particular developmental age can be compared with the chronological age and determined to be within the range or normal, in the "borderline range" of potential significance or in the delayed range, indicating presence of possible handicap. The manual warns of two limitations in using the referral guidelines: (1) they have been constructed based on clinical judgment rather than empirical data, and (2) they account only for individual ages on individual scales rather than for performance on the entire Profile.

Psychometric Properties

Standardization

Specific step-by-step instructions for administering the Developmental Profile II are included in the test manual. The interview format allows the test to be used in a variety of settings, and the instructions include a discussion of how to decide who might best be chosen to answer the questions in each setting. It is emphasized that the meaning of each question must always be preserved, even though the wording can be changed to make any situation more comfortable.

The Developmental Profile II uses standardization data from the original edition published in 1972. The latter was standardized on 3008 children who were tested between June 1970 and March 1972. The children were divided into 16 age groups ranging from 1 month to 12 years, with an average of 225 children per age group. Social class distribution included 11 percent upper, 80 percent middle, and 9 percent lower class. Cultural background included 84 percent white, 14 percent black, and 2 percent "other." Data were collected primarily in urban areas of the states of Washington (9%) and Indiana (91%). Only 9 percent of the subjects in either state were from "small cities" and 2 percent from rural or small town areas.

The results of the standardization study are considered adequate by the researchers for supplying normative data on both sexes from birth to preadolescence. They also concluded that a single set of norms could be considered valid for all social classes. However, there are some limitations in the normative data:

1. They are applicable to white and black children only. Other groups were insufficiently represented in the sample to determine degree of applicability of the derived norms.
2. The majority of subjects were from urban areas. Therefore, the usefulness of the test for children from small towns or rural areas is unknown.
3. The sample contains a strong geographic bias.

Items were considered "normative" for a particular age if they were passed by 70 to 80 percent of the children for that age in the standardization sample. Items were included in the scales if they were passed by approximately 75 percent of the normative population; and they did not

discriminate as a function of sex, race or social class. Following item analysis, 318 items in the original standardized version were reduced to 218. The number of items in the Developmental Profile II was further reduced to 186 by eliminating all items beyond the chronological age of 9 years, and eliminating all items found to be inappropriate, outdated or sexist. No additional analysis of items was done to accomplish this further reduction.

Reliability

To obtain test-retest reliability, each of two interviewers administered the prestandardized version of the Developmental Profile to mothers of 11 children ages 1 month to 9½ years. Interviews were conducted 2 to 3 days apart. Examiners obtained identical scores on 22 percent of the interviews, and were within 1 point of each other on 50 percent, 2 points on 68 percent, and 3 points on 92 percent of the interviews. Differences between raw scores were not statistically significant.

Interobserver reliability was established by 35 Head Start teachers who observed one interview concerning a 4½ year-old-boy. The prestandardized version was used. The teachers' responses were recorded independently and collected immediately; 71 percent had identical scores, 89 percent were within 1 point of the model score, and 97 percent were within 2 points.

Internal consistency was investigated using a modified version (all items below 18 months and above 90 months eliminated) of the Developmental Profile on a sample of 1050 children [6]. Internal consistency coefficients were .79 for the Physical Scale, .78 for the Self-Help Scale, .82 for the Social Scale, .87 for the Academic Scale, and .83 for the Communication Scale. Internal consistency coefficients were also calculated for a group of 72 children in a Head Start program who were tested with both the original and modified versions of the Developmental Profile. Coefficients ranged from .87 to .95. These studies indicate a high degree of correspondence between the original and modified versions, and a high degree of homogeneity among items on each scale.

Validity

Content validity was addressed during development of the Developmental Profile through thorough literature search for appropriate items and item placement, and extensive field testing.

Criterion validity has been investigated by comparing (1) parents estimates of developmental level with other forms of assessment, and (2) Developmental Profile II results with other test outcomes. The ability of the Developmental Profile II to discriminate among groups has also been investigated [4]. The studies comparing parent report with other evaluation methods suggest that parents basically provide accurate developmental information. Differences are usually in the direction of overestimation of abilities. Discrepancy between estimated and observed performance is greatest for children who have physical problems. Studies investigating relationship of the Developmental Profile II with other measures concentrate primarily on the comparability of the IQ Equivalency Score (based on Academic Scale only) with IQ scores resulting from testing with the Stanford-Binet. Moderate to high validity coefficients between the two scores have been reported, but the IQ equivalency score should be interpreted with caution. Caution is recommended because the samples in studies used to investigate it is small, the number of items on which it is based is small, it is a ratio score (meaning that the standard deviation will vary from one age level to the next), and it tends to overestimate IQ scores for children below the norm and underestimate them for children above the norm. A cut-off score for screening purposes can be determined using the IQ equivalency score. The error of prediction is 15 points (on either side of the obtained IQ Equivalency Score) according to one study [7].

Construct validity has been investigated through study of convergent and discriminant validity, and through intervention studies. Limited support for convergent validity (significant correlations between measures designed to assess the same construct) has been demonstrated [7]. The same study could not demonstrate evidence of discriminant validity, but a number of confounding factors (the two measures compared may have tapped different constructs, study sample was restricted, scoring differences and possible method bias) leave this open to further investigation. Several studies reported in the manual used the Developmental Profile II to measure effectiveness of intervention. These studies demonstrate that the instrument is sensitive to growth and change over time and that it can be useful in planning and evaluating programs of individual instruction.

Guidelines for Use in a Clinical Setting

This test could conceivably be used for a child of any appropriate age, i.e., birth to 9½ years, since it is not dependent on observation of physical, cognitive, or language skill performance. It is dependent, however, on certain qualities of parents and caretakers such as their observation skills and cognitive understanding.

The Developmental Profile II is a screening test, and the results must never be interpreted as diagnostic. It is nicely used in conjunction with screening tests that do not result in an estimate of cognitive skills. It should be noted, however, that the Intelligence Quotient Equivalence (IQE) score tends to overestimate IQs of mentally retarded children and to underestimate IQs of above-average children.

In general, clinical observations do not result from this parent interview test. It frequently is of use to determine the observation skills of the parent or caretaker in preparation for intervention planning, and that opportunity is provided to some extent by this instrument. While many of the test items can be converted to direct observation items, this test is most useful in obtaining a general idea of areas of particular strengths and weaknesses of a child, and in determining a general level of cognitive understanding.

Table 5-6. The Developmental Profile: Summary of results of five validation studies

Profile scale used	Sample number	Version of developmental profile	Criterion test	Correlations
Variety of scores and combinations of scores from Developmental Profile	18 mentally retarded children	Prestandardized version administered by teachers	Stanford-Binet (SB)	.55 between SB MA and average functioning age (average age of the 5 scale scores) .80 between SB MA and a mental age score (derived by averaging academic and communication scale age) .84 between SB MA and Profile's Academic Age (these data provided initial formula for deriving IQE score)
Academic Scale	54 mentally retarded children	Poststandardized final version of Developmental Profile I Academic Scale (filled out by teachers)	IQ Test (unidentified) during previous year	.85 between IQ and IQE (tended to overestimate IQ of mentally retarded children)
	16 children with normal intelligence (average IQ, 119)	Poststandardized final version of Developmental Profile I Academic Scale (based on interview of mothers)	Stanford-Binet	.49 between IQ and IQE (tended to underestimate IQ of above average children), statistically significant
Physical Scale	53 children ages 2–11 years	Prestandardized version of Developmental Profile I	Dental age	.96 between dental age and physical scale Preschool age children = .89 (statistically significant) Elementary school age = .48 (statistically significant) Older children = .10 (nonsignificant)
Interview Version versus Performance Observation version of Developmental Profile I (to determine accuracy of the mother's interview)	100 children (55 males, 45 females, 88 whites, 12 blacks) ages 3 mo to 12 yr	197 items from standardized version which could be observed as well as obtained from the interview	Actual testing versus interview information	Overall agreement of 84% between standardized version and mother's report, and 86% between final version of Developmental Profile I and mother's report

Key: MA, mental age; IQ, intelligence quotient; IQE, intelligence quotient equivalency score.
Source: Adapted from G. D. Alpern and M. S. Shearer (revision authors). *Manual: Developmental Profile II*. Aspen, Colorado: Psychological Development Publications, 1980.

Review

The Developmental Profile II is one of the few screening instruments available with which general development of children up to age 9 years can be assessed. The interview format is sometimes extremely useful when children are uncooperative or cannot be present for extended periods of in-person testing.

The most recent edition of the manual (1985) incorporates findings from several studies in addition to those upon which the initial version of the scale was based. This increased evidence of reliability and validity is a welcome addition. The instrument is considered to be able to identify developmental ages of black and white urban mid-Americans of all social classes [4]. Table 5-6 provides a summary of findings from some of the early validation studies. However, it should be recognized that more confidence could be placed in the referral guidelines if they were based on empirically determined data rather than on clinical judgment only, and if they were based on overall scale performance rather than on individual ages for individual scales. It is extremely important to keep in mind that the IQ Equivalence Score tends to overestimate IQs of mentally retarded children and to underestimate IQs of children with above-average IQs.

REFERENCES

1. Alpern, G. D. The Developmental Profile: Review of the Instrument and Recent Research. In W. K. Frankenburg et al. (eds.), *Proceedings: Second International Conference on Developmental Screening.* Santa Fe, N.M.: 1977.
2. Alpern, G. D., and Boll, T. J. *Developmental Profile Manual.* Indianapolis: Psychological Development Publications, 1972.
3. Alpern, G. D., and Shearer, M. S. (revision authors). *Manual: Developmental Profile II.* Aspen, Col.: Psychological Development Publications, 1980.
4. Alpern, G. D., Boll, T. J., and Shearer, M. S. *Developmental Profile II: Manual.* Los Angeles: Western Psychological Services, 1985.
5. Boll, T. J., and Alpern, G. D. The Developmental Profile: A new instrument to measure child development through interviews. *J. Clin. Child Psychol.* 4 : 26, 1975.
6. Lawhon, D. A. *A Summarative Evaluation of the Aids to Early Learning 1976–1977.* Charleston, W.V.: Appalachia Educational Laboratory, 1977.
7. Macmann, G. M., and Barnett, D. W. An analysis of the Construct Validity of two measures of Adaptive Behavior. *J. Psychoeduc. Assess.* 2 : 239, 1984.
8. Stangler, S., Huber, C., and Routh, D. *Screening Growth and Development of Preschool Children: A Guide for Test Selection.* New York: McGraw-Hill, 1980.

VINELAND ADAPTIVE BEHAVIOR SCALES

Descriptive Information

Test Identification

The title of this test is *Vineland Adaptive Behavior Scales* (Vineland), 1984. The test is a revision of the Vineland Social Maturity Scale by Edgar A. Doll. The authors of the Vineland are Sara S. Sparrow, Ph.D., David A. Balla, Ph.D., and Domenic V. Cicchetti, Ph.D. Dr. Sparrow is Associate Professor of Psychology and Chief Psychologist, Child Study Center, Yale University. The late Dr. Balla (1939–1982) was Associate Professor of Psychology at the Child Study Center and Research Associate in the Department of Psychology, Yale University. Dr. Cicchetti is Research Scientist in the Department of Psychiatry, Yale University School of Medicine, and Senior Research Psychologist and Biostatistician, Psychology Service, Veterans Administration Medical Center, West Haven, Connecticut.

American Guidance Service, Inc. (Circle Pines, Minnesota 55014) publishes this test. The Vineland Scales are available in three versions: Interview Edition, Survey Form; Interview Edition, Expanded Form; and Classroom Edition (1984). Materials that can be purchased include manuals and test forms for all three versions, some in both English and Spanish. Supplementary materials that are also available include

1. Cassette tape of sample interviews using the Survey or Expanded Form.
2. Automated System for Scoring and Interpreting Standardized Tests (ASSIST)—microcomputer software packages with methods for score conversion, profiling, and record management of all three versions.
3. Technical and Interpretive Manual, which supplies detailed statistical data gathered during development and standardization of all

three versions (study summaries, case studies, methods for application of test results).
4. Reports to Parents for all three versions, which summarize and explain derived scores in relation to strengths and weaknesses for the individual being evaluated. Cost of the complete Interview Edition (Survey and Expanded Form starter sets) is $63–$70. Survey Form starter set alone lists for $25–$28. Expanded Form starter set alone lists for $41–$46. The Classroom Edition starter set costs $19–$21. More complete information concerning cost can be obtained from the publisher.

Age and Type of Client

Both the Survey Form and the Expanded Form are designed for all children from birth to 18 years 11 months, or low-functioning adults (Motor Skills Scale is designed for children from birth to 5 years 11 months and selected others). The Classroom Edition is designed for students between 3 years and 12 years 11 months of age.

Purpose

The Vineland is designed to assess personal and social sufficiency of nonhandicapped and handicapped individuals from birth to adulthood. It is administered by semistructured interview with a caregiver or person who knows the client well. Each of the three versions of the revised Vineland measures adaptive behavior in four domains: communication (receptive, expressive, written), daily living skills (personal, domestic, community), socialization (interpersonal relationships, play and leisure time, coping skills) and motor skills (gross motor, fine motor). An optionally administered domain of maladaptive behavior (for individuals 5 years 0 months and older) is included in the Survey and Expanded Forms. This scale is the same for each form.

*Time Required to
Administer and Score the Test*

The Survey Form can be administered in 20 to 60 minutes, the Expanded Form in 60 to 90 minutes, and the Classroom Edition in 20 minutes.

Evaluator

The revised Vineland is to be administered by professionals with graduate degrees and specific experience and training both in assessment of individuals and in test interpretation. A background in human development and behavior and in tests and measurements, and experience with developmental disabilities is also expected. Additional qualifications include training in interview techniques, experience in administration and interpretation of adaptive behavior scales, desirable interviewer personality (professional manner, ability to develop rapport with the respondent), and a thorough knowledge of the test. Specific disciplines identified as appropriate are psychology and social work, but it is obvious that appropriate users can be members of many professional disciplines. The revised Vineland should not be used by nonprofessionals. Trained examiners are not required for administration of the Classroom Edition. However, a "qualified professional" is needed to determine and interpret derived scores.

Historical Perspective Of Test Construction

Development and Source of Test Items

Items for the revised Vineland were developed following an analysis of the items on the Vineland Social Maturity Scale and other adaptive behavior scales (unidentified), intensive review of the literature on child development, and an analysis of the authors' clinical and research experience. They were developed to assess adaptive behavior in four domains felt to accurately categorize daily activities of most individuals: communication, daily living skills, socialization, and motor skills. Approximately 3000 items were generated and subjected to the following criteria to determine retention or rejection:

1. Representative of activities necessary for personal and social sufficiency.
2. Of lasting relevance.
3. Easily understandable by respondent, regardless of educational, social, or cultural background.
4. Applicable to most individuals, regardless of background or geographic location.
5. Readily amenable to objective scoring procedures.
6. Easily translatable into educational, habilitative, or treatment program objectives.

Items were reduced to 800 after application of the criteria, then pilot-tested in the New Haven, Connecticut, area and further reduced to 529. These 529 items became the basis for a "national tryout" of the Interview Edition of the revised Vineland. Purposes of the national tryout included

1. Obtain the item difficulty of discrimination data on the national sample of children to construct the standardized version of the revised Vineland.
2. Refine the method of administration.
3. Establish scoring criteria.

The national tryout was conducted from July to November 1980 on a sample of 723 individuals from Minnesota, New York, North Carolina, Louisiana, Arizona, and New Mexico. All socioeconomic categories as well as white and ethnic groups were included. All subjects also received the Peabody Picture Vocabulary Test-Revised (mean score, 103.6; standard deviation, 14.6).

Following the national tryout, the two versions of the Interview Edition (Survey Form and Expanded Form) of the revised Vineland were developed, and the maladaptive behavior domain added. Criteria for item inclusion in the Survey Form included

1. Contribution to an adaptive behavior instrument which was equally sensitive (as much as possible) at all ages from birth to adulthood, and which adequately measured performance in the four original domains.
2. Representative of all clusters in the Expanded Form (by including at least the final item in each cluster representing highest performance).

The final number of items in the standardization version of the Survey Form was 301 (265 adaptive behavior items, 36 maladaptive behavior items). The Expanded Form consists of 577 items (541 adaptive behavior items, 36 maladaptive items), thus helping to pinpoint specific behavior contributing to strengths and weaknesses in each domain.

Review of the Literature in Terms of Test Use

The revised Vineland is useful whenever an assessment of daily functioning is required, whether it be in a clinical, educational, or research setting. Its primary clinical use is predicted to be as a "major or ancillary diagnostic tool" [2]. Assessment of adaptive behavior is necessary to substantiate deficits prior to diagnosis of mental retardation, and to acquire a comprehensive picture of the abilities of many nonhandicapped individuals as well. The test can also be used in clinical settings (1) to compare information about adaptive behavior and intelligence (especially when used along with the Kaufman Assessment Battery for Children reviewed in Chap. 8 of this text, since there is substantial overlap in the two standardization samples), and (2) to assess adaptive behavior in different settings and from different points of view (when either form of the interview version is used with the teacher-completed Classroom Edition).

A second important way in which all scales of the revised Vineland can be used, especially the

Expanded Form, is to develop individual educational, habilitative, and treatment programs. Many such programs stress skills necessary for personal and social sufficiency, and the revised Vineland is capable of indicating strengths and weaknesses in specific areas of adaptive behavior. The Expanded Form actually offers step-by-step guidelines for developing an individual program. All three versions are useful for monitoring individual progress and/or evaluating program success.

Finally, the revised Vineland is useful in conducting many kinds of research, including studies concerning infant development and parent-child relationships as well as mental and physical handicaps. It is particularly useful in longitudinal studies since such a large age range is covered by the test.

Adaptive behavior is a component of all behavior. Therefore, this scale is conceivably useful to most disciplines working with various aspects of behavior of a large variety of handicapped or nonhandicapped individuals of many ages.

Theoretical Constructs and Implications for Intervention

Adaptive behavior is defined in the revised Vineland as ". . . the performance of the daily activities required for personal and social sufficiency" [2]. Three important principles inherent in this definition include

1. Adaptive behavior is age-related, meaning that it is expected to become more complex as individuals grow older.
2. Adaptive behavior is defined by the expectations of other people, meaning that one's adequacy of adaptive behavior is judged by those living, working, and interacting with any individual.
3. Adaptive behavior is defined by typical performance, not by ability, meaning that when ability is present it must be demonstrated when required [2].

Early attempts to define mental retardation included consideration of adaptive behavior skills. When use of intelligence tests became popular, the perceived importance of incorporating adaptive behavior lessened. Edgar Doll, author of the original Vineland Social Maturity Scale, understood the significance of objective measurement of adaptive behavior in defining mental retardation. Among his many contributions to measurement of adaptive behavior were the concepts that

1. Adaptive behavior is developmental in nature.
2. Adaptive behavior is multidimensional (encompasses a wide range of areas, or domains).
3. Administration of adaptive behavior scales requires presence of a respondent who knows the client well, but does not require actual presence of the client whose behavior is being assessed.

During the 1960s and 1970s, attention was again given to incorporating adaptive behavior into the definition of mental retardation. It is now formally included in the definition, and in legislation concerning mentally retarded individuals such as the Rehabilitation Act of 1973 (law promoting education, training, and employment of handicapped persons) and the Education for All Handicapped Children of 1975 (Pub. L. 94–142). This law has multiple impacts on intervention, particularly in instances where state or federal money is used in assessment, intervention, and/or research programs.

Content and Test Administration

Content

All three of the revised Vineland Adaptive Behavior Scales (Survey and Expanded Forms of the Interview Edition, and the Classroom Edition) test in four adaptive behavior domains: communication, daily living skills, socialization, and motor skills. Both the Survey and Expanded Forms contain a maladaptive behavior domain (assessment of activities which may interfere with adaptive functioning) for individuals 5 years of age and older; administration of this domain is optional.

The Survey Form contains a total of 297 test items: 261 within the adaptive behavior domains and 36 within the maladaptive behavior domain. Each domain contains several subdomains into which items are categorized. Table 5-7 indicates the number of items within each subdomain. Items are organized in order of difficulty within each domain.

The Expanded Form contains 577 items, 297 of which are from the Survey Form. Each domain contains several subdomains. Items are arranged according to a variety of activities within each subdomain in clusters of two to eight. Table 5-8 indicates the various subdomains and the number of items in each. Chronological ages at which clusters of activities are expected to occur are indicated on the test form.

The Classroom Edition contains 244 items. Some items are from either the Survey or Expanded Forms, and some are related to basic academic functioning. Items are grouped according to different areas of content within the same domains and subdomains as on the other two forms.

There is no test kit available for use with the revised Vineland. Since it is administered in a semistructured interview, no equipment other than the manual, test form, and a pencil is necessary.

The Survey Form of the Interview Edition has two separate booklets in which results are recorded: a Record Booklet (in which individual test performance is scored) and a Report to Parents Booklet (for summarizing scores and indicating strengths and weaknesses). The Expanded Form of the Interview Edition includes four booklets: an Item Booklet, a Score Summary and Profile Booklet, a Program Planning Report Booklet, and a Report to Parents Booklet. The Item Booklet is where individual test performance is scored. The Score Summary and Profile Booklet is used for interpreting raw data. Its purpose is to pinpoint the clusters of abilities within domains and subdomains that describe activities that should be included in individual program

Table 5-7. Number of items per domain and subdomain in the survey form of the interview edition of the Vineland Adaptive Behavior Scales

Domain	Subdomain	Number of items
Adaptive Behaviors		
Communication	Receptive	13
	Expressive	31
	Written	23
	Total =	67
Daily Living Skills	Personal	39
	Domestic	21
	Community	32
	Total =	92
Socialization	Interpersonal relationships	28
	Play and leisure time	20
	Coping skills	18
	Total =	66
Motor Skills	Gross motor	20
	Fine motor	16
	Total =	36
Maladaptive Behavior		36

Source: Adapted from S. Sparrow, D. Balla, and D. Cicchetti. *Vineland Adaptive Behavior Scales, Interview Edition: Expanded Form Manual.* Circle Pines, Minnesota: American Guidance Service, 1984.

Table 5-8. Domains, subdomains, activities, and number of items in the expanded form of the Interview Edition of the Vineland Adaptive Behavior Scales

Domain	Subdomain	Activity	Number of items
Communication	Receptive	Beginning to Understand	6
		Beginning to Listen	3
		Pointing to Body Parts	4
		Following Instructions	5
		Listening and Attending	5
		Total =	23
	Expressive	Beginning Affective Expression	5
		Prespeech Sounds	3
		Prespeech Nonverbal Expression	3
		Beginning to Talk	5
		Vocabulary	3
		Talking in Sentences	4
		Using Names	4
		Asking Questions	6
		Using Abstract Concepts	4
		Relating Experiences	5
		Using Prepositions	5
		Using Function Words	5
		Articulating	4
		Reciting	4
		Using Plural Nouns and Verbal Tense	6
		Giving Information About Self	7

Table 5-8 (continued)

Domain	Subdomain	Activity	Number of items
Communication— *(continued)*		Expressing Complex Ideas	3
		Total =	76
	Written	Identifying Letters and Words	7
		Beginning to Read	4
		Beginning to Write	5
		Printing and Cursive	4
		Using Reading Materials	4
		Reading Books, Newspapers, and Magazines	5
		Writing Letters and Reports	5
		Total =	34
		Total in Domain =	133
Daily Living Skills	Personal	Eating	6
		Removing Clothing	3
		Bathing with Assistance	3
		Toilet Training	7
		Drinking	6
		Brushing Teeth	4
		Washing Hands and Face	5
		Toileting Tasks	4
		Caring for Nose	5
		Fastening Fasteners	5
		Putting on Shoes	6
		Bathing Without Assistance	3
		Using Tableware	8
		Putting on Clothes	7
		Wearing Clothing Appropriate for Weather	4
		Beginning Health Care	3
		Caring for Hair	5
		Caring for Fingernails	3
		Advanced Health Care	3
		Total =	90
	Domestic	Beginning Housecleaning	3
		Putting Things Away	4
		Beginning Food Preparation	4
		Using Tools	2
		Clearing and Setting Table	6
		Using Kitchen Appliances	3
		Using Equipment and Household Cleaning Products	2
		Making Bed	4
		Advanced Housecleaning	4
		Household Repairs and Maintenance	2
		Cooking	4
		Caring for Clothes	3
		Sewing	4
		Total =	45
	Community	Safety at Home	4
		Beginning Telephone Use	6
		Safety on Streets and Roads	4
		Understanding Money	5

Table 5-8 (continued)

Domain	Subdomain	Activity	Number of items
Daily Living Skills— *(continued)*		Left-Right Orientation	4
		Restaurant Skills	3
		Telling Time: Days, Months, Years	7
		Telling Time: Hours and Minutes	5
		Making Change	4
		Advanced Telephone Use	6
		Saving Money	3
		Earning Money	3
		Budgeting	5
		Job Skills	5
		Managing Money	2
		Total =	66
		Total in Domain =	201
Socialization	Interpersonal Relationships	Beginning Responsiveness	6
		Expressing Emotion	4
		Responding to Familiar People	3
		Imitating Phrases and Movements	4
		Recognizing Emotions	3
		Identifying Others	4
		Responding to Social Communication	3
		Friendship	5
		Giving Gifts	4
		Imitating Social Communication	3
		Cooperative Interactions	3
		Belonging to Groups	4
		Dating	4
		Total =	50
	Play and Leisure Time	Playing with Toys	4
		Interest in Environment	5
		Playing with Others	3
		Make-Believe Activities	4
		Sharing and Cooperating	4
		Watching Television	3
		Following Game Rules	4
		Playing Games	4
		Beginning Group Activities	3
		Hobbies	3
		Extracurricular and Nonschool Activities	2
		Using Television and Radio for Entertainment and Information	4
		Going Places with Friends Independently	5
		Total =	48
	Coping Skills	Following Rules	4
		Beginning Politeness	3
		Using Manners in Conversation	3
		Being Responsible for Time	2
		Being Sensitive to Others	3
		Keeping Secrets or Confidences	4
		Using Table Manners	5

Table 5-8 (continued)

Domain	Subdomain	Activity	Number of items
Socialization— *(continued)*		Controlling Impulses	4
		Apologizing	4
		Borrowing and Returning	2
		Making and Keeping Appointments	2
		Total =	36
		Total in Domain =	134
Motor Skills	Gross Motor	Sitting	4
		Beginning Mobility	3
		Walking	5
		Running	4
		Jumping	3
		Using Stairs	7
		Climbing	4
		Hopping	3
		Throwing and Catching Balls	5
		Riding Tricycle and Bicycle	4
		Total =	42
	Fine Motor	Using Both Hands	6
		Picking up Objects and Building with Blocks	4
		Completing Puzzles	4
		Drawing	7
		Opening Drawers and Doors	5
		Using Scissors	5
		Total =	31
		Total in Domain =	73
Maladaptive Behavior		Total =	36

Source: Adapted from S. Sparrow, D. Balla, and D. Cicchetti. *Vineland Adaptive Behavior Scales, Interview Edition: Survey Form Manual.* Circle Pines, Minnesota: American Guidance Service, 1984.

plans, or activities which the individual should be performing but is not. Program planning profiles can be completed for some or all domains and subdomains. The Program Planning Report Booklet can be used as the client's educational, habilitative, or treatment program plan. The booklet contains space for recording program goals, objectives, methods of implementation, methods of program evaluation, and mastery criteria for each objective. The Report to Parents Booklet is the same as that used for the Survey Form.

The Classroom Edition is also scored in individual test booklets. Responses are recorded in each domain and subdomain according to whether the performance has been observed or estimated. The test booklet contains features similar to those contained in booklets for the Survey and Expanded Forms of the Interview Edition.

Setting and Equipment

The Survey and Expanded Forms of the Interview Edition of the revised Vineland Adaptive Behavior Scales can be administered in any setting that is conducive to an interview. The Classroom Edition questionnaire can be completed independently by the teacher in a setting of choice. The presence of comfortable chairs, one for the respondent and one for the interviewer, is required.

Administrative Procedures

The Survey and Expanded Forms of the Interview Edition are to be completed by conducting a semistructured interview. The respondent should be the person (usually parent or caregiver) who knows the client best. In some cases, more than one respondent may be necessary to give accurate information in all domains. If this is the case, only one respondent should be interviewed for any one domain. Every effort should be made to find one respondent who can answer the questions in all domains since there are no normative data based on use of multiple respondents.

The Classroom Edition is to be completed by the classroom teacher. Teachers complete the questionnaire independently. Scores are given for each item in the edition, and are assigned based on definite knowledge of performance (observed performance) or on knowledge of behavior in other areas (estimated performance).

Administration directions are presented in detail in the manuals. They are clear and easily understood. Items and scoring criteria are, in general, clearly stated [1, 2]. Instructions specifically state that items are not to be read directly, either to or by the respondent. The interviewer is to begin with general questions, *and follow with further probes as necessary,* to elicit more specific information. Domains are to be administered in the order presented in the manuals and test booklet, beginning with communication and

ending with motor skills. The interviewer must determine at what age level to begin discussion. It is not necessary to begin with the first item in any one subdomain. Decisions of this sort are based on familiarity with items around a logical starting age level.

Administration of the revised Vineland is somewhat complex and requires practice and familiarity with the items and interview techniques. Nothing is administered directly to the client in question, and there are no difficult procedures to be carried out. Items are easily presented and responses easily recorded. Appropriate "additional probing" can be difficult when a caregiver does not understand a question.

Scoring

Directions for scoring results of the revised Vineland are clearly stated, and the steps can be followed without confusion. Completing the scoring procedure, however, is sometimes considered complex. There are five possible ways each item on the revised scales can be scored:

  2 = The activity is usually or habitually performed.
  1 = The activity is sometimes performed, or with partial success.
  0 = The activity is never performed.
  N = (no opportunity) The activity is not performed because of limiting external circumstances.
  DK = (don't know) Respondent has no knowledge of the client's performance.

Designations of N and DK are not permitted when scoring the maladaptive behavior domain. More in-depth interpretations of each designation are included in the manuals [1, 2]. Where appropriate, special instructions such as "Do Not Score 1" are included.

Basal scores (highest seven consecutive items scored "2" in each domain) and ceiling scores (lowest seven consecutive items scored "0" in each domain) are established when using the Survey Form. Basal scores only are established for the Expanded Form. Ceiling scores are not established for the Expanded Form because items are arranged in developmental order within clusters rather than in entire domains. Basal and ceiling scores may be established at any time during administration of a domain. Since items are not necessarily administered in order of appearance, the interviewer cannot begin with a certain starting item and proceed forward or backward. After each domain is administered, it is essential to check that appropriate basal and ceiling scores have been established. Raw scores are calculated for each subdomain and transferred to the score summary grid located on the back of the Survey Form Record Book and Expanded Form Score Summary and Profile Book. Transferring the scores can become a significant source of error since they must first be summed from numbers on several pages, then transferred to the back page, and finally summed once again to obtain raw scores.

Administration of the revised Vineland Interview Edition results in a series of derived scores (converted raw scores that have uniform meaning from domain to domain, or subdomain to subdomain, for individuals of all ages) that are based on performance of the national standardization sample and performance of supplementary norm groups (see section on standardization). Derived scores obtained for each of the four adaptive behavior domains include standard scores, bands of error, national percentile ranks, stanines, adaptive levels, and age equivalents. Conversion tables for calculating each of these scores are contained in the manual appendixes. A score profile, located on the back of the Survey Form Record Booklet and Expanded Form Score Summary and Profile Booklet, can be completed to visualize the domain and composite scores in a graphic display. Derived scores are not available for the adaptive behavior com-

posite; it is obtained from the average of the three or four subdomain standard scores.

Standard scores are not available for the maladaptive behavior domain. A raw score is obtained and, using a table, is converted to a "maladaptive level."

The various scores obtained can be interpreted to aid in diagnosis of mental retardation, to assist in educational placement, to provide additional data when comprehensive assessment in conjunction with other measures is desired, to compare the client's performance in one or more domains or subdomains, to assist in planning individual programs to measure changes in adaptive functioning over a span of time, and to help determine need for further assessment [1, 2]. A significant portion of each manual is devoted to the variety of ways in which performance of the revised scales can be interpreted [1, 2].

The revised Vineland is really not considered to be a screening test and, as such, does not have specific guidelines for referral. Cutoff scores for screening are not included. It is primarily expected to be used in conjunction with a variety of diagnostic tests as a way of providing an additional body of data that may be relevant for program planning for individuals with developmental delays. In this way, data from the revised Vineland may help to pinpoint the type of program a client needs to be referred to in order to obtain the most needed intervention. Many of the professionals administering the revised Vineland would be involved in carrying out program planning based on test results rather than using the results as indicators of need for referral.

Psychometric Properties

Standardization

A clearly outlined, step-by-step procedure for test administration is included in the manuals for the revised Vineland Adaptive Behavior Scales.

Instructions are clearly stated and, even though the procedure is somewhat complex, should allow the test to be administered in a standardized fashion. It should be recalled that interview questions are not intended to be read directly to or by the respondent, making it essential that the interviewer be thoroughly familiar with the items and their intent in order to be able to follow the standardized procedures.

The revised Vineland Adaptive Behavior Scales were standardized on a national, representative sample of 3000 individuals from birth through 18 years, 11 months of age, and on a supplementary sample of handicapped individuals. Data from the same samples were used for standardization information for both the Survey and Expanded Forms of the Interview Version. Data regarding the national standardization sample were collected between September 1981 and May 1982, at 35 sites in 24 states. Data regarding the supplementary sample were collected between September 1982 and November 1982 (number of states and sites not identified). Categories of handicapped individuals included a combined sample of ambulatory and nonambulatory mentally retarded adult residents of residential facilities, only ambulatory mentally retarded adult residents of residential facilities, mentally retarded adult clients of nonresidential facilities, emotionally disturbed child residents of residential facilities, visually handicapped child residents of residential facilities, and hearing-impaired child residents of residential facilities. Table 5-9 contains more-detailed information regarding demographic data for the national sample, and Table 5-10 contains additional available information about the supplementary sample.

The Classroom Edition was standardized on a nationally representative sample of 3000 students ages 3 years through 12 years 11 months. Stratification variables included sex, race or ethnic group, community size, geographic region, and level of parent education.

Derived scores for the Survey Form were developed using data from two types of normative groups: the national standardization sample and seven supplementary norm groups of handicapped individuals. Procedures used for developing derived scores are explained in the manuals, and the various norms tables are contained in Appendix B of the manuals.

Development of optional scoring procedures (prorated sum of domain standard scores to be used when data from one domain is missing, estimated scores for motor skills domain in clients 6 years of age and older) and of procedures for investigating significant differences between domain standard scores are described in the manuals [1, 2].

Norms for the Expanded Form of the Interview Edition were generated from data collected in the national standardization program for the Survey Form. Rasch-Wright calibration estimates were used to generate these norms. Appropriate reference tables are contained in the manual for the Expanded Form.

Reliability

Three types of reliability are reported for the revised Vineland: split-half (internal consistency), test-retest reliability, and interrater reliability (internal reliability).

Split-half, or internal consistency, reliability coefficients were based on items *actually administered* in each adaptive behavior domain and subdomain. Correlation coefficients obtained for the Survey Form were also used to estimate split-half reliability coefficients for the Expanded Form. Coefficients for all domains and subdomains on both forms were considered adequate to excellent by the authors for interpretation of individual performance. Ranges of coefficients calculated are presented in Table 5-11.

Test-retest reliability was examined by administering the Survey Form twice to parents or caregivers of 484 individuals from ages 6 months to 18 years 11 months. The sample was divided into six age groups (years–months): 0–6 to 2–11, 3–0 to 4–11, 5–0 to 6–11, 7–0 to 9–11, 10–0 to 13–11, and 14–0 to 18–11. The same interview-

Table 5-9. The Revised Vineland Adaptive Behavior Scales:
Demographic characteristics of the national standardization sample

Characteristic	National sample
Number of age groups	15 (yearly increments from birth through 11 years 11 months, and 2-year increments from 12 years 0 months to 18 years 11 months; there were a total of 200 individuals per age group)
Sex and age	1500 females (96–101/age group) 1500 males (99–104/age group)
Geographic region and age	18.6% (*n* = 557) from the Northeast (25–45/age group) 29.4% (*n* = 884) from the North Central U.S. (47–70/age group) 33.1% (*n* = 993) from the South (51–98/age group) 18.8% (*n* = 566) from the West (27–46/age group) Percentages from each region closely approximated percentages of U.S. population in each region
Parent education and age	15.4% had less than a high school education (16–41/age group) 45.4% were high school graduates (76–100/age group) 20.9% had 1–3 years of college or technical school (31–56/age group) 18.3% had 4 or more years of college (27–47/age group) Percentages for each group came within 5 percentage points or less of those representing the U.S. population Data are also available for parent education by geographical region; Vineland sample data approximate U.S. population data within a range of approximately 10 or fewer percentage points
Race or ethnic group and age*	73.7% white (136–157/age group) 15.1% black (23–37/age group) 8.6% Hispanic (11–24/age group) 2.6% other: native Americans, Alaskan natives, Asians, Pacific Islanders, all other groups not classified as white, black, or Hispanic (2–9/age group)
Community size and age	30% were from "central cities" with populations of 50,000 or more (46–70/age group) 40% were from suburbs or small towns with populations of 2500–49,999 (66–103/age group) 30% were from rural areas with populations of 2499 or less (48–80/age group) Percentages of each community size closely approximated percentages for U.S. population
Categories of educational placement (percent)	Regular classroom (96.1%) Speech-impaired (0.6%) Learning disabled (1.3%) Mentally retarded (0.5%) Emotionally disturbed (0.2%) Other (other health impairments, orthopedically impaired, multihandicapped, visually handicapped, hard-of-hearing and deaf) (0.4%) Gifted and talented (0.9%)

*Of the total group, 26.3% were minorities (43–64/age group). Percentages for each group came within 1 or less percentage point of those representing the U.S. population. Data are also available for race or ethnic group by geographic region. Vineland sample data approximate U.S. population data within a range of approximately 6 or fewer percentage points. Additional data are available for race or ethnic group and parent education. Vineland sample data approximate U.S. population data within a range of approximately 25 or fewer percentage points. Fewer individuals in the Vineland sample had less than a high school education compared with the U.S. as a whole, and, in most cases, more of the Vineland sample had high school educations and beyond than the U.S. population as a whole. Greatest differences were in the Hispanic and "other" groups. Source: Adapted from S. Sparrow, D. Balla, and D. Cicchetti. *Vineland Adaptive Behavior Scales, Interview Edition: Expanded Form Manual.* Circle Pines, Minnesota: American Guidance Service, 1984.

Table 5-10. The Revised Vineland Adaptive Behavior Scales: Supplementary norm group samples by age group

Age group	Ambulatory and nonambulatory mentally retarded residents	Ambulatory mentally retarded residents	Nonambulatory mentally retarded residents	Mentally retarded nonresidents
40 years or younger	765	569	196	80
Older than 40 years	291	218	73	10
Total N	1056	787	269	90

Age group	Emotionally disturbed residents	Age group	Visually handicapped residents	Hearing-impaired residents
9-0-10-5	15	6-0-7-5	24	33
10-6-11-5	18	7-6-8-5	24	41
11-6-12-5	20	8-6-9-5	24	52
12-6-13-5	27	9-6-10-5	34	43
13-6-14-5	23	10-6-11-5	40	67
14-6-15-6	31	11-6-12-11	39	87
Total N	134	Total N	185	323

Source: Adapted from S. Sparrow, D. Balla, and D. Cicchetti. Vineland Adaptive Behavior Scales, Interview Edition: Expanded Form Manual. Circle Pines, Minnesota: American Guidance Service, 1984.

Table 5-11. Reported reliability values for the Revised Vineland Adaptive Behavior Scales

Type of reliability	Category for which reported	Range of coefficients
Internal consistency (split-half reliability)	Survey Form domains and adaptive behavior composites by age for standardization sample	Median range, .83–.94
	Survey Form subdomains by age for standardization sample	Median range, .69–.84
	Expanded Form domains and adaptive behavior composites by age (based on Survey Form values) for standardization sample	Median range, .86–.97
	Expanded Form subdomains by age for standardization sample	Median range, .84–.88
	Survey Form domains and adaptive behavior composite for supplementary norm groups	Range, .76–.99
	Survey Form subdomains by supplementary norm groups	Range, .76–.99
	Expanded Form domains and adaptive behavior composite for supplementary norm groups	Range, .76–.99
	Expanded Form subdomains for supplementary norm groups	Range, .89–.99
Test-retest reliability coefficients	Survey Form adaptive behavior domains and adaptive behavior composite for standardization sample	Range, .76–.93
	Survey Form maladaptive behavior domain—Part I raw scores for standardization sample	Range, .84–.89
Interrater reliability coefficients	Survey Form adaptive behavior domains and adaptive behavior composite for standardization sample	Range, .62–.78
	Survey Form maladaptive behavior domain—Part I raw scores for standardization sample (ages 5 and over); results apply to both Survey and Expanded Forms since domain is identical in both	Range, .74

Source: Adapted from S. Sparrow, D. Balla, and D. Cicchetti. *Vineland Adaptive Behavior Scales, Interview Edition: Expanded Form Manual.* Circle Pines, Minnesota: American Guidance Service, 1984.

er readministered the scale following an interval of 2 to 4 weeks (mean, 17 days). The range of test-retest reliability coefficients is presented in Table 5-11, and is considered good to very good by the authors. Estimated coefficients were not computed for the Expanded Form, and it is suggested that values for the Survey Form be considered as "lower bound" estimates for the Expanded Form.

Interrater reliability was examined for the Survey Form by having 160 parents or caregivers of individuals in the standardization sample interviewed twice by separate examiners. Ages of individuals in this group ranged from 6 months to 18 years 11 months. The time interval between the two test administrations ranged from 1 to 14 days (mean, 8 days). With the exception of a moderate correlation of .62 for the socialization domain standard scores, interrater reliability coefficients are considered quite good by the authors. The range of coefficients is presented in Table 5-11. Coefficients were not calculated for the Expanded Form, and it is suggested that values for the Survey Form be considered a "lower bound" estimate for the Expanded Form.

Standard errors of measurement have also been calculated for both the Survey and Expanded Forms of the revised Vineland Interview Edition. These measurements were used to compute the bands of error for standard scores (probability that the individual's true score falls within a particular confidence interval).

Validity

Three types of validity are reported for the revised Vineland: construct, content, and criterion-related validity.

Construct validity data establish the degree to which the underlying construct or trait said to be measured by the scale is actually measured [2]. Three types of construct validity data are presented in the manual. The first relates to developmental progressions of Vineland scores. Increasing mean raw scores obtained for 15 age groups in the standardization sample across four behavior domains indicate that adaptive behavior, as measured by the Vineland, is age-related while maladaptive behavior is not. The second type of construct validity relates to factor analysis of domains and subdomains. Results of factor analysis indicated that the Adaptive Behavior Composite is an appropriate index to use in interpretation of Vineland results, and confirmed (in general) the organization of subdomains into their respective domains. The third type of construct validity involved exploration profiles of scores for the supplementary norm groups of handicapped individuals. This exploration basically confirmed expected differences in adaptive behavior between the standardization sample and the supplementary groups.

Content validity indicates that a scale adequately samples the universe of behaviors defining the constructs measured by the scale [2]. Content validity is felt to be supported by the thorough procedures used in the original development of items.

The relationship between the revised Vineland and other measures of significance (both Adaptive Behavior Scales and Intelligence Scales) was investigated to obtain *criterion-related validity*. As expected, higher correlations were found between the revised Vineland and other measures of adaptive behavior than with measures of intelligence (supporting the assumption that Adaptive Behavior Scales measure different things than Intelligence and/or Achievement Scales). These correlations were only moderate-

ly high, however, thus providing evidence that the revised Vineland is not simply duplicating already existing measures. Higher correlations were found between the Vineland communication domain and intelligence and/or language-based tests, probably related to the communication domain content, which is most similar to content measured by cognitive and language tests. Table 5-12 contains a summary of correlations between the revised Vineland and other measures.

Validation data are based on administration of the Survey Form. Adjusted validity coefficients were developed for the Expanded Form from the same data. Selected Survey Form validity coefficients between .20 and .80 were used to compute expected validity coefficients for the Expanded Form for each domain and the Adaptive Behavior Composite. Coefficients for the Expanded Form would be expected to differ only slightly from those for the Survey Form. Expanded Form coefficients are presented in tabular form in the manual [2]. Further information regarding technical aspects of the test's validation may be found by consulting the manuals or the *Vineland Technical and Interpretive Manual* [3].

Guidelines for Use in a Clinical Setting

The revised Vineland Adaptive Behavior Scales can be used to assess adaptive behavior skills of most any client, across a large span of ages, of normal or abnormal intelligence. Since it is not dependent on observed skill performance, there are relatively few situations in which data about adaptive behavior could not be obtained. It is important to be sure that the person selected to respond to questions knows the individual about whom data are being gathered well. If administration of the motor skills domain is desired, the individual must be 5 years 11 months of age or younger, or must have some form of motor handicap. When administration of the maladaptive behavior domain is desired, the individual must be 5 years of age or older.

*Table 5-12. Summary of correlations between the
Revised Vineland Adaptive Behavior Scales and other measures*

Test	Correlation
Original Vineland Social Maturity Scale	.55 between adaptive behavior composite and social quotient (389 individuals in national standardization sample)
	.97 total of raw scores for four domains in revised Vineland and total raw score in original Vineland (30 mentally retarded institutionalized adults)
	.88 (partial correlation, removing effect of chronological age) between revised and original total raw scores (35 hearing-impaired children in residential settings)
Adaptive Behavior Inventory for Children (ABIC)	.58 between adaptive behavior composite and ABIC average scaled scores
AAMD Adaptive Behavior Scale	.40 to .70 between raw scores of the four Vineland adaptive behavior domains and raw scores for subdomains of AAMD adaptive behavior scale Part I (30 severely retarded adults and 30 profoundly retarded adults, all in residential settings)
Intelligence Tests Kaufman Assessment Battery for Children (KABC)	Correlations between Vineland adaptive behavior domain and/or adaptive behavior composite scores and five Global Scale standard scores of the KABC are presented in tabular form in the Survey Form Manual; they range between .07 and .52 (719 individuals aged 2 6/12–2 11/12 from the national standardization sample)
Peabody Picture Vocabulary Test-Revised (PPVT-R) (classified as an intelligence test in Vineland manuals)	Correlations between Vineland adaptive behavior domains and adaptive behavior composite scores, and PPVT-R standard scores range from .12–.37 (2018 individuals aged 2 6/12–18 11/12 in the national standardization sample)
Variety of intelligence tests (including Stanford-Binet, WAIS, WAIS-R, Leiter, Slosson, PPVT or PPVT-R, WISC or WISC-R, Hayes-Binet, Perkins-Binet) administered to various supplementary norm groups	Correlations between Vineland domain and/or adaptive behavior composite scores and these various intelligence tests are given in tabular form in the Survey Form Manual

Key: AAMD, American Association on Mental Deficiency; WAIS, Wechsler Adult Intelligence Scale; WISC, Wechsler Intelligence Scale for Children.
Sources: Adapted from S. Sparrow, D. Balla, and D. Cicchetti. *Vineland Adaptive Behavior Scales, Interview Edition: Survey Form Manual.* Circle Pines, Minnesota: American Guidance Service, 1984; and from S. Sparrow, D. Balla, and D. Cicchetti. *Vineland Adaptive Behavior Scales, Interview Edition: Expanded Form Manual.* Circle Pines, Minnesota: American Guidance Service, 1984.

It is essential to recall that a label of mental retardation cannot be applied without testing adaptive behavior in conjunction with intelligence. The revised Vineland, with its updated norming for various groups and restructured format, gives information that is highly complementary to that obtained by intelligence testing. Its applicability across age groups makes it one of the most versatile adaptive behavior scales available.

In general, direct clinical observations would not be expected to result from this parent or caretaker interview test. The value of the data resulting from administration of the revised Vineland can be significant, however. The variety of uses to which the three formats of the test lend themselves is great. With appropriate planning and test format selection, the clinician can obtain data ranging from usefulness in general assessment to in-depth program planning and intervention.

Review

The revised Vineland Adaptive Behavior Scales were designed to assess personal and social sufficiency of nonhandicapped and handicapped individuals from birth to adulthood. The scales are a revision of the Vineland Social Maturity Scale by Edgar Doll. Its intended use is primarily diagnostic, although it has some potential to be used in a screening capacity. Strengths of the revised Vineland include the extremely complete statistical data. The manuals contain detailed information about the standardization process to which the scales were subjected, and clear step-by-step directions for administration, scoring, and interpretation. Standardization was conducted on a large, nationally representative sample (3000 individuals), and the test is one of the most carefully normed instruments in use. Supplemental normative data on some populations with handicaps are also available. There are a variety of ways to use the revised Vineland, all of which are well outlined in the manuals.

The manuals for the revised Vineland Adap-

tive Behavior Scales are large and complex. They are very complete, but the extensive information included makes access to anything specific a time-consuming task. One helpful feature of the manual concerns the information about supplemental norms. All information concerning these additional groups is printed in blue, thus making it easy to distinguish from that regarding the national sample, which is printed in black.

The criteria regarding experience in interviewing and familiarity with content concerning growth and development must be adhered to. The semistructure interview format assumes such knowledge and experience, and lack of it is likely to lead to administration errors.

Even though scoring booklets are designed to facilitate scoring of individual items (color-coded, three-column system), the format predisposes to errors in transferring results to the back page (Summary Sheet). Individual item scores must be summed, at times from numbers on several pages, increasing opportunity for errors. Awareness of such possibilities is required by the examiner.

Clinical use of the Vineland has indicated that it can be difficult to interpret age equivalents to parents in a meaningful way. Parents and examiners often observe that children can do more or less than what is predicted by the earned age equivalent, possibly because the Vineland is particularly sensitive to parent bias in reporting, to administration and scoring errors, or to some other as yet unidentified reason. This aspect of test use may benefit from further study. The revised version of the Vineland is a recent test, and a variety of questions should be expected. A great deal of research has gone into this test, and its extensive statistical data should make it a valuable contribution.

REFERENCES

1. Sparrow, S., Balla, D., and Cicchetti, D. *Vineland Adaptive Behavior Scales, Interview Edition: Survey Form Manual*. Circle Pines, Minn.: American Guidance Service, 1984.

2. Sparrow, S., Balla, D., and Cicchetti, D. *Vineland Adaptive Behavior Scales, Interview Edition: Expanded Form Manual.* Circle Pines, Minn.: American Guidance Service, 1984.
3. Sparrow, S., Balla, D., and Cicchetti, D. *Vineland Adaptive Behavior Scales: Technical and Interpretive Manual.* Circle Pines, Minn.: American Guidance Service, 1984.

Tests Requiring Parent Report And Examiner Observation

GESELL PRESCHOOL TEST

Descriptive Information

Test Identification

The title of this test is *Gesell Preschool Test for Evaluating Motor, Adaptive, Language, and Personal-Social Behavior in Children Ages 2½–6* (Gesell Preschool Test), 1980 [2, 8]. This test is an updated version of the original 1928 Gesell Preschool Tests [2]. Its authors are Louise Bates Ames, Ph.D., Clyde Gillespie, B.S., Jacqueline Haines, A.B., and Frances L. Ilg, M.D. At the time the Gesell Preschool Test was published (1980), all four authors were working at the Gesell Institute of Human Development in New Haven, Connecticut. Programs for Education, Inc. (P.O. Box 167, Rosemont, New Jersey 08556) publishes the test.

Cost of a start-up package of basic materials (test manual, recording sheets, developmental schedules, cubes, bean bag, picture vocabulary booklet, letters and numbers, three-hole form board, color forms, copy forms, pellets and bottle, typical response cards, carrying case) is $129–$150. Cost of a complete Set of Materials (all of the above, plus cassette tape presentation about the developmental approach used by the Gesell Institute; *The Gesell Institute's Child From One to Six* [2]) is between $145–$170. Cost of the Preschool Test Kit (consists of reusable materials *only* and is useful for situations where more than one examiner will be using the kit) is $75–$90. Shipping and handling cost 10 percent additional.

Age and Type of Client

The Gesell Preschool Test is designed to be used for any child between 2½ and 6 years of age.

Purpose

The Preschool Test battery, through a series of individual test situations, measures relative maturity in motor, adaptive, language, and personal-social behavior. The intent of the test is to describe the age level at which a child is functioning (developmental level, behavior age) as well as relative strengths and weaknesses. The test battery is not intended to result in completely objective measurements such as an intelligence test would. A developmental quotient (DQ) can be calculated. The test battery is felt to be particularly useful in helping to prevent school failure by assuring that a child's behavior is at a level commensurate with expectations for the placement being considered.

Time Required to Administer and Score Test

The amount of time necessary to administer this test is designated at 40 minutes [2]. The time required is likely to vary with the child's age and ability to cooperate. The amount of time needed to score the test varies between 15 and 30 minutes.

Evaluator

The Gesell Preschool Test is designated for use by early childhood specialists, educators, medical and psychiatric practitioners, psychologists, caregivers, case workers, nursery school teachers, and by personnel at institutions and agencies. The authors feel that the test is appropriate for use by nearly everyone involved with young children. People who are not trained professionals can make appropriate use of resulting information. It should be recalled that no test will yield accurate and useful information unless it is properly administered. Special attention to training should be given for test users who do not have professional backgrounds. This test is designated as a screening or diagnostic test, or as a basis for early intervention, depending on ". . .qualifications of the examiner" [2].

Historical Perspective of Test Construction

Development and Source of Test Items

Most items on the Gesell Preschool Test are currently included in the developmental portion of the Revised Gesell and Amatruda Developmental and Neurological Examination for the same age group (i.e., 2½–6 year olds) [9]. The authors of the Preschool Test state that some new tests have been added to the battery and others dropped, but give no particular source for specific item development. However, some information regarding the source of the items on the Revised Developmental and Neurological Examination is available.

The original scales were devised based on research documenting characteristic behavior traits of 34 advancing levels of maturity from birth to 10 years of age. Approximately 3000 behavior items were available for classification into growth gradients and normative developmental schedules. Primary attention was given to the first 5 years of life. The basic research was concerned with normal mental growth, and subjects were studied at lunar month intervals in several ways, including standardized behavioral examinations, naturalistic observations, home visits, and parent interviews [4–6]. Cinema records were used as a recording device because ". . . cinema captures the morphology of the behavior in its original integrity" [8]. Developmental data were collected in four major fields of behavior: motor, adaptive, language, and personal-social. The resulting scales ranged from birth to 72 months and were divided into five sections: adaptive, gross motor, fine motor, language, and personal-social. Most of the items tested for in-

clusion in the revised scales came from the original Gesell material. Some items were adapted from other tests, and some were actually devised by the revision authors. The format of the scales is identical. A total of 489 items were included in the revised scales: from 56 to 145 per behavior area across all ages, from 1 to 14 per behavior area for any one age, and from 13 to 36 across all behavior areas for any one age [9].

Review of the Literature in Terms of Test Use

The authors of the Gesell Preschool Test have described several "practical" uses for the test:

1. Determination of the difference between immaturity and mental retardation.
2. Representation of neurological function (since behavior is considered a function of structure).
3. Providing parents with a "general orientation" to reasonable expectations at various ages.
4. Providing information for adoptive families regarding endowment and potential of the new family member.
5. Determination of correct school placement by behavior age as opposed to just chronological age, IQ, or reading ability.
6. Assessment as opposed to testing (resulting in classification, educational programming, decision making, and intervention as opposed to a numerical score) [1].

The test provides a variety of information and seems useful to a wide variety of professionals. The information may provide a general picture of a child's overall behavioral maturity, or it may isolate strengths and weaknesses that might be used in specific treatment settings. The test is considered appropriate for administration by some nonprofessionals, and care must be taken that these people have been properly trained before results of their testing are used to make significant decisions.

Theoretical Constructs and Implications for Intervention

The Gesell Preschool Test is based on many of the same theoretical constructs as previous work by members of the Gesell Institute. Primary among them is the concept of growth.

Growth . . . becomes a key concept for the interpretation of individual differences. There are laws of sequence and maturation which account for the general similarities and basic trends of child development. But no two children . . . grow up in exactly the same way. Each child has a temperament and a style of growth which are as characteristic of individuality as the lineaments of his countenance [7].

Specifically, emphasis is placed on the process and products of early mental growth. *Mental growth* is described as a progressive morphogenesis of patterns of behavior. By envisioning the mind as a growing system, it should be easier to observe and comprehend determinants of the behavior of children. Essentially normal infants will develop normally unless some noxious organic or sociocultural event occurs.

The work that preceded formation of the developmental schedules was an attempt to capture a survey of the dynamic growth process in four basic fields of behavior: motor characteristics, adaptive behavior, language behavior, and personal-social behavior [7].

Behavior develops. Normal behavior assumes characteristic patterns as it develops. The principles and practice of developmental diagnosis rest on these simple, far-reaching propositions. Developmental diagnosis consists of a discriminating observation of behavior patterns and their appraisal by comparison with normal behavior patterns [10].

It is emphasized that while behavioral tests are designed to establish normality, to reveal minor deviations in otherwise healthy children, and to define the maturity and integrity of the central nervous system, they must always be interpreted in light of adequate social and medical history and appropriate laboratory investigation.

The authors of the Gesell Preschool Test believe that behavior is largely determined by inherited biological factors and develops in a patterned, predictable, and measurable way. They believe that growth characteristics are the "end-product expressions" of an interaction between intrinsic (inherited, biological) and extrinsic (environmental) determinants.

Further, the test represents the concept of equilibrium/disequilibrium (reciprocal interweaving).

. . . in any growing behavior (or area of behavior), it is possible to identify paired-but-opposed types of responses that occur in repeated alternation until the behavior has reached its final or complete stages, spiraling upward as it progresses [1].

Whether a child is in a stage of equilibrium or disequilibrium may contribute to evidence of maturity and to readiness for school.

Research conducted at the Gesell Institute suggests that behavior in elderly people tends to change in similar ways to that of young children, but in reverse sequence. Behavior usually remains stable until 65 to 70 years of age, and then begins either to become less effective or less active, or it may begin to deteriorate. Behavior of many senile adults is similar to that of 3 to 5 year olds, and can be measured on the Preschool Test.

The Gesell Preschool Test is a behavior (or developmental) examination that reveals the approximate age (based on normative data) achieved by the behavior (match, below, or above chronological age). It results in a DQ rather than an IQ. In general, IQs result from measurement of purely intellectual abilities (usually more verbally based) as opposed to the developmental test, which results in measurement of four fields of behavior (motor, adaptive, language, personal-social) [1].

Implications for intervention using the Gesell Preschool Test can be significant. In addition to the "orientation" guidance for parents and the results from which intervention programs can be planned, school placement based on behavioral readiness (as assessed by the test) is possible. School systems that have tried using the test as a basis for school placement report smaller numbers of children requiring remedial help, and sharp performance contrasts in abilities between children placed in first grade according to developmental readiness and those placed according to chronological age alone [1].

Content and Test Administration

Content

The Gesell Preschool Test provides an examination of behavior in four areas: motor, adaptive, language, and personal-social development. The test is arranged in age increments of 6 months (2½–6 years). There are a total of 218 items on the test (3–11/behavioral area/age, and 16–34/total test/age).

The battery contains 13 separate tests (Cube Test, Interview Questions, Paper and Pencil Tests, Incomplete Man, Preposition Discrimination, Digit Repetition, Picture Vocabulary, Comprehensive Questions, Color Forms, Action-Agent Language Indicator, Three-Hole Form Board, Identification of Letters and Numbers, and Motor). Varying numbers of tests are printed on each of eight separate test forms (one side only). A ninth separate page is a face sheet on which a behavioral summary, recommendations, and comments may be recorded. There is also a blank sheet of green paper on which to present cube formations and for tests requiring the child to demonstrate pencil skills.

Results of testing are recorded in a folder on which the Gesell Developmental Schedules are printed. This schedule is a revision of the Developmental Schedules based on work done during development of this test, and is slightly different from other versions currently in use.

Equipment necessary to administer the Gesell Preschool Test includes 10 red wooden cubes, a number 2½ pencil, copy form cards, picture vocabulary book (from Stanford-Binet Intelligence Test), color forms (five colored cardboard shapes), three-shape form board, cards with letters or numbers, pellets and bottle, and a bean bag. All materials except the pencil can be purchased in a test kit. The test manual, along with testing and recording forms, may be purchased with the test kit. Additional items that can be purchased but are not required include a set of typical response cards for the Incomplete Man and Copy Form Tests, a cassette tape on which the developmental approach used at the Gesell Institute is discussed, and the textbook *The Gesell Institute's Child from One to Six: Evaluating the Behavior of the Preschool Child* [1].

Results of the Preschool Test are recorded onto a form on which the developmental schedules appropriate for the entire 2½ to 6 year age range are printed (Fig. 5-7). This form allows examiners to see immediately how the behavior of any child compares with that of children the same age, younger or older. Even though the items have not been recently revised, behaviors for 2-year-old children have been included as guidelines for examiners seeing behaviors at a less than 2½ year level. Performance that is even or uneven, as well as whether behavioral successes are scattered across areas, can be determined with the format of these recording forms. The back of the folder in which results are recorded contains an examiner's checklist of significant testing and nontesting behavior (Fig. 5-8).

Setting and Equipment

The Gesell Preschool Test can be administered in nearly any setting as long as some privacy and comfort can be obtained. There must be enough floor space to allow for jumping over a 27-in. distance, and for catching or throwing a bean bag. A table and chair appropriate to the child's size are necessary since much of the testing involves table-top activities. A chair for the examiner is also required. Finally, a stopwatch or other timing device with a second hand is useful.

Administration Procedures

The Gesell Preschool Test requires direct observation of and interaction with the child being tested. While there is no stated stipulation that a parent or caretaker may not be in the room, the great majority of test items cannot be completed on the basis of report. Items in the motor, adaptive, and language areas are completed following direct testing of the child. *Most* items in the personal-social area require conducting a parent interview [1]. The test manual is organized according to the 13 separate tests included in the battery, and instructions appropriate for all age levels are completed for one test before beginning the next.

Directions are given in detail, complete with examples of what to say and what to observe. In general, directions for each of the several tests in the battery contain sections on required test materials, general directions, procedure to follow, and descriptions of normative age responses. Descriptions of individual item administration are quite clear.

Directions for administering the Preschool Test, while not difficult, are complex, primarily because so much information (directions for several subtests within many of the 13 tests in the battery) about so many age groups (2½ –6 years) is presented together. Many examples of normative performance are described, but some subjective judgment regarding quality of performance is required. This test requires familiarity and experience by the examiner before it can be properly administered.

Scoring

Directions for scoring responses are briefly and succinctly stated as follows:

    + = Succeeds
  + + = Performs at level higher than
         expected for age
    ± = Questionable success
    − = Failure

Symbols representing the appropriate response are placed in the vertical columns directly to the left of each item on the score sheet (see Fig. 5-7). When completed, the examiner should be able to interpret whether behavior is age-appropriate or not, as well as where strengths or weaknesses lie. Since no numerical score can be used to interpret "normality" or "abnormality," judgment based on knowledge, experience, and appropriate test use must be made. Use of the developmental quotient can aid in this process, but this aspect of the scoring procedure makes it a complex one to use and underscores the need for examiners to be knowledgeable and properly trained in test use.

The Preschool Test results in interpretation of a child's behavior as mature or immature (a personality profile) rather than in designation of an intelligence level. With experience, examiners can determine age levels at which individual children are responding and obtain an overall behavior age or identification of particular strengths and weaknesses. A DQ can be calculated by determining an overall behavior age in months, dividing by chronological age in months and multiplying by 100. It takes experience to accurately determine behavior age since it is not based on a specific numerical test score.

The Preschool Test is described as being useful as a screening test (in addition to a diagnostic test or for early intervention planning), but there is no description of just how to use it in this way. No suggestions for any kind of cutoff scores or performances below which a child should definitely be referred for more complete developmental services are included. The closest the authors come to suggesting cutoff scores is a statement in the manual that any child more than 2 years behind chronological age peers should receive special help [8]. This value may be difficult to assess without a numerical scoring system. Each school, agency, and institution would have to determine the types of profiles they would consider in need of various types of referrals. Once again, care would be required in se-

Age	Motor	Adaptive	Language	Personal-Social
2	Walks: runs well, no falling Stairs: walks up and down alone Large ball: (no dem.) kicks Cubes: tower of 6-7 Book: turns pages singly	Cubes: tower of 6-7 Drawing: imitates V stroke Formboard: places blocks on separately (G) Formboard: adapts after 4 trials Color Forms: does not identify any	Speech: jargon discarded Speech: 3 word sentence Speech: uses I, me, you Picture Vocabulary: 2 + correct	Toilet: may verbalize needs fairly consistently Play: domestic mimicry Play: hands cup full of cubes Play: parallel play predominates Feeding: inhibits turning spoon Dressing: pulls on simple garment Commun: verbalizes immed. experiences Commun: refers to self by name Commun: comprehends & asks for "another" Temperament: gentle, easy
2½	Stands: tries, on 1 foot Cubes: tower of 10 Drawing: holds crayon by fingers	Cubes: tower of 10 Cubes: aligns 2 or more, train Drawing: imitates V & H strokes Drawing: scribbles to circular stroke Inc. Man: adds 1 part Formboard: inserts 3 blocks on presentation Formboard: adapts repeatedly, error Color Forms: places 1	Interview: gives first name Interview: tells sex (G) Prepositions: obeys 1-2 Picture Vocab: 7 correct Action Agent: 3 correct	Play: pushes toy with good steering Play: helps put things away Commun: refers to self by pronoun "me" rather than by name Commun: repetition in speech and other activity Self help: can put on own coat (not necessarily fasten) Temperament: opposite extremes
3	Walks on tiptoe, 2 or more steps Stands on 1 foot, momentary balance Skips: tries Rides tricycle using pedals Stairs: alternates feet going up Jumps down: lands on feet (G) Broad jump: distance 12" Pellets: 10 into bottle in 26" (G); 24" (B)	Cubes: adds chimney to train Cubes: imitates bridge Copy Forms: copies circle Copy Forms: imitates cross Inc. Man: adds 3 parts Formboard: adapts, no errors or immediate correction of error Color Forms: places 3 Counts with correct pointing: 3 objs. Pellets: 10 into bottle in 26" (G); 24" (B)	Speech: uses plurals Interview: tells age (G) Interview: tells sex (B) Prepositions: obeys 3 Digits: repeats 3 (1 of 3 trials) Picture Vocab: 11 correct Comprehension Question A: answers 1 Action Agent: 6-7 correct Picture Vocab: 11 correct	Feeding: feeds self, little spilling Feeding: pours well from pitcher Dressing: puts on shoes Dressing: unbuttons front and side buttons Commun: asks questions rhetorically Commun: understands taking turns Commun: knows a few rhymes Temperament: cooperative
3½	Stands on 1 foot 2" or more Jumps: both feet leave floor Broad jump: distance 19" Jumps down, lands on feet (B) Hops on one foot: succeeds (G) Pellets: 10 into bottle in 23"	Cubes: builds bridge from model Copy Forms: copies cross Inc. Man: adds 4 parts Inc. Man: eyes better than a scribble Pellets: 10 into bottle in 23"	Interview: gives no. of siblings Prepositions: 4 correct Digits: repeats 3 (2 of 3 trials) Picture Vocab: 12 correct Comprehension Quest. A: answers 2 Action Agent: 12 correct	Dressing: washes, dries, hands, face Play: associate play replaces parallel Commun: calls self "I" Commun: asks "How" questions Toileting: seldom has "accidents" Temperament: vulnerable
4	Stands on 1 foot 2-7" Stairs: walks down, foot to a step Skips: on one foot Jumps: run, or standing broad jump Broad jump: 20" Bean bag catch: any method Pellets: 10 into bottle in 23"	Cubes: imitates gate or better (G) Copy Forms: imitates square or better Inc. Man: adds 5 parts Inc. Man: arm straight out from body or better Pellets: 10 into bottle in 23" Counts 4 objects	Interview: gives own age (B) Prepositions: 5 correct Digits: repeats 3 (3 of 3 trials) Digits: repeats 4 (1 of 3 trials) Picture Vocab: 14 correct Comprehension Quest. B: 1 correct Action Agent: 14 correct	Dressing: buttons clothing Dressing: washes & dries face & hands, brushes teeth Dresses: dresses & undresses, supervised Dressing: laces shoes Dressing: distinguishes front & back

Age	Motor	Adaptive	Language	Personal-Social
				children Play: builds buildings with blocks Develop: goes on errands outside home (no crossing streets) Develop: tends to go out-of-bounds Commun: asks "Why" questions Temperament: expansive
4½	Hops on one foot: succeeds (B) Broad jump: 24" Bean bag: overhand throw: succeeds (G) Bean bag catch: hands vs. chest or better (B) Pellets: 10 into bottle in 20"	Cubes: makes gate from model Copy Forms: copies square recognizably Copy Forms: divided rectangle—ladder design, lines straight Inc. Man: adds 7 parts Letters: 1,2 recognizable Numbers: 1,2 recognizable Counts: 4 obj. & answers "How many?" Pellets: 10 into bottle in 20"	Articulation: not infantile Interview: gives names of siblings Digits: repeats 4 (2 of 3 trials) Comprehension Quest A: 3 correct Action Agent: 16 correct	Commun: calls attention to own performance Commun: relates fanciful tales Play: shows off dramatically Temperament: unpredictable
5	Stands on one foot 9" or more Walks on tiptoe: 5 or more steps Skips: using feet alternately Broad jump: 27" distance Pellets: 10 into bottle in 18"	Cubes: 6 cube steps with dem. Copy Forms: copies triangle ± Copy Forms: all forms on 1 page Copy Forms: divided rect. ladder design, side lines slanted Inc. Man: adds 8 parts Name: prints first name Counts: 10 objects correctly Calculates: within 5 Pellets: 10 into bottle in 18"	Interview: gives first & last name Picture Vocab: 15 correct Comprehension Quest. B: 2 correct Action Agent: 17 correct	Dressing: ties a bow knot Dressing: dresses & undresses with little assistance Commun: asks meaning of words Play: dresses up in adult clothes Temperament: gentle, friendly
5½	Stands on one foot 12" Bean bag overhand: succeeds (B) Bean bag catch: hands vs. chest or better (G)	Cubes: 10 cube steps with or without dem. (G) Copy Forms: copies triangle recognizably Copy Forms: divided rectangular H line crosses V, angled lines may cross V Copy Forms: diamond—1 or 2 sides correct Inc. Man: eyes match in size Inc. Man: arm points upward Counts: 12 objects correctly	Interview: knows month of birthday Action Agent: 18-19 correct Digits: repeats 4 (3 of 3 trials)	Money: identifies pennies & nickels Play: understands games like tag and hide and seek Temperament: breaking up
6	Stands on each foot alternately Broad jump: distance 32" Bean bag: advanced throwing Bean bag catch: hands only Pellets: 10 into bottle in 16"	Cubes: 10 cube steps with or without dem. (B) Copy Forms: divided rect. 3 lines may cross center V line Copy Forms copies diamond, oddly shaped (good shape not till 7 yrs.) Inc. Man: adds 9 parts Inc. Man: adds 2 or 3 parts at neck Name: prints first and last (G) (normative at 6½) Adds and subtracts within 10 (normative at 6½) Pellets: 10 into bottle in 16" Counts 13 + objects	Interview: knows day and month of birthday (normative at 6½) Digits: repeats 5 (1 of 3 trials) Picture Vocab: 16 correct Action Agent: 19 correct	Dressing: ties shoe laces Commun: differentiates A.M. and P.M. Commun: knows right and left (3 of 3 or complete reversal) Commun: recites numbers to 30's Temperament: oppositional, emotional

Fig. 5-7. The Gesell Preschool Test for evaluating motor, adaptive, language, and personal-social behavior in children ages 2 ½ to 6 (Gesell Developmental Schedules). (Copyright © 1979 by Gesell Institute of Human Development. Reprinted by permission.)

I. Physical data

Hair color_____

Distinguishing features _____

II. Behaviors noted

1. Separation from mother
   - ☐ easily separated
   - ☐ will not let go of mother's hand
   - ☐ sits on mother's lap
   - ☐ stands next to mother
   - ☐ other _____

2. Activity Level
   - ☐ seated but legs swinging, arms moving, etc.
   - ☐ seated but no overflow of behavior
   - ☐ seated but does not remain so (runs around)
   - ☐ talks incessantly
   - ☐ little verbal overflow
   - ☐ plays with pencil (or other test materials)
   - ☐ other _____

III. Testing Session

1. Posture
   - ☐ pencil grasp
   - ☐ body shifts
   - ☐ other _____

2. Manner of following directions
   - ☐ understands with ease
   - ☐ needs frequent redirection
   - ☐ other _____

3. Physical activity
   - ☐ arm movement
   - ☐ leg movement
   - ☐ tongue movement
   - ☐ other _____

4. Speech
   - ☐ fluent and articulate
   - ☐ muddled
   - ☐ infantile
   - ☐ other _____

5. Language
   - ☐ expresses self well
   - ☐ thought processing problems
   - ☐ other _____

IV. Personality

☐ shy	☐ verbal	☐ expressive	☐ ability to inhibit
☐ outgoing	☐ quiet	☐ talkative	☐ self-confident

V. Use of results

_____

_____

_____

_____

Preschool Test page 10

Fig. 5-8. Examiner's Checklist for the Gesell Preschool Test. (Copyright © 1979 by Gesell Institute of Human Development. Reprinted by permission.)

lection of experienced professionals to make such decisions.

Psychometric Properties

Standardization

Specific directions for standard administration of the Preschool Test are included in the test manual and in the textbook, *The Gesell Institute's Child from One to Six: Evaluating the Behavior of the Preschool Child* [2, 8]. They are clearly stated and are easily followed. The only section not requiring standardized administration is the Personal-Social section of the test. Some data for scoring this section comes from direct observation of child performance, but most is based on an interview with the parent or caretaker. A detailed list of appropriate questions is provided in the textbook but not in the test manual, leaving the examiner the choice of either using the developmental schedules (on which results are scored) as the basis for guiding the interview or obtaining the textbook. The authors state that they have collected data regarding the value of the parent or caretaker filling out a personal-social checklist as opposed to conducting a complete interview, but the data are not reported.

A new cohort of children was studied for this revision of the original 1928 Gesell Preschool Test. The authors state that more care was taken to assure that subjects were representative of the gamut of socioeconomic levels. The demographic characteristics of the sample, as well as characteristics not described by the authors, are included in Table 5-13.

Normative data are presented in both the test manual and the textbook, but in different formats. Recall that the test manual presents all testing directions, across all ages, for each of the 13 tests in the battery separately. In other words, all directions for administering Cube Tests are given in one section, followed by all directions for administering the Interview Questions, etc. In each of these sections, normative behavior for each age range is described and is used as the basis for

scoring the child's responses. The textbook is organized according to the four behavioral areas tested (motor, adaptive, language, personal-social). The individual subtests of the 13 tests that relate to each behavioral area are described within that section, and the norms for each skill across all age groups are listed. Normative data indicate that, on this test, girls generally accomplish most measurable abilities approximately 6 months earlier than boys. Reference is made to comparison of performance of the current sample of children with the original cohort from which norms for the original version were obtained. A table with this comparative information is included in the textbook [1]. On 59 percent of the measures (30 of 51 comparisons) compared, behaviors were attained at exactly the same ages by the two groups of children. In 18 of the 21 remaining comparisons, present subjects were 6 months more advanced than the original group at the same ages. The authors conclude that, in certain respects, today's children (both sexes) are slightly more advanced developmentally when compared with children tested in the 1930s.

Reliability

No information about reliability is discussed in either the test manual or the textbook.

Validity

No information about validation studies is described in detail in the test manual or in the textbook.

Guidelines for Use in a Clinical Setting

The Preschool Test is conceivably a valuable instrument to use with any child of appropriate age for whom an estimate of overall behavioral maturity is required. While individual strengths and weaknesses can be assessed, the test does not result in specific numerical scores, which may be required for certain types of school (or

Table 5-13. Demographic characteristics of standardization population sample for the Gesell Preschool Test

Category	Characteristics
Geographic location	Connecticut
Racial characteristics	"Nearly all Caucasian"
Total number in sample	640 children (320 boys, 320 girls between 2½ and 6 years of age)
	80 children (40 boys, 40 girls) at each 6-month level between 2½ and 6 years
Sex	50% male, 50% female
Characteristics not indicated	Source of subjects
	Criteria for inclusion in study
	Study period
	Mean length of parental education

other educational setting) placement. Behavioral maturity is considered by the authors to be a significant factor in decisions regarding when to begin school and most appropriate classroom settings.

There is no description of how this test relates to others except the comparison with an earlier version of itself (described under normative data). It is not really intended to be predictive of IQ, and examiners should not expect to use it in this fashion. Nonetheless, the authors do consider it to be useful as both a screening and diagnostic measure. The Preschool Test should be expected to add an estimate of behavioral maturity to specific information provided by other instruments, potentially making application of the more specific results more usable to both child and school system.

The Preschool Test provides a good, structured way to approach observation of a child's overall developmental status. Such observation may result in anticipatory guidance for parents, early intervention through formal or informal stimulation programs, or appropriate school (or other educational setting) placement. Since it does not yield the numerical results so often required for school placement, its special value would lie in increasingly appropriate use being made of such results by augmenting decisions with an assessment of overall behavioral maturity. When using the Preschool Test as a guide for

school placement, the authors present the following generalizations:

1. Boys can be expected to develop more slowly than girls during the early years (and may be as many as 6 months slower between ages 5 and 7 years).
2. Girls should be at least 5 years old and boys 5½ years old before entering kindergarten; girls should be at least 6 years old and boys 6½ years old before entering first grade (any other ages should receive critical screening for behavioral maturity).
3. Any children more than 2 years behind their chronological age mates should be placed in some kind of special class or group where they can receive individual attention.
4. Behavioral maturity should influence classroom placement even when children test as intellectually advanced.
5. Changes in classroom placement should be considered as problems in maturity become evident, rather than waiting until the end of a school year.

The Preschool Test manual and the textbook contain good descriptions of expected behaviors of children in each of the age groups tested. They also contain descriptions of how children of these ages may be expected to act in the testing situation. Attention is called to the fact that, with maturity, both test responses and patterns of refusal to participate in testing change. Therefore, the patterns of both "overflow behaviors" (those in which the child engages even though they are not part of the structured testing) and actual refusals can aid in determining behavioral maturity.

Review

The Gesell Preschool Test is designed to result in an estimate of behavioral maturity of children 2½ to 6 years old. Information is gathered in four areas: motor, adaptive, language, and personal-social. A DQ can be obtained. The authors cite a number of potential uses of information regarding behavioral maturity, and particularly stress its importance in decisions about school placement.

The value of the Preschool Test lies in the complete assessment that is possible with its proper use. The test enables the examiner to recognize individual differences that should be attended to, even when development is within normal limits. The test is the result of many years of experience by distinguished workers in the field of child development and represents a combination of experience and empirical testing. A complete testing kit is available and comes with a carrying case, making the test easily transportable. The testing folder contains the Gesell Developmental Schedules (format on which test results are indicated) so that strengths and weaknesses in both individual skills and behavioral areas can easily be displayed.

The Preschool Test, like many of the other Gesell instruments, is complex to administer. While directions are clear and materials easy to use, the test format requires significant experience for effective administration. Some particularly useful information, such as how to calculate the DQ and how much time the test takes to administer, are contained in sources other than the manual (i.e., textbook, catalog). Other information seems scattered. Individual tests within the

battery are printed on several loose pages, requiring the examiner to be adept at maneuvering papers while carrying out test items. (It is recommended that the individual test forms be stapled into the test folder after use.) The Personal-Social Interview format is nonstandardized (the examiner may choose between using a list of specific questions, using the developmental schedule items as a general guide, or using general observation), raising the possibility that abilities in this area are less well surveyed. And, as in previous versions of Gesell instruments, characteristics of race, geography, socioeconomic status, reliability, and validity are limited, constituting a considerable weakness for this well-known test.

The idea of testing behavioral maturity should be considered seriously. The lack of a numerical test score makes examiner experience and judgment particularly important in test administration. With proper education and experience, information gathered about behavioral maturity could positively affect decisions about proper school placement and intervention for many young children.

REFERENCES

1. Ames, L. B., et al. *The Gesell Institute's Child From One to Six: Evaluating the Behavior of the Preschool Child.* New York: Harper & Row, 1979.
2. Gesell Early Childhood Tests, Films and Books for Professionals and Parents: Your Guide to Materials for the Nationwide Movement for School Success (Catalog). Flemington, N.J.: Programs for Education, Inc., 1985.
3. Gesell, A. *Infancy and Human Growth.* New York: Macmillan, 1928.
4. Gesell, A. *An Atlas of Infant Behavior: A Systematic Delineation of the Forms and Early Growth of Human Behavior Patterns. Volume One: Normative Series.* New Haven: Yale University Press, 1934.
5. Gesell, A. *An Atlas of Infant Behavior: A Systematic Delineation of the Forms and Early Growth of Human Behavior Patterns. Volume Two: Naturalistic Series.* New Haven: Yale University Press, 1934.

6. Gesell, A. *Infant Development: The Embryology of Early Human Behavior*. New York: Harper & Brothers, 1952.

7. Gesell, A., et al. *The First Five Years of Life: A Guide to the Study of the Preschool Child*. New York: Harper & Brothers, 1940.

8. Haines, J., Ames, L. B., and Gillespie, C. *The Gesell Preschool Test Manual for Use in Conjunction with the Gesell Preschool Test and Kit*. Lumberville, Pa.: Modern Learning Press, 1980.

9. Knobeloch, H., and Pasamanick, B. (eds.). *Gesell and Amatruda's Developmental Diagnosis: The Evaluation and Management of Normal and Abnormal Neuropsychologic Development in Infancy and Early Childhood* (3rd ed.). New York: Harper & Row, 1974.

10. Knobeloch, H., Stevens, F., and Malone, A. *Manual of Developmental Diagnosis: The Administration and Interpretation of the Revised Gesell and Amatruda Developmental and Neurologic Examination*. Hagerstown, Md.: Harper & Row, 1980.

LEARNING ACCOMPLISHMENT PROFILE-DIAGNOSTIC EDITION

Descriptive Information

Test Identification

The title of this test is *Learning Accomplishment Profile-Diagnostic Edition* (LAP-D), 1977. Its authors are David Wilson LeMay, M.Ed., Patricia M. Griffin, M.Ed., and Anne R. Sanford, M.Ed. Although not stated in the literature provided with the LAP-D manual, the authors of this instrument have backgrounds and experience in education. All were working with the Chapel Hill Training Outreach Project, in North Carolina, at the time of test development. Kaplan Press (P.O. Box 5128, Winston-Salem, North Carolina 27113) publishes this test. The LAP-Diagnostic Edition Kit sells for $325–$375; the LAP-D Scoring Booklet (20 per package), $20–$30; and Individual Education Plan (IEP) Forms (20 per package), $30–$40.

Age and Type of Client

The LAP-D was designed for administration to young handicapped and normal children 12 to 72 months of age.

Purpose

The LAP-D is a diagnostic-prescriptive assessment tool based on the theoretical foundation of task analysis. Its purpose is to "enable the examiner/teacher to develop appropriate instructional objectives and strategies" [1]. This tool has three major functions: (1) evaluation of a child's entry skills, (2) evaluation of the child's exit skills, and (3) validation of the instructional program. The LAP-D contains scales in Gross Motor, Fine Motor, Cognitive, Language, and Self-Help. Individual Educational Program (IEP) Forms are available and are directly correlated with the LAP-D, providing a means for planning educational goals and objectives.

Time Required to Administer and Score Test

Administration time for the LAP-D is approximately 1½ to 2 hours. Scoring time is about 10 to 15 minutes.

Evaluator

The LAP-D does not specify the qualifications of the evaluator, although the "teacher" is frequently mentioned. Any professional experienced in pediatric testing should be able to administer the test. No specific training requirements are outlined.

Historical Perspective of Test Construction

Development and Source of Test Items

The following criteria were used for the inclusion of items in the LAP-D: (1) the test should sample representative behaviors; (2) using the task analysis theory that learning is sequential, items should represent a hierarchy from simple to complex; (3) items should represent important milestones; (4) objects should be clearly stated; and (5) items should easily translate into instructional programming.

The authors drew items from the literature relating to normal child development (Gesell, Bayley, Ilg and Ames, Cattell, Frankenburg and Dobbs, Doll, Terman); these items were representative of skills mastered during the preschool years. Task analysis was done to isolate prerequisite skills for each test item so that these items could be presented in a progressively complex sequence. One of the goals of this instrument was easy translation into instructional programming; thus, the items were written with clear objectives so IEP goals could be easily ascertained.

Review of Literature in Terms of Test Use

There is no published literature reviewing this instrument.

Theoretical Constructs and Implications for Intervention

The LAP-D is theoretically based on the task analysis model of diagnostic-prescriptive education. "In the task analysis model, skill development is viewed as a continuum, moving upward from fundamental and instinctive behaviors to complex and learned behaviors" [1]. Each skill included is accompanied by prerequisite steps, which are arranged on a hierarchical pattern from simple to complex. The task analysis model allows for assessment of a child in behavioral terms of observed or not observed skills. No assumption can be made regarding the cause of a child's level of abilities. The authors state "it is unnecessary if not detrimental for the teacher to have identification tags (labels) to attach to each child" [1]. The LAP-D is therefore a "nonlabeling" tool that translates assessment into educational objectives.

Content and Administration

Content

The LAP-D is divided into five scales and thirteen subscales. The five scales include Gross Motor, Fine Motor, Cognitive, Language, and Self-Help.

The Gross Motor Scale is divided into two subscales: Body Movement and Object Movement. Body Movement involves balance and locomotion. It contains 48 items with 3-month increments from 6 to 30 months, with two to three items per increment. The 36- to 72-month levels are divided into 6-month increments, with four to six items per increment. The Object Movement Subscale involves the reception and propulsion of objects. It contains 31 items with 3-month increments from 3 to 24 months and one to four items per increment. The 24- to 72-month levels are divided into 6-month increments, with one to four items per increment.

The Fine Motor Scale is also divided into two subscales: Manipulation and Writing. The Manipulation Subscale assesses the child's ability to interact with various materials with the exception of pencils. The Writing Subscale assesses the child's skill with pencils in drawing and writing tasks. The Manipulation Subscale contains 43 items with 3-month increments from 6 to 36 months, and 6-month increments from 36 to 72 months. The majority of the increments include one to four items in each, with eight items at the 36-month level. The Writing Subscale contains 37 items with 3-month intervals from the 12- to 18-month level with two items per interval, and 6-month intervals from the 24- to 72-month level with three to six items per interval.

The Cognitive Scale is divided into Matching (reading prerequisites) and Counting (arithmetic prerequisites). The Matching Subscale contains 27 items in 6-month increments, with the majority of levels having one to three items and three levels (48-month, 54-month, and 72-month) having five to six items. The Counting Subscale contains 28 items in 6-month intervals from 36 to 72 months of age, with one to four items per level up to 66 months and eight to ten items per level in 66- and 72-month levels.

The Language Scale is divided into the two subscales of Naming (expressive language) and Comprehension (receptive language). The Naming Subscale contains 29 items in 3- to 6-month increments, with one to two items in the 15- to 48-month increments and four to seven items in the higher increments. The Comprehension Subscale contains 27 items and is divided into 3- to 6-month increments from 6 to 72 months, with one to four items per increment.

The Self-Help Scale is divided into the five subscales of Eating, Dressing, Grooming, Toileting, and Self-Direction. The Eating Subscale contains eight items from 3 to 18 months, with one to two items per 3-month increment. The Dressing Subscale contains 23 items in 6-month increments from the 24- to 42-month level with one item in each increment, except for the 36-month level which has four items. The Grooming Subscale contains seven items in 6-month increments from 24 to 42 months, with one item per increment, except for 36 months which has four items. The Toileting Subscale contains nine items in 6-month increments from 12 to 48 months, with one to two items per increment. The Self-Direction Subscale contains six items from the 24- to 42-month level in 6-month increments, with one to two items per increment.

Most of the items in the LAP-D are familiar to examiners who have assessed developmental skills in preschoolers because the items were attained from other developmental tests and the normal development literature. Examples of items at the 48-month level are (1) Gross Motor: body movement (stands on tiptoes, walks backward), object movement (throws ball overhand, catches bean bag); (2) Fine Motor: manipulation (laces sewing cards, six-piece puzzle), writing (copies cross, draws three-part person); (3) Cognitive: matching (matches object pictures, matches complex patterns), counting (counts 10 cubes, points to numerals); (4) Language: naming

(names missing part, names eight actions), comprehension (responds to four prepositions, relates pictures to story); and (5) Self-Help (sample items presented at different age levels): 18 months—eating (lifts and returns cup), 24 months—dressing (removes coat), 24 months—grooming (washes hands with assistance), 30 months—self-direction (picks up toys when prompted), 36 months—toileting (pulls down pants unassisted).

The LAP-D Test Kit available from Kaplan Press includes the examiner's manual, scoring booklets, and all the items necessary (41 items) to administer the assessment tool, with the exception of food items. A metal carrying case is provided for storage. Color-coded bags for small items are included for ease of administration and storage. The test manual is contained in a loose-leaf flip easel. Additional scoring booklets can be purchased separately.

The test manual is contained in a loose-leaf easel for easy administration and contains the test items, procedure for administration, and criteria for scoring. The test scoring booklet includes space for item scoring, comment area for each item, and pre- and postscoring space. An assessment profile provides a visual display of the child's pre- and posttest scores according to the percentage of items passed. This assessment profile provides a criterion-referenced table for determining individual gains. It does not provide specific information on level of functioning or strength and weakness patterns.

Setting and Equipment

The suggested environment for the administration of the LAP-D is a quiet, well-lit room, a low table, and two chairs (one child-sized). It is recommended that distractions be held to a minimum. A large area is required for the Gross Motor Scale, which can be administered outdoors. Measurements needed for the Gross Motor Scale should be done prior to administration of the scale. All materials are contained in the test kit except for food items, blank paper, and writing implements.

Administration Procedures

The LAP-D is administered in a one-to-one situation. It is easily administered given good organization of materials by the examiner. The examiner's manual suggests that the child be seated to the left of the examiner, with the materials to the right of the examiner on a low chair or the floor, out of the child's view. The test manual specifies the procedures and verbal directions for each item to be administered. The directions are easily understood, clear, and concise.

Scoring

Recording procedures are provided in a concise manner. Each of the subscales is administered, with each item being scored by stated criteria on a pass/fail format. All items in each subscale are not administered due to basal/ceiling rules. The basal level is reached when a child passes three consecutive items. The ceiling is established when the child fails three items in a five-item span. The scores of the passed items are totaled in each subscale to yield the total score. The total score is converted into a percentage representing the number of items passed out of the possible number of test items. This score provides a criterion-referenced method for determining improvements in the child's performance over time.

The developmental age of each item is also located in the test manual and the scoring booklet. A chart is included in the examiner's manual and provides the developmental age associated with the test item and the source of the test item.

The purpose of the LAP-D is to evaluate a child's entry and exit skills (i.e., the child's skills before and after the intervention program) and to provide information of the effects of this program. The criterion-referenced percentage scores provide the ability to compare a child's pretest performance with that child's posttest performance. A general developmental age can be estimated. Therefore, the interpretation of test information involves the child's entry skills and exit skills. The authors strongly state that the LAP-D cannot be used for identifying neurological, psychological, intellectual, motor, or linguistic dysfunction. No etiologies can be ascertained by this instrument. A child should also not be labeled or placed in a special class due to the results of the LAP-D in isolation. If a child demonstrates a serious delay on the LAP-D, a more in-depth evaluation by experienced pediatric professionals is warranted. However, little guidance is provided as to whom referrals should be made, and "serious" delay is not defined.

Psychometric Properties

Standardization

The test manual contains specific instructions necessary for administration of items in a standard fashion. Kaplan Press provides special training workshops on the administration of the LAP-D. A numbered LAP-D certificate is awarded on completion of a workshop.

The sample size of the normative population was 35 children. Of the 35 children, 20 were male (57.1%) and 15 female (42.9%). Seventeen of the children were black (48.6%), and 18 (51.4%) were white. Age ranges were divided into 16 below 46 months of age and 19 above 46 months of age. The children were between 30 and 73 months of age, with the mean age of 46.63 months and a standard deviation of 11.7 months. No information is available regarding date of administration, socioeconomic status, setting, specific age intervals, or geographic location.

No specific normative data are available. In the Examiner's Manual it is reported that "older children performed consistently better than did younger children in all of the scales of the test" [1]. Instructions are provided in the Examiner's

Manual for construction of local norms using the measures of central tendency.

Reliability

Test-retest reliability was obtained by three examiners who tested the 35 children from the normative sample. The length of time between testings is not reported. The test-retest reliability data are reported by subscales, and the total test reliability was found to be .98.

Validity

No validity studies are available on this assessment tool.

Guidelines for Use in a Clinical Setting

The LAP-D assesses children from 12 to 72 months in fine motor, gross motor, cognitive, language, and self-help areas. The pretest provides information regarding entry skills. An educational program is then designed for that child. The posttest provides information on level of exit skills, gains made, and information on the effectiveness of an educational program. The manual encourages the examiner to note emerging skills so that the development of the educational program can be more specific and appropriate for the child. Other clinical observations could be made depending on the professional background and experience of the examiner.

This test is not appropriate for diagnosis of specific dysfunction, etiology, labeling, or placement in special classes. The degree of physical, cognitive, receptive, and expressive language required by this instrument is directly dependent on the subscale being administered. Directions are given verbally, although demonstration accompanies most items, reducing the level of receptive language required. Examiners are encouraged to use nonverbal instructions when verbal instructions are not understood.

The LAP-D in conjunction with the LAP-R provides an assessment system that allows for objective evaluation of a child's progress and the effects of the educational program (LAP-D) and an ongoing assessment of a child's progress and activities for inclusion into the educational program (LAP-D). The LAP-R allows the teacher to continually assess a child's mastery level through daily observation or direct item administration. The LAP-D requires a more standardized approach to testing, with pre- and posttesting being its most appropriate use. The differences between the LAP-R and LAP-D have been minimized due to the inclusion of definable behavioral objectives and scoring criteria in the LAP-R. It is recommended that the LAP-D be used with other developmental scales or assessment tools because it provides information only on a child's progress and has no ability to diagnose dysfunction or etiology.

Review

The LAP-D is an assessment tool of general development for 1 to 6 year olds. It covers the areas of gross motor, fine motor, cognitive, language, and self-help. It can be administered by a variety of professionals but was specifically developed for teachers. The three major functions of this assessment tool are evaluation of entry skills, evaluation of exit skills, and validation of instructional program. This assessment tool easily translates into individual education goals and objectives. Educational goals that directly correlate with LAP-D test items are provided. The stated population for the LAP-D is normal and young handicapped children. The information provided with this tool does not elaborate on the definitions or type of handicapping conditions which would or would not be appropriate for this type of assessment. The LAP-D cannot be used for identifying neurological, psychological, intellectual, motor, or linguistic dysfunction. No etiologies can be ascertained. A child should not be labeled or placed in a special class due to the results of the LAP-D. Children who demonstrate serious delays on this tool should be evaluated by experienced pediatric professionals with in-depth assessment tests.

The small number of children included in the reliability study seriously impedes one's ability to generalize the results to the general population. Therefore, much caution should be exercised regarding its use and interpretation. The authors feel locally constructed norms provide more appropriate information regarding the results of this tool for individual children. Using each child's pre- and posttest scores, the examiner can evaluate a child's progress and the effects of the educational program. No standard scores or specific age equivalences can be ascertained.

REFERENCE

1. LeMay, D. W., Griffin, P. M., and Sanford, A. R. *Learning Accomplishment Profile-Diagnostic Edition (Revised) Examiner's Manual.* Winston-Salem, N.C.: Kaplan Press, 1977.

LEARNING ACCOMPLISHMENT PROFILE, REVISED EDITION

Descriptive Information

Test Identification

The title of this test is *Learning Accomplishment Profile, Revised Edition* (LAP-R), 1981. The original edition, published in 1974, is entitled Learning Accomplishment Profile. The revised edition of the LAP contains behavioral objectives instead of general descriptions of developmental milestones. Its authors are Anne R. Sanford, M.Ed., and Janet G. Zelman, M.Ed. Although not stated in the literature provided with the LAP-R, the authors of this instrument have backgrounds and experience in education. Both were working with the Chapel Hill Training Outreach Project in North Carolina. Kaplan Press (P.O. Box 5128, Winston-Salem, North Carolina 27113) publishes this test. The LAP-R Administration/Scoring Form costs $5–$10; and the Learning Activity Cards, $35–$45.

Age and Type of Client

The LAP-R was designed for administration to young handicapped and normal children between 36 and 72 months of age. Specific information regarding the type of handicapping condition this tool is appropriate for is not stated.

Purpose

The stated purpose of this instrument is to provide teachers with "a criterion-referenced tool for systematic assessment of a child's skills" [1]. Skill areas tested include gross motor, fine motor, prewriting, cognitive, language, self-help, and personal-social. This instrument enables the identification of developmental learning objectives and ongoing measurement of progress. Individualized education plans can be generated by use of the Learning Activity Cards that are correlated with the LAP-R.

Time Required to Administer and Score Test

Assessment time for the LAP-R is not stated; for examiners with experience in administration of this tool, the time is estimated at 2 to 2½ hours. Scoring is relatively simple and takes approximately 15 minutes.

Evaluator

The LAP-R does not specify the qualifications of the evaluator, although the "teacher and para-professional" are mentioned. Any professional experienced in pediatric testing should be able to administer this tool. There are no specific training requirements outlined.

Historical Perspective of Test Construction

Development and Source of Test Items

The test items for the LAP-R were drawn from several pediatric assessment tools (Alpern-Boll,

Bangs, Bayley, Caplan, Cattell, Communicative Evaluation Chart, Coley, Cohen and Gross, Doll, Frankenburg, Gesell, Hurlock, Illingworth, Knoblock and Pasamanick, Merrill-Palmer Scale, Preschool Language Scale, Sharp and Loumeau, Sheridan, Sequenced Inventory of Communication Development, Slosson, Skills Sequence Checklist, Sequential Testing and Educational Programming, Stott, Terman, Vammoer, Weiss, and Lilywhite). Each item specifies the assessment tool from which it originated.

Review of Literature in Terms of Test Use

There is no published literature reviewing this instrument.

Theoretical Constructs and Implications for Intervention

The LAP-R is based on theories underlying normal growth and development; in addition, the test is based on theories used to develop the 27 pediatric assessment tools (listed above), from which the test items were drawn. Therefore, it appears that the LAP-R is based on numerous theories of child development. This tool was constructed due to the authors' concern regarding the dichotomy between professional diagnosis and classroom or educational intervention. Sanford and Zelman felt that a criterion-referenced tool was needed to assist teachers in assessment and educational planning of each student. The authors suggest using the LAP-R to assess children and then using the Learning Activity Cards for educational planning.

Content and Test Administration

Content

The LAP-R assesses the areas of gross motor, fine motor, prewriting, cognitive, language (receptive and expressive), self-help, and personal-social. Although the LAP-R includes some assessment items below the 36-month level, the focus

of this tool is 36 to 72 months of age. Other assessment tools are recommended for children functioning under 36 months. There are a total of 379 assessment items.

The Gross Motor Index contains 56 items (10 of the items for skills below the 36-month level) with yearly increments from 36 to 72 months, with approximately 10 to 12 items per increment.

The Fine Motor Index contains 42 items (nine items below the 36-month level) with 6-month increments, six to nine items per increment with the exceptions of two to three items for the 54- and 72-month levels.

The Prewriting Index contains 36 items (10 items below the 36-month level) with 6-month increments, three to five items per increment.

The Cognitive Index contains 90 items (eight items below the 36-month level) with 6-month increments, eight to ten items for the 36- to 54-month levels and 13 to 19 items for the 60- to 72-month levels.

The Language Index contains 55 items (15 items below the 36-month level) with 6-month increments, four to five items in the 42-, 54-, and 72-month levels and nine items in the 36-, 48-, and 60-month levels. There are 18 receptive language items and approximately 37 expressive language items.

The Self-Help Index includes 60 items (11 items below the 36-month level) with 6-month increments, 14 items in the 36- and 48-month levels and four to six items in each of the remaining levels.

The Personal-Social Index includes 40 items (six items below the 36-month level) with 6-month increments, nine items at the 36- and 48-month levels and two to five items in each of the remaining levels.

Professionals experienced in developmental pediatric assessment will be familiar with most of the 379 items in this tool. Examples of items at the 48-month level are (1) Gross Motor: walks on circular line, stands on 1 foot for 5 seconds, and throws ball overhand (10 feet); (2) Fine Motor: places small objects into bottle, folds and creases paper, and completes three-piece puzzle; (3) Prewriting: copies cross, holds paint brush with fingers instead of fist, and draws a person with two body parts; (4) Cognitive: matches four colors, points to rough and smooth textures, and counts by rote to 10; (5) Language: tells use of objects, repeats 12-syllable sentence, and uses prepositions; (6) Self-Help: puts on socks, buttons front buttons, and serves food to self; and (7) Personal-Social: tells age, participates in make-believe play, and plays cooperatively with other children.

The test materials available from Kaplan Press include only the test booklets and activity cards. No test equipment is provided. The equipment necessary for administration of this tool is extensive. Many of the materials are usually found in preschool settings but many would need to be purchased or made.

The LAP-R test booklet contains the test items, directions, scoring criteria, and scoring form. One booklet is designed for use with one child. The format of the booklet is easy to read and understand. Each section (or index) begins with a listing of test items in that index, allowing the administrator to easily determine what skills are being tested. Each test item references the original assessment tool from which it was drawn.

The charts are provided for the examiner to fill in, displaying the results of the child's performance. The Initial Assessment Chart provides space for documentation of strength and weakness patterns in each skill index from the first assessment. The Assessment Review Chart provides space for strength and weakness information in each skill index after reassessment. The Individual Education Program provides a format for writing the child's educational program. The Profile Chart provides a bar graph for identification of skill levels attained and strength and weakness patterns.

Setting and Equipment

Administration of the LAP-R requires a relatively quiet room that has enough space for a child to perform gross motor items. Furniture should include a child-sized table and chair. Since the LAP-R does not include any of the materials needed, all materials should be gathered and organized before administration of this instrument.

Administration Procedures

The LAP-R can either be administered in a one-to-one situation or be used as an ongoing assessment tool with daily observations serving as the information used to score the test. It requires observation and scoring of the child's specific responses to each item.

Unlike the original version of the LAP, the LAP-R provides specific administration directions, allowing for a more standardized approach in item presentation. The directions are easily understood, clear, and concise. The procedure is not complex once the examiner becomes familiar with the format.

Scoring

Recording procedures are provided in a short, concise manner. Each of the seven skill areas is administered, and each item is scored by stated criteria on a pass (+)/fail (−) method. The basal level is determined when a child has demonstrated acquisition of eight consecutive items in an index. The ceiling is established when the child is unable to pass three items in a five-item sequence. Each skill area is administered using the basal/ceiling format.

The information gained from the LAP-R refers to specific skills demonstrated or not demonstrated. The purpose of the instrument is to provide a direct correlation between assessment and educational programs. A strength and weakness pattern can be ascertained. No standard scores, quotients, or age equivalences are provided by this tool, although a basic idea of functional age level can be estimated because skills are broken down into age groupings. Caution must be exercised regarding the use of approximate age groupings since this test was drawn from numerous tests that vary greatly in developmental age equivalencies.

Psychometric Properties

The LAP-R is not a norm-referenced assessment tool. No studies have been done regarding reliability and validity of this tool.

Guidelines for Use in a Clinical Setting

The LAP-R evaluates seven areas of skills expected of the 3- to 6-year-old child. If the examiner's goal of testing is to develop an educational plan with specific activities, this tool may be helpful. If a standard score or specific age equivalency is desired, the LAP-R would not be appropriate. The booklet provides space for the examiner's comments regarding a child's performance on each item. It is possible to make valuable clinical observations, depending on the professional background and experiences of the examiner.

The LAP-R can be used in conjunction with the Learning Accomplishment Profile-Diagnostic (LAP-D is reviewed in this chapter). The LAP-D provides an evaluation of a child's progress and the effects of the educational program. The LAP-R provides an ongoing assessment and specific activities to be included in the child's educational program. The differences between the LAP-R and the LAP-D have been minimized due to the inclusion of definable behavioral objectives and scoring criteria in the LAP-R. Both tools should be used with other developmental assessment tools because they cannot diagnose dysfunction or etiology.

Review

The LAP-R is a criterion-referenced tool for 3 to 6 year olds that covers the areas of gross motor, fine motor, prewriting, cognitive, language, self-help, and personal/social. It can be administered by a variety of professionals, but was specifically developed for teachers to provide a means of assessing a child for the purpose of educational programming. The stated population for the LAP-R is normal and young handicapped children. The information provided with this tool does not elaborate on the definition or type of handicapping conditions that would or would not be appropriate for this test. Anne Sanford (author) states in the introduction that it is the responsibility of the test administrator "to analyze each item to ascertain its appropriateness for individual children" [1]. No guidelines are provided for item adaptation or elimination. Item analysis is even more important in the development of the educational program so that inappropriate goals for the child's handicap can easily be identified. Sanford states "It is essential that no LAP-R item be considered a 'sacred' step in individual programming. Constant awareness of the child's specific handicapping condition mandates flexibility and creativity in the selection of materials and design of procedures which will not penalize the youngster" [1].

This test is not norm-referenced, nor have there been any reliability or validity data collected on it. Therefore, caution should be exercised regarding its use and interpretation. The opportunity for variability of results is great. Due to the lack of studies, the examiner must question the validity of the test and test items and the reliability of the instrument. The therapist attempting to evaluate the motor skills of a child will probably not find this assessment tool particularly helpful since it does not provide standard scores, age equivalencies, or diagnostic information.

REFERENCE

1. Sanford, A. R., and Zelman, J. G. *Learning Accomplishment Profile-Revised Edition.* Winston-Salem, N.C.: Kaplan Press, 1981.

VULPÉ ASSESSMENT BATTERY

Descriptive Information

Test Identification

The title of this test is *Vulpé Assessment Battery,* Second Edition (Vulpé), 1977. The original edition, published in 1969, is entitled Home Care and Management of the Mentally Retarded Child and the Assessment Battery. The author of the Vulpé Assessment Battery is Shirley German Vulpé, with contributions by Ellen Rollins and Janet Wilson. Vulpé has a combined Canadian occupational therapy and physical therapy degree. Ellen Rollins' professional background and education is in clinical and developmental psychology. Janet Wilson's professional background and training is in physical therapy. The National Institute on Mental Retardation (Canadian Association for the Mentally Retarded, Kinsmen, NIMR Building, York University Campus, 4700 Keele St., Downsview [Toronto], Ontario M3₅-1F3) publishes this test. (Price not available.)

Age and Type of Client

The Vulpé was designed for administration to normal, at-risk, or atypically developing children between birth and 6 years of age.

Purpose

The purpose of this tool is to provide the evaluator with (1) a comprehensive developmental assessment, (2) a sequential teaching approach, (3) an indication of program goals, and (4) an accountability system for individual programs.

Time Required to Administer and Score Test

The manual estimates administration time to be approximately 1 hour. It is not necessary for the administration to be completed in one setting, nor is it necessary for the entire battery to be administered to each child.

Evaluator

The battery was designed for administration by people with a variety of training and professional backgrounds. The author suggests that it is appropriate for specific professionals to administer specific sections of the battery (e.g., a speech and language therapist should administer the Oral Reflex and Language Sections).

Historical Perspective of Test Construction

Development and Source of Test Items

The items for the Vulpé Assessment Battery were drawn from many pediatric assessment tools. Vulpé extensively reviewed available pediatric assessments and child development information, selecting items that represented developmental stages. The author found that there was great variability among the tools in reporting the age level at which a skill should be accomplished; she chose to use the youngest reported age level for placement of items in this tool. Each item is referenced according to the assessment tool or body of knowledge from which it was drawn (188 references).

Review of Literature in Terms of Test Use

The author provides an extensive review of the literature in the manual on many different topics. Examples of areas summarized include effectiveness of early intervention; role of the environment, caregivers, and professionals; and effects of the handicapped child on families. Many aspects of the scales are also referenced and summarized. A total of 347 references are provided and divided into 17 subject areas. No literature reviewing the use of the Vulpé is available.

Theoretical Constructs and Implications for Intervention

The Vulpé Assessment Battery is based on theories underlying normal growth and development as well as on multiple theories provided in the review of the literature for the development of the assessment battery. The basic approach of this battery relates to the need for early intervention; therefore, assessment of children as young as possible is recommended. The author feels this approach will enable the examiner to develop intervention programs that relate to a child's strengths and weaknesses and therefore maximize his or her learning potential.

Content and Administration

Content

The Vulpé Assessment Battery is divided into eight sections and 26 subsections. The eight sections include Basic Senses and Functions, Gross Motor, Fine Motor, Language, Cognitive, Organization of Behaviors, Activities of Daily Living, and Environment.

The Basic Senses and Functions Section contains 16 items and deals with the central nervous system's ability to process visual, auditory, olfactory, proprioceptive, and vestibular information. Items involved with motor planning, balance, muscle strength, range of motion, and reflex status are also included. If a child demonstrates deficits or abnormalities in balance, muscle strength, reflex maturation, and motor planning, the examiner is instructed to refer to Appendix A. Appendix A contains a Developmental Reflex Test and lists cross-references of assessment items in other sections that would provide more information about balance, muscle strength, and motor planning. The author states that this section should be administered first, as deficits in this area will affect the child's performance on the remainder of the assessment battery. Examples of items from Basic Senses and Functions Section: observe child's response to cellophane, a bell, and a voice; observe child's response to being touched with a piece of cotton.

The Gross Motor Section contains 206 items. Basic behaviors assessed include standing, jumping, walking, running, hopping, and skipping. Cross-referencing is provided in the areas of muscle strength, balance, and motor planning. Examples (3- to 3½-year level): balancing on 1 foot for 2 seconds, walking backward 10 feet.

The Fine Motor Section contains 177 items. Skills assessed include eye movements, eye-hand coordination, manipulation, and interaction with toys and utensils. Examples (3- to 4-year level): copying a drawing of a square, 10-block tower.

The Language Section contains 241 items. It is divided into two subsections: receptive and expressive language.

The Receptive Language Subsection contains 81 items pertaining to hearing sounds, understanding sounds, understanding words in context, and comprehension of sentences. Examples (30- to 33-month level): understanding common adjectives, understanding of negatives.

The Expressive Language Subsection contains 160 items pertaining to babbling, jargon, use of one to two word sentences, and free expression. Examples (30- to 33-month level): retelling simple facts of a story, counts to 3.

The Cognitive Processes and Specific Concepts Section contains 245 items and is divided into 13 subsections.

The Color Concept Subsection (nine items) involves discriminating, matching, sorting, and naming colors. Examples (2½- to 3-year level): sorting colors, naming one color.

The Shape Concept Subsection (22 items) includes three-dimensional and two-dimensional shape discriminations. Examples (3- to 3½-year level): matching squares, imitation of drawing a circle.

The Size Concept Subsection (six items) involves size discrimination and understanding of labels pertaining to size. Examples (2½- to 3-year level): ability to graduate six sizes, understanding the concept of "bigger."

The Body Concept Subsection (32 items) includes body parts, functions, and emotions. Examples (2½- to 3-year level): knowledge of 10 body parts, verbal expression of emotions.

The Object Concept Subsection (17 items) involves object permanence to categorization of objects. Examples (1½- to 3-year level): identification of objects from parts, identification of objects by function.

The Space Concept Subsection (36 items) includes the relationship of body and space and understanding of spatial verbal concepts. Examples (2½- to 3-year level): understanding of the concept of "behind," relationship of parts to whole (jig-saw puzzle).

The Time Concept Subsection (16 items) involves the sequencing of events and the understanding of present, past, and future. Examples (3- to 4-year level): distinction of night and day, understanding of "today, yesterday, and tomorrow."

The Amount and Number Concept Subsection (22 items) includes the understanding of quantities. Examples (2½- to 3-year level): tells age, counts two objects.

The Visual Memory Subsection (12 items) looks at the child's ability to retain visual information up to an 18-month level. Examples: remembering places of household objects, selection of picture from memory.

The Auditory Discrimination Subsection (12 items) involves the child's ability to discriminate sounds and words. Examples (4- to 5-year level): discrimination of own language errors, discrimination of rhyming words.

The Auditory Attention, Comprehension, and Memory Subsection (25 items) involves the child's ability to remember auditory information. Examples (2½- to 3-year level): follows three-step command, repeats seven-syllable sentence.

The Cause/Effect Concept Subsection (12 items) involves the child's ability to understand cause and effect up to the 24-month level. Examples (4- to 6-month level): relationship of motor activity to obtaining object, using objects to act on other objects.

The Categorizing/Combining Scheme Subsection (24 items) involves the organization of information. Examples (3- to 4-year level): combining concept of object with its opposite, combining concept of object pictured with object category.

The Organization of Behavior Section involves the child's ability to organize behavioral responses to the environment. It contains 79 items and is divided into four subsections.

The Attention and Goal Orientation Subsection contains 18 items relating to the child's ability to maintain attention, direct activity, and

achieve goals. Examples (3- to 4-year level): adaptive attention to activities of daily living—can eat, dress independently, sustained play with another child for 30 minutes.

The Internal Behavior Control Related to Recognition and Response to Environmental Limits Subsection contains 20 items. The developmental sequence of this subsection originates at the child's ability (1) to control his or her internal state and motor behavior, (2) to recognize behavioral limits, and (3) to independently control behavior. Examples (12- to 18-month level): Child repeats behaviors that previously elicited and maintained social interaction, the child stops an activity when requested.

The Problem Solving and Learning Patterns Subsection contains 17 items ranging from a child's ability to solve concrete problems to abstract problem solving. Learning patterns involve the techniques children use to acquire knowledge (e.g., visually, auditorily). Examples (3- to 4-year level): verbal problem solving (child asks questions to solve problems), imagination and independent thought (child frequently discusses "What if?" situations).

The Dependence/Independence Subsection contains 24 items. This subsection relates to the child's development from total dependence to independent functioning. Examples (16- to 24-month level): uses words to indicate needs, independent behavior in absence of familiar adult.

The Activities of Daily Living Section contains 222 items and is divided into seven subsections: feeding, dressing, toileting, grooming, sleeping, play, and social interaction.

> Feeding (47 items). Examples (4- to 5-year level): chooses own menu, sets table, and serves self.
> Dressing (32 items). Examples (3- to 4-year level): puts shoes on correct feet, buttons shirt.
> Social Interaction (48 items). Examples (2- to 2½-year level): offers help to others, shares, and takes turns.
> Play (50 items). Examples (3- to 3½-year level):

predominance of social group play over parallel play, interest in excursions.

Sleeping (16 items). Examples (12- to 18-month level): child sleeps for 10 to 12 hours at night, child has one or two naps of 1 to 4 hours during the day.

Toileting (17 items). Examples (2½- to 3-year level): distinguishes between bowel and bladder function, anticipates toilet needs in time to get to bathroom.

Grooming (12 items). Examples (3- to 4-year level): Brushes teeth independently, blows nose independently.

The Environment Section is organized differently than the previous sections. Assessment questions are provided with a discussion of specific variables pertaining to the question. This assists the examiner in organizing the material related to the question. Information is obtained through observation and by interviewing the caregivers. The author relates that value judgments should not be made, but that this section provides some structure for acquiring the knowledge needed for appropriate programming for the child. The Environment Section contains 44 questions and is divided into seven subsections.

Setting (seven questions). Example: Does the environment contain things to facilitate gross motor movements?

Educational or Institutional Setting (three questions). Example: "What personnel have the most contact with the children?" Discussion: educational experience of personnel, knowledge of child, knowledge of child's educational program.

Caregiving Personnel—Basic Characteristics (eight questions). Example: Does caregiver derive pleasure from young children?

Caregiver—Knowledge of Interactive Aspects of Child Development (three questions). Example: Is the caregiver aware that children frequently initiate and direct caregivers' response?

Caregiver—Knowledge of Own Role in Devel-

opmental Process (two questions). Example: Is the caregiver aware of his or her control over experiences to which the child is exposed?

Caregiver—Knowledge of Developmental Needs of Children (11 questions). Example: Is caregiver aware that children's behaviors are influenced by a reward system—praise/ encouragement and punishment/ignoring?

Caregiver—Teaching and Behavior Management Techniques (10 questions). Example: Does the caregiver talk to a child at a level the child can understand?

Setting and Equipment

The suggested environment for the administration of this battery is a quiet room with a child-sized table and chairs, room for a mat for younger children, and room for gross motor activities for older children. Only the Vulpé Assessment Battery Book/Manual is available for purchase. An extensive list of equipment needed for administration of this battery is provided in Appendix E. The equipment should be gathered and organized prior to the assessment. The manual and/or scoring sheets, paper, and pencils are also necessary.

Administration Procedures

The administration format is variable. Information is gathered through caregiver report, observation of the child's behavior and environment, facilitating behaviors by setting up the environment, and direct administration of specific items. The author states it is not necessary to administer all the sections if reliable information is already known in some areas. It is also not necessary to complete the assessment in one session. The manual/administration sheets provide guidelines regarding the administration of each item and/or how the information may be obtained. The potential for variability in administration is great.

The manual provides specific administration instructions and verbal directions for some items. It suggests possible methods for ascertaining the relevant information for other items. It is suggested that items should initially be presented at the child's estimated mental age. If mental age is unknown, discussion of the child's level with a caregiver may be useful for deciding entry level. Also, a screening format using a few items at each age level may be helpful in providing an entry level. Once entry level is established, the examiner is instructed to administer items until the child fails all items in an age level.

The examiner should be familiar with the test items and organize the materials and presentation sequence prior to administration. Due to the extensive amount of information that can be obtained from this battery, administration can be a fairly complex procedure.

Scoring

The author developed a scoring procedure called the Performance Analysis System. Its purpose was to provide an objective method for "(1) assessing a child's performance in a task, (2) exploring which teaching techniques the child learns most readily, (3) scoring the assessment results, (4) applying these results to an individualized learning program, and (5) recording progress in developmental activities" [2].

The scoring method provides a systematic procedure for adjusting the environment, the task, and/or the presentation of the task to ascertain the child's competencies and learning styles. In the manual, the author states the scoring directions with much discussion on each aspect of the scoring procedure and documentation of the viability of this system. The author acknowledges that the use of the variations of the scoring system is very much dependent on the skill of the examiner, which increases the potential for variable results.

The scoring system involves assigning one of seven possible scores for each item administered. The seven scores are as follows:

1. A *no* score is given if the child displays no interest or motivation to complete the task.
2. An *attention* score is given if the child attends or demonstrates interest in the task but does not actively participate in completion of the task.
3. A *physical assistance* score is given when a child actively participates in the activity once assistance is provided by physical support to the child, physical support with materials, modifications of environment, and/or modification of media.
4. A *social/emotional assistance* score is used when the child participates in the task when more reassurance and/or reinforcement are provided by the examiner.
5. A *verbal assistance* score is given when a child's response changes with more verbal cues or if the directions are repeated.
6. An *independent score* is used when the child is successful in completion of the task in a familiar environment with no assistance provided.
7. A *transfer* score is given if the child can successfully complete a task in different environments with different materials.

The examiner is also to take into account an activity analysis for each task and the child's information processing style. Activity analysis involves looking at the components of an activity, and the interactive aspects of developmental tasks. "For example, performance of a fine motor task may rely on abilities in reflex control, gross motor skill, social adaptive behavior, behavioral organizational skills, cognitive appreciation of the task, and/or auditory language abilities" [2]. The suggested information processing model is input, integration, feedback, assimilation, and output. Some discussion of these aspects is provided in the manual. Space is provided on the scoring sheet for comments and elaboration of the child's performance. Most test items have criteria established for successful completion of the task. The scoring system is fairly complex due to the numerous variables evaluated, the potential amount of information each test item can provide, and the cross-referencing system. "Assessment items are cross-referenced if they appear in more than one section. This eliminates the need of testing an item more than once and also indicates that the activity requires skills in more than one developmental area" [2].

The amount of information potentially gained from this battery is extensive. Its purpose is to provide a direct link between assessment and educational programs. No standard scores, quotients, or age equivalences can be ascertained, although a basic idea of functioning age level can be estimated since skills are grouped by age levels. This estimate can provide information on the relative strengths and weaknesses a child possesses. Descriptive information regarding a child's learning patterns can be gained from the scoring system. The cross-referencing of items can provide the examiner with common linkages between skill areas. The author provides a format for writing a report and a format for developing a program plan from this assessment battery. These formats provide the examiner with assistance in organizing the information gained.

Psychometric Properties

The Vulpé Assessment Battery is a criterion-referenced evaluation instrument. There have been no published studies regarding reliability and validity of this tool.

Guidelines for Use in a Clinical Setting

The Vulpé assesses children from birth to 6 years of age in eight skill areas. If the examiner's goal of testing is to gain extensive descriptive information about a child, to define relative strength and weaknesses, and/or to develop a habilitation program, this tool will be very helpful. If a standard score or specific age equivalency is desired, this tool would not be appropriate. The Vulpé can also assist the examiner in identifying other tests or diagnostic procedures that may be helpful in understanding the child's abilities and dis-

abilities; however, the Vulpé does not diagnose dysfunction or etiology. The scoring sheet provides space for the examiner's comments regarding a child's performance on each item. The Vulpé provides a structure and organization for making clinical observations through the scoring system. It is possible to make valuable clinical observations, although much would depend on the professional background and experiences of the examiners.

Review

The Vulpé Assessment Battery is a comprehensive assessment tool for children from birth to 6 years of age that evaluates the areas of basic senses and functions, gross motor, fine motor, language, cognitive, organization of behavior, activities of daily living, and environment. It can be administered by a variety of professionals, but some sections could provide more comprehensive information if evaluated by a professional trained in that area. For example, the occupational and/or physical therapist could most likely make better use of the gross and fine motor sections in conjunction with the Developmental Reflex Test and the cross-referencing of motor planning, muscle strength, balance, and range of motion items. Due to the unique scoring system, item adaptation is systematized and provides basic information regarding the child's learning style, but organizing this information can be a complex procedure. Development of an educational program can be derived from information obtained from the assessment. This test is not norm-referenced, nor has there been any reliability or validity data collected on it. Therefore, caution should be exercised regarding its use and interpretation. The opportunity for variability of results is great.

REFERENCES

1. Taylor, R. L. *Assessment of Exceptional Students: Educational and Psychological Procedures.* Englewood Cliffs, N.J.: Prentice-Hall, 1984.

2. Vulpé, S. *Vulpé Assessment Battery* (2nd ed.). Downsview, Ontario: National Institute on Mental Retardation, 1977.

Tests for Visually Impaired Children

REYNELL-ZINKIN SCALES: DEVELOPMENTAL SCALES FOR YOUNG VISUALLY HANDICAPPED CHILDREN

Descriptive Information

Test Identification

The title of this test is *Reynell-Zinkin Scales: Developmental Scales for Young Visually Handicapped Children—Part 1: Mental Development* (Reynell-Zinkin Scales), 1979. Its authors are Joan Reynell and Pamela Zinkin. No specific information is provided regarding the authors' educational or experiential background, although it is stated that work on the scales began in 1970 at the Wolfson Centre, Institute of Child Health, London, England. NFER Publishing Company (Darville House, 2 Oxford Road East, Windsor Berkshire SL4, IDF England) publishes this test. (Price not available.)

Age and Type of Client

This scale was designed for administration to multihandicapped visually impaired and blind children between the approximate ages of birth and 5 years.

Purpose

The Reynell-Zinkin Scales were developed "to enable professional people, concerned with young visually handicapped children, to have some guidelines for assessment and developmental advice" [2]. The authors feel that the strength of these scales is the developmental information provided for use in ascertaining appropriate instructional goals.

Time Required to Administer and Score Test

Time required to administer the test is approximately 1 hour; scoring requires approximately 5 minutes.

Evaluator

The authors state that the examiners "should have a sound understanding of early intellectual development and some understanding of how this deviates in visually handicapped children" [2]. They suggest doctors, psychologists, and teachers of visually impaired children as appropriate examiners.

Historical Background of Test Construction

Development and Source of Test Items

The Reynell-Zinkin Scales were developed due to the lack of appropriate assessment tools for the visually impaired. In its development, the authors desired items that provided information on cognitive processes versus specific skill acquisition. Their developmental hierarchy is based on works by other professionals (specific professionals or literature not stated) and their own observations. Many items in the Social Adaptation Scale are adapted from the items in the Social Maturity Scale for Blind Preschool Children by Maxfield and Bucholz.

Review of Literature

There are no studies published in the United States using this assessment tool. A critique of this test is available in *The Ninth Mental Measurements Yearbook* [1].

Theoretical Constructs and Implications for Intervention

The authors' purpose in item selection was to include items that provided information on mental processes, not specific skill acquisition. They

used information from child development literature (unspecified) and their own observations.
Their intent is to provide professionals with
guidelines as to the developmental progression a
visually impaired child may follow. Also, the use
of the scales should allow the professional to
provide instructional advice to parents or caretakers of these children.

Content and Administration

Content

The Reynell-Zinkin Scales are divided into five
subscales. The Social Adaptation Subscale includes six items of social interaction and 12
items in self-help. Many of the items in this subscale are related to those found in the Social Maturity Scale for Blind Preschool Children by
Maxfield and Bucholz. The authors state that this
subscale has the "lowest intellectual components" [2] and tends to rely on specific instruction
previously provided to the child. Examples of
items: recognition of familiar voice, demands personal attention, removes simple garment, and eats
with spoon.

The Sensorimotor Understanding Subscale
contains 20 items involving the child's understanding of objects and the relationship of one
object to another. It also contains three items
pertaining to the function of objects. Examples
of items: explorative manipulation of shape, extensive search for lost object, sorts beads into
big and small, and appropriate use of brush, cup,
spoon.

The Exploration of Environment Subscale
contains 12 items involved with the child's understanding and exploration of environmental
space. Examples of items: exploration of furniture, finds door of room, directed purposeful locomotion (i.e., "Sit down at table."), and goes
about immediate neighborhood.

The Response to Sound and Verbal Comprehension Subscale involves the child's response
to sound, understanding of words, and ability to
follow oral directions. It contains 36 items and is

divided into four sections. Examples of items:
Section 1—reaches for source of sound in correct direction, appropriate response to familiar
phrase or words; Section 2—puts spoon in cup,
puts the fork on the plate; Section 3—"Which
object do we drink out of?," "Find two things
we use for eating dinner"; Section 4—"Show me
the longest pencil," "Put the short pencil in the
biggest cup."

The Expressive Language Subscale contains
two major divisions: structure and content. The
structure area uses sounds, words, and phrases
appropriately in expression and contains 22
items. Examples of items: six to twelve meaningful words, appropriate use of prepositions, and
use of complete sentences.

The content area involves the child providing
verbal descriptions of the use of objects or descriptions of actions. This area contains 18
items. Examples of items: "What is this for?"
(point to a telephone), and "What happened?"
(put child's hand on car and push it along).

A Communication Subscale is also available,
although it does not include age equivalences.
The authors felt it may provide helpful information on children who are unable to communicate
through verbal expression due to auditory and/
or motor handicaps. It is divided in two sections
—receptive and expressive communication with
10 items per section. Examples of items: receptive—appropriate response to any familiar communication pattern, responds to three or more
signs or gestures; expressive—makes wants
known by any deliberate communication, uses
three or more signs or gestures appropriately.

Setting and Equipment

No specifications are provided regarding the
physical setting for this assessment tool. As with
most assessments, an area free of distractions
with child-sized tables and chairs or the child's
specific seating equipment would be appropriate.

The test kit includes only a manual. The examiner must obtain the necessary materials from
the equipment list in Appendix Two. The scale

was developed in Britain, and the equipment list includes many items specific to the British culture, for example, "bricks" and "sweets." The examiner may be very confused in regard to the actual list of test items. These discrepancies can result in great variability in items used in this assessment tool.

Administration Procedure

The administration format is variable. Information is gathered through parental report, observation of the child's behavior, facilitating behaviors by setting up the environment, and direct administration of specific items. The manual provides specific administration instructions and verbal directions for some items. It suggests possible methods for ascertaining the relevant information for other items. This scale was not necessarily designed for each item in a subscale to be administered in succession. Example: item number 5 in subscale Exploration of Environment—finding the door of a room. The authors suggest that this item be administered at the end of testing session as all are ready to leave. Therefore, the examiner should be familiar with the test items and organize the materials and presentation sequence prior to administration. If this is accomplished, the Reynell-Zinkin Scales is not particularly complex. However, the scales are somewhat cumbersome, with the potential for great variability in administration.

Scoring

The manual provides specific scoring directions for some items but gives vague directions for others. This provides the potential for great variability between examiners. The Record Sheet provides space for scoring but not instructions for each item, so the manual is necessary for the scoring criteria.

Each of the subscales is administered and each item is scored on a pass/fail basis. Criteria for when to appropriately stop administering a subscale is not provided. Therefore, it is left to the examiner's discretion regarding when a child has demonstrated his or her highest abilities. A raw score of 1 is given to each passed item. The raw score is then added up for each subscale and converted to an age equivalent by using tables located in the manual. There are tables for the blind, partially sighted, and sighted. The examiner must decide which table would be the most appropriate for the specific child. It is suggested that if a child uses visually guided movement to reach for a toy, the Partially Sighted Table is used; and if a child uses tactile exploration to reach for a toy, the Blind Table is used. The authors suggest that the Sighted Table may provide helpful information with the sighted severely mentally handicapped population and in comparing the performance of visually impaired children with that of their sighted peers.

The authors suggest that "the age score tables may be useful in the following ways: (1) as an indication of the rate of progress of an individual child, (2) as an indication of specific areas of difficulty at any stage, and (3) to compare the rate of development of a particular child with that of others in a comparable visual category" [2]. Interpretive information should include guidelines for the child's instructional program.

Psychometric Properties

Standardization

For determination of the age equivalents used in the manual's tables, 109 children were tested; 42 of those children were tested two or more times for 203 complete test administrations. The time intervals between assessments for children tested more than once ranged from 3 months to 1 year. Ninety-seven testings were done on blind children, and 86 were completed on partially sighted children. Of the 109 children, 17 were additionally diagnosed with mild cerebral palsy and 8 were hearing-impaired. A wide range of intellectual abilities was represented. No other specific information was provided. For determination of age scores, ages were divided into 3-month intervals from 0 to 5 years. The mean score at each interval was plotted on a graph and "the curves smoothed statistically" [2]. In a review in *The Ninth Mental Measurements Yearbook,* Hart felt that it was difficult to determine the validity of the scores due to small sample size and the lack of specific information reported [1].

Reliability

No reliability studies have been done.

Validity

No validity studies have been done.

Guidelines for Use in a Clinical Setting

The Reynell-Zinkin Scales assess visually impaired multihandicapped children from 0 to 5 years of age in several areas of development. Since very few assessment tools are available for this population, clinicians may find this tool useful in gathering general information and clinical observations. The extent and specificity of the observations depend on the examiner's professional background and experience.

Review

The Reynell-Zinkin Scales are used as an assessment tool for evaluation of the mental development of multihandicapped visually impaired children between 0 and 5 years of age. The instrument is divided into five subscales: Social Adaptation, Sensorimotor Understanding, Exploration of Environment, Response to Sound and Verbal Comprehension, and Expressive Language. The purpose of the scales is to provide professionals with guidelines to the mental development of this population and assist them in providing appropriate recommendations for the children's instructional program. Clinicians who evaluate and work with the multihandicapped visually impaired are well aware of the lack of developmental information available for this population. The Reynell-Zinkin Scales appear to be sensitive to the visually impaired child, with many test items having particular relevance to the visually impaired child's development (e.g., Exploration of Environment Subscale, Response to Sound and Verbal Comprehension Subscale). There are relatively few items on each scale, and each item yields a fairly wide age equivalent; therefore, only very gross approximations of age levels is possible. Questions regarding item placement and progress in age equivalences, administration and scoring ambiguities, and no standardization, reliability, or validity studies make these scales basically useful only for descriptive information. A detailed account of the child's performance and clinical observations will provide the examiner with information and clues to the programmatic needs of the child.

REFERENCES

1. Hart, V. Review of Reynell-Zinkin Scales: Developmental Scales for Young Visually Handicapped Children. *Part 1. Mental Development Manual.* In J. V. Mitchel (ed.), *The Ninth Mental Measurements Yearbook* (on-line data base). Lincoln, Nebr.: Buros Institute of Mental Measurement, 1985. (AN0916-2456)
2. Reynell, J., and Zinkin, P. Reynell-Zinkin Scales: Developmental Scales for Young Visually Handicapped Children. *Part 1. Mental Development Manual.* Windsor, England: NFER Publishing Co., 1979.

A SOCIAL MATURITY SCALE FOR BLIND PRESCHOOL CHILDREN

Descriptive Information

Test Identification

The title of this test is *A Social Maturity Scale for Blind Preschool Children* (Social Maturity Scale), 1957. Its authors are Kathryn E. Maxfield, Ph.D., and Sandra Bucholz, M.A. Dr. Maxfield was at the City College of New York at the time of publication of this test. No additional information is included in the manual regarding Sandra Bucholz. American Foundation for the Blind (15

West 16th St., New York, New York 10011) publishes the test at a cost of $6–$7 for the manual, $0.20–$0.25 for a single copy of the record blank, $2–$3 for 10 copies, and $5–$6 for 25 copies.

Age and Type of Client

The Social Maturity Scale for Blind Preschool Children is appropriate for use with visually impaired children between birth and 6 years of age.

Purpose

The test is an inventory that provides an objective means for determining present status or progress of blind children in acquisition of personal and social independence and competence [3]. It is not an intelligence test. Emphasis is placed on what young blind children *habitually* do in everyday activities as opposed to what they *can* do.

Time Required to Administer and Score Test

No specific amount of administration time is stated or recommended. Interviewers are expected to be skilled enough to be able to direct conversation and complete the scale within "reasonable time limits." Experience indicates that 15 to 30 minutes is usually required. Scoring takes 10 to 15 minutes.

Evaluator

Professionals from any discipline can administer the Social Maturity Scale for Blind Preschool Children; no particular disciplines are identified as being appropriate or inappropriate. The authors do state that the scale is most effectively used by those who have had considerable experience in psychological testing of young children and in diagnostic interviewing of both parents and children. It is of particular advantage to have familiarity with the Vineland Social Maturity

Scale (1936 edition) on which the original version of the Maxfield-Bucholz Scale is based.

The authors do not discuss the use of the Social Maturity Scale for Blind Preschool Children by nonprofessionals. However, the suggestion that it is best used by those familiar with psychological testing, as well as the need to be able to develop good interviewing rapport with parents and children, suggests that considerable training would be required before reliable use could be expected by nonprofessionals.

Historical Perspective of Test Construction

Development and Source of Test Items

Ninety-five items comprise the current version of the inventory. Eighty of these items have been adapted from items on the Vineland Social Maturity Scale (1936 edition) in a format known as the Maxfield-Fjeld Adaptation of the Vineland Social Maturity Scale [2, 4]. Eight items are the result of splitting several Maxfield-Fjeld items, and seven are new items. Organization of the Maxfield-Bucholz Scale is based on data and statistical analysis provided by Dr. Samuel P. Hayes, developer of the Interim Hayes-Binet Intelligence Test for the Blind. Administration of the scale results in assignment of a social quotient (SQ), which represents the relationship between chronological age (CA) and social age (SA).

Review of Literature in Terms of Test Use

The Social Maturity Scale is intended to be used as an interview scale. The adult being interviewed must know the child well, since actual performance rather than apparent "inherent ability" is reported. Performance of some items can be observed if necessary. Final judgment regarding strengths and weaknesses should be reserved, when possible, until the scale has been applied more than one time. Determination of the number of times the scale should be applied is based on factors such as the child's health, previous opportunities for developmental experience, SQ, and the ability of the informer to respond with apparent accuracy to the questions. The scale is best used if administered at 6-month intervals during the first 2 years and at 9- to 12-month intervals through 6 years of age. The results can then be used to place children in appropriate developmental and/or educational programs, or to plan intervention activities. When it is impossible to administer the scale so frequently, especially when only one administration is possible, clinical judgment must be combined with scale results to make decisions regarding placement or intervention.

As stated previously, the Social Maturity Scale for Blind Preschool Children is not an intelligence test. It is an inventory of social competence, based on the concept of social maturation. Results can be used in a compatible fashion with IQ tests, but should not be interpreted as measures of cognitive ability.

A variety of professionals working with young visually impaired children have the expertise to apply the clinical judgment necessary for appropriate use of the Social Maturity Scale for Blind Preschool Children. It would be possible to train nonprofessional personnel to administer the scale by interview, but use of clinical judgment when results are ambiguous is inappropriate for nonprofessionals.

Theoretical Constructs and Implications for Intervention

The Social Maturity Scale is based on the concept of social maturation. This concept implies growing competence in performance of activities involving personal independence and social adjustment, both increasing in complexity with chronological age. The level of expectancy is based on performance of other blind children in the same chronological age range. Results are intended to reflect what a visually impaired child *actually* does with day-to-day social and personal independence skills, not on what *possible* performance is.

Although not specifically stated in the test manual, the Social Maturity Scale has several possible implications for intervention. Its usefulness for individual program planning, based on the child's strengths, weaknesses, and overall performance level, is obvious. Its usefulness for placement in the most appropriate classroom setting is also apparent. The scale could conceivably be used for curriculum planning and revision since it is based on normative data for a particular group of children. Certainly it would be useful for some individual and group evaluation over a specified period of time, such as a school year, and may actually point out need for curriculum change if used in this fashion.

Content and Test Administration

Content

The Social Maturity Scale tests, through interview, in the areas of general self-help skills, self-help dressing skills, self-help eating skills, communication skills, socialization skills, locomotion skills, and occupation skills. The seven scales contain a total of 95 items. There are 10 to 20 items at each year level between 0 and 6, and from 0 to 10 items per category at any 1-year level. There is no commercially available test kit. No testing equipment other than the manual, test form, and a pencil is really necessary since it is an interview test. When examiners wish to validate a reported skill by actual demonstration, appropriate equipment found in the home or testing environment may be used.

This scale is scored in individual test booklets. Items are arranged by chronological age so that all items in each of the seven categories for any 1-year increment are grouped together. Categories to which each item belongs are coded beside each as follows:

G = General self-help skills
D = Self-help dressing
E = Self-help eating
C = Communication

S = Socialization
L = Locomotion
O = Occupation

The front of the test booklet contains identifying information and space to record information about degree of vision, prognosis, and other relevant information. An extra page is included at the end of the booklet for notes.

Testing results in recording the number of items passed for each year of chronological age. Total social age, as well as a social quotient, can then be determined by using a conversion table included in the manual.

Setting and Equipment

The Social Maturity Scale for Blind Preschool Children can be administered in any setting conducive to interview. The presence of two comfortable chairs, one for the interviewer and one for the interviewee, is required. If the child is present, presence of suitable attractive toys would be a wise addition to the interview setting.

Administrative Procedures

The Social Maturity Scale is an interview test that may be responded to by any person, usually the mother, who knows the child well. Direct observation of the child can be carried out when necessary, but requires the examiner to have several suitable toys available.

Administration Procedure

Directions for scale item administration are presented in detail in the manual. The authors state that items are seldom directly quoted, but that examiners must have sufficient interviewing skills to present specific examples for the informant to respond to when necessary. The importance of gaining rapport with the informant is repeatedly emphasized.

Administration of this scale is not particularly complex. It is not required that any item be ad-

ministered directly to the child, and there is no complex equipment to operate. The examiner must, however, make use of past experience, knowledge of child development, and clinical judgment to decide at which age level to begin testing. Although it is not clearly stated in the manual, similarity to the 1936 edition of the Vineland Social Maturity Scale would indicate that testing proceeds until there are no more items receiving full or partial credit.

Scoring

Directions for recording responses to individual items are clearly stated and easily followed. Directions for scoring results of the scale are completely stated, but the language is somewhat cumbersome.

Scoring the Social Maturity Scale is somewhat complex. Responses can be scored in several ways, including receiving full, partial, or no credit, by indicating that the item was formerly performed or is not currently performed due to special circumstances. The number of items passed for each year, including partial credit, are then totaled. Social age values for each year level are calculated from tables included in the manual. Social age values are dependent on the number of items passed at each year level.

Administration of the Social Maturity Scale results in assignment of a social quotient. This quotient is determined, as on the Vineland Social Maturity Scale, by converting chronological ages to years and tenths of years as illustrated in the manual. Resulting social quotients can be used to compare performance of visually impaired children against that of other visually impaired children of the same chronological age. It is important to follow scoring guidelines carefully so that visually impaired children with additional handicaps do not receive unduly depressed scores without recognition that delays may be the result of handicaps other than blindness (e.g., mental retardation, cerebral palsy).

The authors do not state whether they consider the scale best used as a screening or diagnostic test, although they do note specifically that it is not an intelligence test. There are no guidelines for referral included, and very little is stated or implied about how the results can be used other than to determine social competence of young, blind children.

Psychometric Properties

Standardization

Specific, step-by-step instructions for administering the Social Maturity Scale are included in the test manual. Although the questions need not be directly quoted from the manual, it is emphasized that experience with developmental testing and with interviewing will aid the examiner in preserving the intent of each question. Instructions for standardized scoring and interpretation are also present.

Children in the standardization sample were all visually impaired and were classified primarily as having or as not having retrolental fibroplasia. The dates between which standardization data were collected are not specified. Since the manual was published in 1957, data collection

occurred prior to that time. A summary of demographic characteristics is contained in Table 5-14.

When considering normative data, it is essential to remember that the Social Maturity Scale for Blind Preschool Children was organized using data gathered on children with impaired vision. Growing use of the Maxfield-Fjeld Scale [4] had indicated a need for revision: items needed reworking or relocating, some needed to be eliminated, and some things needed to be added. Therefore, a study was organized and a total of 484 children were recruited, but 86 were excluded for a variety of reasons. Resulting normative data are based on 605 ratings of 398 children (several children were examined at more than one chronological age, and each examination was treated as a separate subject). There is no statement in the manual regarding who actually carried out the examinations. Based on data from this study, the Maxfield-Fjeld Scale was reorganized and changed to become the present Maxfield-Bucholz Scale. Items were placed in descending order for each year level according to those falling within the 35 to 65 percent passing range. This range was felt to adequately separate the age levels as well as make allowance for on-

Table 5-14. Summary of characteristics of the standardization population for a social maturity scale for blind preschool children

Data characteristics	Standardization population characteristics
Geographical location	Primarily Middle and North Atlantic States (New York, New Jersey, Massachusetts, Connecticut) and North Central States (Illinois, Minnesota)
Criteria for inclusion in study	Attendance at one of the following service-oriented programs: New York Association for the Blind (The Lighthouse) (256 children) New Jersey State Commission for the Blind (66 children) Boston Nursery for Blind Babies (80 children) Connecticut State Board of Education of the Blind (26 children) University of Chicago Project (49 children) Minneapolis Society for the Blind (7 children)
Racial characteristics	Unspecified
Mean educational levels of parents	Data based on some parents from the New York Lighthouse Program and the Boston Nursery for Blind Babies Program only. Statistically treatable data not available. More parents of children with retro-

Table 5-14 (continued)

Data characteristics	Standardization population characteristics
Mean educational levels of parents— *(continued)*	lental fibroplasia (RLF) reported graduating from high school, but a greater proportion of non-RLF children's parents didn't report school attendance

Diagnostic characteristics	Cause of blindness
	    60% of cases in premature babies with RLF
	    Most non-RLFs had cataracts or optic atrophy
	Degree of vision (primarily based on legal definition of blindness, and not reported for all children)
	    None or light perception (LP)
	    More than LP
	    Vision unknown
	Based on data from the New York Association for the Blind, the New Jersey State Commission for the Blind, the Connecticut State Board of Education of the Blind and the Boston Nursery for Blind Babies, the following percentages were found in each category
	    Among RLFs
	        Vision unknown = 24%
	        More than LP = 64%
	        None or LP = 12%
	    Among non-RLFs
	        Vision unknown = 23%
	        More than LP = 48%
	        None or LP = 29%
	Degree of prematurity
	    By birthweight
	        Among RLFs
	            4 pounds or under = 92%
	            Over 4 pounds = 8%
	        Among non-RLFs
	            4 pounds or under = 13%
	            over 4 pounds = 87%
	    By gestational age
	        Among RLFs
	            87% born during 6th or 7th month
	        Among non-RLFs
	            80% were full-term

Total number of subjects in sample	398
Total number of ratings on all subjects (when one child was tested at more than one chronological age, each rating was treated as a separate case)	605
Total number of ratings at each year level	(see table below)

Year level	0–1	1–2	2–3	3–4	4–5	5–6	
Number	50	134	148	120	96	57	Total = 605

Population limitations resulted in no children below age 5 months and only "a few" at ages 7–8 months; the oldest child was 5 years 11 months.

Source: Adapted from K. E. Maxfield and S. Bucholz. *A Social Maturity Scale for Blind Preschool Children: A Guide to Its Use.* New York: American Foundation for the Blind, Inc., 1957.

going social maturation within each 12-month period. An attempt was made to make the norms for the Maxfield-Bucholz Scale as close as possible to norms for sighted children, and to be sure there was a suitable distribution within categories, by including a few items slightly above and below the 35 to 65 percent passing range. A last check on item placement was made by calculating the mean and standard deviation of the ages at which each item was passed. Finally, additional items were chosen to fill gaps that existed at the 5- to 6-year level due to original items at that level being found to be more appropriately included at the 4- to 5-year level. A table is included in the manual that indicates percent of total sample passing each item at each year level on the Maxfield-Bucholz Scale, and the comparative placement of the same item on the Maxfield-Fjeld Scale [3].

Reliability

No studies of reliability are reported in the manual. The authors state that a true measure of reliability can be made only after a scale has been used with sufficient numbers of children at varying age levels. They feel their population is too small in terms of differing social background, in heredity, in developmental opportunities, and in eye conditions.

Validity

No validity studies are reported in the manual. Difficulties with internal consistency, based on varying number of items per category, presence of new items that were not part of the parent scale, and lack of subjects under 6 months of age, are acknowledged. The authors state that validity would be likely to surpass that of the Maxfield-Fjeld Scale through use of scale construction techniques such as the percent-passing technique (using the 35 to 65 percent passing range as the criteria for item inclusion in most categories).

Guidelines for Clinical Use

This scale could be used for any visually impaired child between birth and 6 years of age since it is dependent on informant interview rather than on child performance. It is always wise to recall that, while most parents or others knowing a child well are able to report behavior quite accurately, examiners must be alert for situations where it is apparent that direct observation of the child is necessary.

This scale can be used in conjunction with other screening and diagnostic scales for visually impaired children that do not concentrate primarily on measurement of acquisition of personal and social independence. The Reynell-Zinkin Developmental Scales for Young Visually Handicapped Children, Part I: Mental Development includes a section on social adaptation that includes similar items but with further qualitative breakdown [5]. Other sections in the Reynell-Zinkin Scales include sensorimotor understanding, exploration of environment, response to sound, and verbal comprehension of expressive language. The Reynell-Zinkin Scales have not been standardized, and what statistical investigation has been done has actually involved comparisons with the Maxfield-Bucholz. Even so, use of the Maxfield-Bucholz as a screening device could give information that would be useful in deciding whether further assessment with a broader instrument would be beneficial.

The Perkins-Binet Tests of Intelligence for the Blind are intended to be age-level scales of intelligence that approximate the Stanford-Binet Scale, Form L-M, in structure and content [1]. There are two forms: one for subjects with usable vision and one for those with nonusable vision. It is appropriate for individuals 3 to 18 years of age. Normative data are based on legally blind subjects. Mental ages and intelligence quotients result from test administration. The Perkins-Binet Scales do not tap the developing acquisition of personal and social independence and competence, and the Maxfield-Bucholz could be considered a companion for measurement of social adaptation. It is possible, however, that examiners would want a broader-based scale, such as the Reynell-Zinkin, as a companion scale. The Maxfield-Bucholz could still be used as a screening measure to indicate preliminary information about general level of social skills.

In general, direct clinical observations do not result from use of this scale since it relies on informant interview. It may be of some value to determine how accurate the behavior observation skills of the informant are in order to plan intervention, and this information can be supplied to some extent by use of this scale. Results of the Social Maturity Scale for Blind Preschool Children are useful in ways similar to results of the Vineland Social Maturity Scale: to gain some idea of the personal and social strengths and weaknesses of blind children in order to plan for further diagnosis and/or intervention.

Review

The Social Maturity Scale for Blind Preschool Children is intended to provide an objective means for determining present status or progress of blind children in acquisition of personal and social independence and competence. It is not clearly stated whether its intended use is in a screening or diagnostic capacity. The interview format makes it more widely applicable in situations where children are resistant to direct testing, and where collecting information regarding personal and social independence and competence is vital to planning for appropriate intervention. The present scale is relatively old and has not been standardized as an entity separate from previous versions. There is a significant lack in terms of reliability and validity studies; these studies, along with a clearer indication of the capacity in which the test is to be used, would strengthen the test considerably. Directions for administration are clearly stated, but directions for scoring and test interpretation are somewhat confusing. It is important to recall the authors' reminder that this is a scale to measure

personal and social independence and competence, and not for use to document intellectual capability or emotional adjustment.

REFERENCES

1. Davis, C. J. *Perkins-Binet Test of Intelligence for the Blind.* Watertown, Mass.: Perkins School for the Blind, 1980.
2. Doll, E. *A Measurement of Social Competence: A Manual for the Vineland Social Maturity Scale.* Circle Pines, Minn.: American Guidance Service, 1953.
3. Maxfield, K. E., and Bucholz, S. *A Social Maturity Scale for Blind Preschool Children: A Guide to Its Use.* New York: American Foundation for the Blind, Inc., 1957.
4. Maxfield, K. E., and Fjeld, H. Social Maturity of Visually Handicapped Preschool Children. *Child Dev.* 13 : 1, 1942.
5. Reynell, J. *Manual for the Reynell-Zinkin Scales: Developmental Scales for Young Visually Handicapped Children. Part I: Mental Development.* Windsor, Berkshire SL4, IDF England: NFER Publishing Company, Ltd., 1979.

CHAPTER REVIEW

The developmental tests critiqued in this chapter are defined as tests that provide information about more than two discrete aspects of development. They have been divided into four general categories: screening, parent report, parent report and examiner observation, and tests for the visually impaired:

Screening Tests
    Denver Developmental Screening Test
    Meeting Street School Screening Test
    Miller Assessment for Preschoolers
Tests Requiring Parent Report
    Developmental Profile II (Alpern-Boll)
    Vineland Adaptive Behavior Scales
Tests Requiring Parent Report and Examiner
    Observation
    Gesell Preschool Test
    Learning Accomplishment Profile-
    Diagnostic

Learning Accomplishment Profile-
  Revised
Vulpé Assessment Battery
Tests for Visually Impaired Children
  Reynell-Zinkin Developmental Scales for
    Young Visually Handicapped Children
  A Social Maturity Scale for Blind Preschool
    Children

The tests in each of these categories have
been summarized in Tables 5-15 to 5-18, respectively. The tables allow for a quick perusal of
specific aspects of each test for ease in identification of critical attributes possessed or not possessed by the instruments. Each table contains
information regarding the type of test, age, disability, time required for administration, type of
administration, areas assessed, standardization,
reliability, and validity. This information provides for easy comparison of these critical attributes among the tests in this chapter.

The tests critiqued in this chapter provide
screening information and/or more in-depth assessment information. In both types of tests,
strength and weakness patterns can be ascertained. Most of the tests were developed to be
administered to all types of children and tend to
assess developmental milestones in many areas.
Tests developed for certain disabilities (e.g.,
learning disabled or visually impaired) contain
content areas specific to the disability and tend
to be more specialized. The standardization data
as well as the reliability and validity studies available for each test vary greatly. Therefore, decisions regarding the proper use and interpretation
of the test fall to the examiner. It is clear that
more research is needed, especially in the area of
psychometric properties. However, much information about a child can be collected and interpreted by an examiner who recognizes the
strengths and weaknesses inherent in each test.

Table 5-15. *Characteristics of three developmental screening tests*

Test	Screening	Time to administer	Ages	Disability	Parent report	Task observation	Gross motor	Fine motor	Language	Personal-social	Sensorimotor	Cognitive	Combined abilities	Motor patterning	Visual-perceptual-motor	Standardization	interrater Good (>.80)	Test-retest Good (>.80)	Validity addressed	Predictive
																	Reliability		Validity	
										Areas assessed										
Denver Developmental Screening Test	X	15–30 min	0–6 yr	All	X	X	X	X	X	X						N = 1036 (Denver)	N = 16 X	N = 186 X		X
Meeting Street School Screening Test	X	15–20 min	5 yr– 7 yr 5 mo	Learning disability		X			X					X	X	N = 500 (Providence, R.I.)	N = 2 X	N = ? X	X	X
Miller Assessment for Preschoolers	X	20–30 min	2 yr 9 mo– 5 yr 8 mo	Learning disability		X					X	X	X			N = 1200 (U.S.A.)	N = 40 X	N = 90 X	X	

Table 5-16. *Characteristics of two developmental tests requiring parent report*

Test	Screening/assessment	Time to administer	Ages	Disability	Parent report	Task observation	Gross motor	Fine motor	Self-help	Social	Academic	Communication	Programming	Standardization	interobserver Good (>.80)	Test-retest Good (>.80)	Split-half	Validity
									Areas assessed							Reliability		
Developmental Profile II (Alpern-Boll)	X	20–40 min	0–9 yr	All	X		X	X	X	X	X	X		N = 3008 (91% urban Indiana)	N = 36	N = 11		X
Vineland Adaptive Behavior Scales Survey Form	X	20–60 min	0–18 yr	All	X		X	X	X	X		X		N = 3000 (24 states)	N = 160	N = 484	X	X
Expanded Form	X	60–90 min	0–18 yr	All	X		X	X	X	X		X		N = 3000 (24 states)	N = 160	N = 484		X
Classroom Edition	X	20 min	3–12 yr	All	X (Teacher report)		X	X	X	X		X		N = 3000			X	X

Table 5-17. Characteristics of three developmental assessment tests requiring parent report and observation

Test	Assessment	Time to administer	Ages	Disability	Parent report	Task observation	Gross motor	Fine motor	Self-help	Language	Cognitive	Personal-social	Organization of behavior	Environment	Programming	Standardization	Reliability	Validity
Gesell Preschool Test	X	40 min	2½–6 yr	All	X	X	X	X	X	X		X				N = 640 (Connecticut)		
Learning Accomplishment Profile Revised	X	2–2½ hr	3–6 yr	All		X	X	X	X	X	X				X			
Diagnostic	X	1 hr	1–6 yr	All		X	X	X	X	X	X		X		X			
Vulpé Assessment Battery	X	1 hr	0–6 yr	All	X	X	X	X	X	X	X	X	X	X	X	N = 35		

Table 5-18. Characteristics of two developmental tests for visually impaired children

Test	Screening/assessment	Time to administer	Ages	Disability	Parent report	Task observation	Gross motor	Fine motor	Self-help	Communication	Socialization	Sensorimotor	Exploration of environment	Programming	Standardization	Reliability	Validity
Reynell-Zinkin Developmental Scales for Young Visually Handicapped Children	X	1 hr	0–5 yr	VI	X	X				X	X	X	X	X	On VI children, N = 109 with 203 testings		
Social Maturity Scale for Blind Preschool Children	X	Not stated	0–6 yr	VI	X		X	X	X	X	X				On VI children, N = 398 with 605 testings		

Key: VI, visually impaired.

Sensorimotor Tests

6

Georgia A. DeGangi

The domain of sensorimotor skills encompasses a wide range of skills and operates on a continuum. During the sensorimotor phase of development in the first 2 years of life, the infant learns to detect and interpret information from the senses. This learning process allows for the integration of primitive reflexes, the development of posture and balance, and the development of fine and gross motor skills. The most important sensory channels at this stage of development are the tactile, vestibular, and proprioceptive senses because of their strong neurophysiological connections with the motor system. These three basic senses interact with vision and hearing to allow for an adaptive motor response to sensory input. The infant uses information from these senses to develop motor planning abilities, bilateral motor integration, postural control, body scheme, self-image, reflex integration and balance, and eye-hand coordination. These intermediary skills emerge in the preschool years and lead to refinements in perceptual-motor development, which includes the areas of auditory-language, visual-spatial, and visual-motor skills. These end products are the basis for academic performance. Figure 6-1 presents the developmental components comprising the domain of sensorimotor behaviors.

Typically, children with sensorimotor deficits exhibit delays in fine and gross motor skills and display poor balance, incoordination, lack of hand dominance, and difficulties planning and sequencing movements over time and space. Distractibility, tactile defensiveness, gravitational insecurity, and problems with auditory-language and visual-spatial skills may also be apparent. If the child's problems remain undetected until the school years, difficulties in reading, writing, and mathematics often emerge. Children with learning disabilities that are a result of sensory integrative dysfunction may be identified in the preschool and school-age years. There is growing evidence that sensorimotor deficits are present in other populations, such as the mentally retarded [3] or autistic [4] child. However, these developmentally disabled children with more obvious deficits in cognition, emotional stability, language, and motor abilities present the diagnostician with a more serious dilemma, because the sensorimotor deficit may be masked or complicated by the more predominant handicap.

Since children with sensorimotor deficits are likely to exhibit problems in (1) the processing of vestibular, tactile, and proprioceptive inputs, (2) the development of motor skills, (3) the integration of sensory and motor behaviors, and (4) the development of perceptual-motor skills, instruments designed to test sensorimotor functions should address these various components. A major consideration in selecting an appropriate sensorimotor instrument is whether the test is sensitive to how sensorimotor functions are manifested throughout the developmental continuum. For instance, measures of tactile function in infants may include the baby's behavioral and motor response to having paper placed on his or her face; whereas, in the preschool child, observations of responses to being touched in a play situation may be most appropriate. For a school-aged child, tactile functions are considerably more discriminative, and a test for this age group may include integration of

143

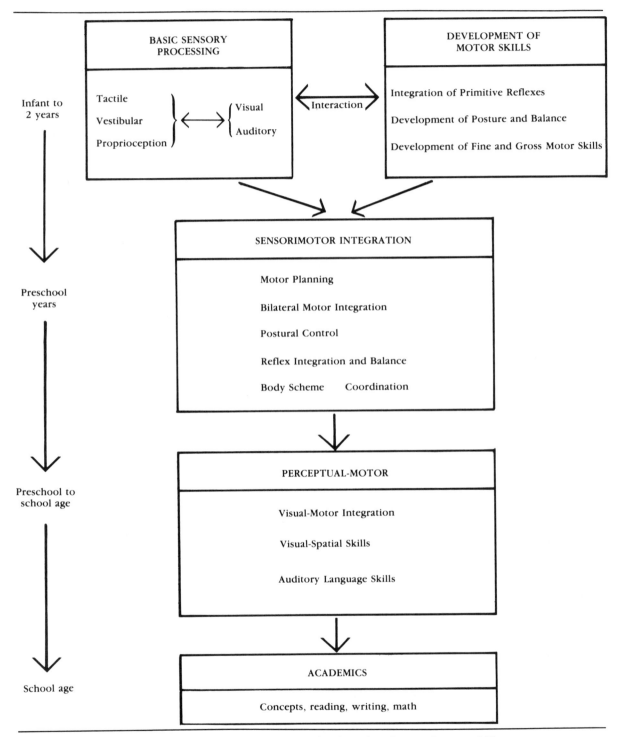

Fig. 6-1. Development of the components comprising the domain of sensorimotor skills.

touch with vision, as in a graphesthesia or stereognosis task.

In addition to considerations based on age, a test should be evaluated for its usage with different disabilities. The presence of sensorimotor deficits has been documented in children with a variety of developmental disabilities. For instance, the presence of vestibular dysfunction has been noted in autistic children [1], in children with communication disorders [6], in emotionally disturbed children [5], and in cerebral-palsied children [7]. Tactile dysfunction has been observed as well in mentally retarded children [2]. Each of these disabilities presents the test examiner with different problems in administering the test items and in evaluating the child's response to the task. Therefore, if a test is not specifically designed for and validated on samples reflecting these different disabilities, judgments regarding the child's performance on a particular sensorimotor test and interpretation of test results are based on the examiner's clinical experience and not on objective data. As a result, there may be wide variations in how responses are recorded and interpreted across different test examiners.

In addition to age and disability considerations, a test examiner should evaluate various characteristics of validity and reliability as they relate specifically to testing the domain of sensorimotor functions. A checklist is provided in Table 6-1 for evaluating the usefulness of a sensorimotor instrument. The criteria presented in this table were also used in critiquing the various instruments described in this chapter.

The instruments presented in this chapter were specifically selected based on their clinical usefulness with various age groups and populations as well as on their prevalence of usage by therapists, psychologists, and teachers. Published, standardized instruments were selected over informal checklists, since the former most often provide reliable and valid measures supporting their use as a sensorimotor instrument. It is recognized that checklists and clinical observations of behaviors associated with sensorimotor deficits have a role in diagnosis, particularly with populations for whom no instruments are available. They are not covered in this chapter, however, because the observations have not been validated on the population for which they were intended to be used and because of their tendency to be subjective in the scoring of observations. Although The Guide to Testing Clinical

Table 6-1. Checklist for evaluating the validity and reliability of sensorimotor tests

A. Validity
 1. Is the domain of sensorimotor behaviors to be measured by the test clearly defined in the test manual?
 2. Do the items on the scale measure sensory and motor integration functions?
 3. Are the items representative of sensorimotor functions for the particular age group for which the scale is designed?
 4. Is the scale appropriate for the intended uses and population? Have test data been collected on the populations for which the instrument is intended?
 5. Are cutoff scores or a range of scores recommended for identifying children with different degrees and types of sensorimotor dysfunction?
 6. How accurately can the scale identify sensorimotor dysfunction? What is the amount of error in misclassifying children?
 7. Do the results derived from the scale lend themselves to developing appropriate treatment or educational programs?
 8. Do the test items discriminate between the performance of normal children and that of children with specific sensorimotor deficits?

B. Reliability
 1. Do the reliability quotients indicate that the scale can be scored and interpreted objectively? How rigorous were the reliability studies? (i.e., did they report a measure of simple agreement or interobserver and test-retest reliability?)
 2. Are the reliability coefficients adequate for interpreting results in the intended manner (i.e., by subtest and total test scores)?
 3. Are reliability studies completed on both individuals for whom the test was intended and a normative sample?

Observations in Kindergartners by Dunn is not a standardized test, it is included in this chapter because it presents a quantifiable method of examining neurophysiological behaviors associated with sensory integrative dysfunction and because this particular set of clinical observations is often used by therapists in diagnosis.

The tests in this chapter include the following:

1. Beery-Buktenica Developmental Test of Visual-Motor Integration
2. Bruininks-Oseretsky Test of Motor Proficiency
3. DeGangi-Berk Test of Sensory Integration
4. The Marianne Frostig Developmental Test of Visual Perception
5. A Guide to Testing Clinical Observations in Kindergartners
6. The Imitation of Gestures
7. Jordan Left-Right Reversal Test
8. Motor-Free Visual Perception Test
9. Peabody Developmental Motor Scales (Revised)
10. The Purdue Perceptual-Motor Survey
11. Quick Neurological Screening Test (Revised)
12. Southern California Postrotary Nystagmus Test
13. Southern California Sensory Integration Tests
14. Test of Visual-Perceptual Skills (Non-Motor)

BEERY-BUKTENICA DEVELOPMENTAL TEST OF VISUAL-MOTOR INTEGRATION

Descriptive Information

Test Identification

The title of this test is *Beery-Buktenica Developmental Test of Visual-Motor Integration* (VMI), 1967. Its authors are Keith E. Beery, Ph.D., and Norman A. Buktenica, Ph.D. Beery is a child psychologist who has worked with the learning disabled. Buktenica is also a psychologist. The Modern Curriculum Press (13900 Prospect Rd., Cleveland, Ohio 44136) publishes the test at a cost of $12–$14 for 15 Short Form VMI tests (for

2–8 year olds), $17–$19 for 15 Long Form VMI tests (for 2–15 year olds), $10–$12 for the test manual, and $11–$13 for the VMI Monograph and Stimulus cards.

Age and Type of Client

The VMI was primarily designed for use with children in their preschool and early elementary school years, although it can be given to children from 2 to 15 years of age. It is designed to screen for children who have potential learning disabilities in the preschool and kindergarten age group. In older children, the test is designed to screen for those who have learning disabilities and neurological impairments.

Purpose

The VMI was constructed as a developmental test of visual-motor integration; it provides age norms and describes the developmental sequence for design copying of geometric forms. The VMI can also be used for research purposes to identify which components are involved in form reproduction, such as spatial orientation of the form. The test is intended as an educational assessment for use in designing appropriate educational programming for children based on their performance on the test. The manual stresses that the VMI should not be used as a diagnostic tool.

Time Required to Administer and Score Test

Although the time required to administer and score the VMI is not provided in the manual, the test can be given in approximately 10 minutes. Scoring takes an additional 5 to 10 minutes once familiar with the scoring criteria.

Evaluator

The VMI should be useful to teachers and special educators, as it is intended to be an educational assessment. The directions for administering the VMI are easy and require no special training. The monograph states that a neurologist may be able to infer a neurological disorder based on a child's performance on form reproduction tasks, but only in conjunction with other behavioral indicators.

Historical Perspective of Test Construction

Development and Source of Test Items

A group of 72 geometric forms were first prepared for preliminary testing with a sample of 600 children between the ages of 2 and 15 years. After item analysis, a developmental sequence of 30 forms was selected. For instance, the first four items include a circle (3-year level), cross (4-year level), diagonal line (4.4-year level), and a square (4.6-year level). Another sample of 600 children was used in the 30-form sequence from which 24 forms were selected for the final edition. Three samples were used for the standardization of the 24-form test format.

Review of Literature in Terms of Test Use

Several studies have been conducted on the use of the VMI with various populations, as a screening instrument of visual-motor integration, and as it compares with the Bender-Gestalt Test for Young Children [4]. The VMI was found useful in testing moderately retarded children ranging in age from 6 to 12 years [5]. In a study by Pryzwansky [9], both individual and group administration of the VMI yielded comparable scores for kindergarten children. In this study, however, reliability between first grade teachers, resource teachers, and a school psychology intern was only fair (.68–.73). The author expressed concerns regarding the clarity of scoring criteria. The ability of the VMI to predict academic achievement was investigated using three samples of kindergarten children and following their academic performance over 3 years [3]. All correlations were statistically significant. The author concluded that the VMI gives a reasonable estimate of future academic performance, although arithmetic was the area best predicted by the VMI.

When the VMI was compared with the Bender-Gestalt Test for Young Children, significant differences were found in age-equivalent scores for students in kindergarten through the third grade [6]. Although the two tests purport to measure the same construct, there was a substantial proportion of unaccounted-for variance in the correlations. The Bender-Gestalt also yielded a higher mean age score than the VMI; the difference between the two mean age scores ranged from 6.8 to 11.2 months. Similar findings were reported by Brown [1], who found a significant difference between the means obtained using the VMI and the Bender-Gestalt. Brown concluded that neither test should be used solely as a measure of visual-motor integration when making diagnostic decisions. The differences in scores obtained on the two tests may reflect differences in the test items and their scoring criteria as well as sampling procedures. In Leton's review of the VMI [7], he states that no indication is made of whether children with visual-motor handicaps were excluded from the sample. If they were excluded, the norms would be biased in a negative direction, which may account for the lower age-equivalent scores obtained on the VMI. On the other hand, Rice [10] in his review notes that the VMI has smaller increments between items than the Bender-Gestalt Test. The difference in age equivalents could also reflect an increased sensitivity to discrete age differences.

Theoretical Constructs and Implications for Intervention

A comprehensive review of the literature is presented in the monograph that accompanies the administration and scoring manual. The major premise underlying this review is that visual perception and motor functions are not necessarily predictive of visual-motor integrative functioning. Problems in visual-motor functions may be a result of either dysfunction in visual perception or an interaction of the visual and motor systems. Much of the theoretical basis of the VMI is based on Kephart's work, which emphasizes the importance of motor and perceptual integration as the basis for higher intellectual functions. Since learning disabilities are closely associated with integrational problems, the reproduction of geometric forms may be a relatively sensitive measure of neurological integrity. Difficulties in reproducing geometric forms is reported by the authors to be associated with poor neurological organization. Further research is needed to document the relationship of neurological dysfunction and visual-motor integration using standardized instruments.

The VMI was specifically developed because of the restricted age ranges in the Gesell Developmental Schedules and the Bender Visual-Motor Gestalt Test, and because these tests must be administered individually. The VMI can be administered in groups, thus making it useful for screening purposes.

Content and Test Administration

Content

The VMI test consists of 24 geometric forms. There are two booklets, one for ages 2 to 8 and the other for ages 2 to 15.

Setting and Equipment

The only equipment necessary for administering the VMI are a booklet, a table and chair, and a sharp pencil. The test can be administered individually or in groups.

Administration Procedures

The VMI is easy to administer. The directions are simple and are read to the child or group of children. The child is requested to draw a form exactly like the one presented in the test booklet. The child may not erase, and testing is discontinued after the child has failed on three consecutive forms.

Scoring

For each form in the VMI there is a page in the manual presenting scoring criteria. Age norms and requirements for passing the item are presented for each form. Age equivalents are presented for males and females ranging in age from 2 years 10 months up through 15 years. The number of passes on the test are added up to the three consecutive failures to attain a raw score, which is then converted to an age-equivalent score.

Psychometric Properties

Standardization

The VMI was initially standardized on 1039 children in 1964; however, the standardization sample was extended to 3090 children in 1981. Three groups of children were used in the 1981 standardization sample: a middle-class suburban group (70.8%), a rural group (7.3%), and a lower middle-class urban group (21.9%), all of whom were from Illinois. The children in the sample were represented across the age ranges of 3 to 14 years, with fairly equal distributions of males and females. Table 1 in the monograph presents the breakdowns by age, sex, and race. All children in the three groups were considered normal intellectually.

Reliability

Interrater reliability was obtained through analysis of variance of the means for 120 subjects. The age ranges for the subjects are not reported. The coefficient was .98 between psychologists and resource teachers, .95 between resource teachers and classroom teachers, and .93 between psychologists and classroom teachers. Test-retest reliability ranged from .63 for a 7-month period between testings [3] to .92 for a 2-week period between testings. Split-half reliability coefficients ranged from .66 to .93, with a median of .79. In the test manual published in 1967, a study of test-retest reliability was completed on mentally retarded children using an interval of 4 to 8 weeks (mean age of 12 years and mean intelligence quotient [IQ] of 51). For this sample, the reliability coefficient was .90. Other studies of test-retest reliability have been conducted with considerably lower coefficients on second, fourth, and sixth graders, ranging from .45 to .75 [11]. Although Beery and Buktenica obtained overall good reliability coefficients in both their 1964 and 1981 studies of reliability, these additional studies lend only fair support to the objectivity of the scoring and stability of test results. In Chissom's review of the VMI [2], he criticizes the unsystematic way in which reliability evidence is presented. The coefficients were obtained on the entire age range, which is considered to be inflated. Although his review pertains to the 1964 standardization, the same problems also pertain to the 1981 reliability studies.

Validity

In the 1967 manual, a number of validity studies are reported. A correlation of .89 was obtained between chronological age and number of items correct for the total suburban group. Correlations between the VMI and The Marianne Frostig Developmental Test of Visual Perception were .80 (Pearson r). The correlation was .55 between the VMI and the Illinois Test of Psycholinguistic Abilities (ITPA); however, it was .80 for the visual-motor sequential subtest on the ITPA. Rice [10] criticizes these studies as being circular in that the constructs being measured by both instruments have yet to be validated and cannot be operationally defined using one another.

In the 1982 manual, other studies of validity are presented. Correlations between the VMI and readiness tests averaged to .50. The correlation between the VMI and the Bender-Gestalt Test ranged from .41 to .82, which indicates fair to moderate overlap in the domain of behaviors measured. The authors report that factor analytic studies support the link between visual-motor integration and handwriting ability. The correlation coefficient between handwriting and the VMI was .42, which denotes a moderate relationship. Correlations between the VMI and mental age on the Primary Mental Abilities Test were .59 for first grade, .37 for fourth grade, and .38 for seventh grade. The authors also report evidence of predictive validity for kindergarten boys identified as "at risk" who later developed reading difficulties. The predictive validity was found to decline as children advanced in grade levels. The authors speculated that children may learn to compensate through verbal language skills for any visual-motor weakness, thus lowering the predictive validity. A study by Painter [8] demonstrated improved performance on the VMI following special education programs that included sensory-motor training. Painter found statistically significant gains on the VMI in the group of 10 kindergarten children who received tutoring over 7 weeks.

Several authors who have reviewed the VMI have criticized its validity on several counts. Chissom [2] states that no extensive predictive validity studies have been conducted using objective criteria. The study reported in the 1982 manual examines the relationship of the VMI to later reading difficulty; however, no studies have been conducted to predict handwriting problems. Leton [7] criticizes the fact that studies were not conducted on children with graphomotor problems and those with learning disabilities. These studies are necessary for diagnostic validity. Leton also questions whether the domain validity is accurately assessing visual-motor behaviors. He views the items as limited in scope and the scoring criteria as deficient in considering such problems as tremor, perseveration, and distortion. None of these problems were remedied in the 1981 standardization.

Guidelines for Use in a Clinical Setting

The VMI is useful in screening children individually or in groups in the area of visual-motor integration. Since results on the VMI may differ (from 6–11 months) from that of the Bender-Gestalt Test, results on the VMI should be considered somewhat deflated and may not accurately diagnose a visual-motor integration problem. Additional testing should also be done to determine if the problem lies in the visual, motor, or visual-motor integration areas. Other tests that can be used in conjunction with the VMI are the Motor-Free Visual Perception Test, the Southern California Sensory Integration Tests (Design Copying and Motor Accuracy-Revised Subtests), and the Test of Visual-Perceptual Skills (Non-Motor).

Review

The VMI is a test of visual-motor integration designed for use with children ranging in age from 2 to 15 years of age. It is particularly useful in screening preschool and elementary school-age children with learning disabilities involving visual-motor integration and can be administered individually or in groups. The test is well standardized but has a limited geographic distribution and is easy to administer, although scoring criteria tend to be somewhat subjective. There is evidence that scores on the VMI correlate with academic performance in the first grade and are also predictive of reading difficulties in kindergarten boys. Consequently, the VMI would be a good test for use in screening kindergartners. Since the Bender-Gestalt Test and the VMI may yield different age-equivalent scores (even though they purport to measure similar domains), decisions regarding children who fall below their chronological age should be reserved until further diagnostic testing has been completed. Likewise, children exhibiting delays on the VMI (e.g., falling 6 months or more below their chronological age) will require more extensive diagnostic testing to determine the nature of their problem, particularly in delineating visual and motor components of visual-motor integration skills. More refined scoring criteria should be developed on the VMI, as well as additional reliability and validity studies, since the instrument has proved useful to educators and since these are areas of weakness that have been identified from previous studies.

REFERENCES

1. Brown, M. J. Comparison of the Developmental Test of Visual-Motor Integration and the Bender-Gestalt Test. *Percept. Mot. Skills* 45 : 981, 1977.
2. Chissom, B. S. Review of the VMI. In O. K. Buros (ed.), *The Seventh Mental Measurements Yearbook (Vol. 2)*. Highland Park, N.J.: Gryphon Press, 1972. P. 867.
3. Klein, A. The validity of the Beery Test of Visual-Motor Integration in predicting achievement in kindergarten, first, and second grades. *Ed. Psychol. Meas.* 38 : 457, 1978.
4. Koppitz, E. M. *The Bender-Gestalt Test for Young Children (Vol. 2)*. New York: Grune & Stratton, 1975.
5. Krauft, V. C., and Krauft, C. C. Structured vs. unstructured visual-motor tests for educable retarded children. *Percept. Mot. Skills* 34 : 691, 1972.
6. Lehman, J., and Breen, M. J. A comparative analysis of the Bender-Gestalt and Beery/Buktenica Tests of Visual-Motor Integration as a function of grade level for regular education students. *Psychol. Sch.* 19 : 52, 1982.
7. Leton, D. A. Review of VMI. In O. K. Buros (ed.), *The Eighth Mental Measurements Yearbook (Vol. 2)*. Highland Park, N.J.: Gryphon Press, 1978. P. 870.
8. Painter, G. The effect of a rhythmic and sensory-motor activity program on perceptual-motor-spatial abilities of kindergarten children. *Excep. Child.* 33 : 113, 1966.
9. Pryzwansky, W. B. The use of the Developmental Test of Visual-Motor Integration as a group screen instrument. *Psychol. Sch.* 14 : 419, 1977.
10. Rice, J. A. Review of the VMI. In O. K. Buros (ed.), *The Eighth Mental Measurements Yearbook (Vol. 2)*. Highland Park, N.J.: Gryphon Press, 1978. P. 870.
11. Ryckman, D. B., and Rentfrow, R. K. The Beery Developmental Test of Visual-Motor Integration: An investigation of reliability. *J. Learn. Disabil.* 4 : 333, 1971.

BRUININKS-OSERETSKY TEST OF MOTOR PROFICIENCY

Descriptive Information

Test Identification

The title of this test is *Bruininks-Oseretsky Test of Motor Proficiency* (BOTMP), 1978. Its author is Robert H. Bruininks, Ph.D. Bruininks is a professor of psychoeducational studies at the University of Minnesota. American Guidance Service (Circle Pines, Minnesota 55014) publishes the test at $178–$185.50. The test kit includes 25 booklets, 25 individual record forms, test equipment, and manual.

Age and Type of Client

The BOTMP was developed for children ranging in age from 4½ to 14½ years of age. It was specifically designed for assessing motor skills in children with serious motor dysfunctions and developmental disabilities.

Purpose

The test was developed for use by educators, clinicians, and researchers (1) in assessing gross and fine motor skills in children as well as neurological development, (2) in making decisions about educational placement or the need for corrective motor training, (3) in developing and evaluating motor training programs (the efficacy of specific treatments or motor curricula and determining which students benefit most from developmental and therapeutic motor input), and (4) as a screening tool.

Time Required to Administer and Score Test

Administration of the entire battery takes approximately 45 to 60 minutes. The Short Form, which is used for screening, requires 15 to 20 minutes to administer and score.

Evaluator

Examiners do not need special training to administer the BOTMP; however, they need to be practiced in giving the directions and administering the particular test items.

Historical Perspective of Test Construction

Development and Source of Test Items

The BOTMP is based in part on the United States adaptation of The Oseretsky Tests of Motor Proficiency [5]. The revised test was initially developed by Dr. Bruininks in 1972, and it reflects changes in content and statistical data.

Review of Literature in Terms of Test Use

The Oseretsky, the original test from which the BOTMP was developed, has been adapted and used with various populations, including mentally retarded children and adults [6] and those with neuromotor dysfunction [8]. The original instrument was used primarily in clinical research because of its length and the difficulty in interpreting results. The revised version of the test has remedied these problems.

Theoretical Constructs and Implications for Intervention

In the revised version of the BOTMP, the author included items that would reflect recent research in the following areas: (1) Maintenance of body posture is necessary for skilled motor acts; (2) Integration of visual-perceptual skills with refined motor responses is critical for reading and writing skills; and (3) Precision and speed of fine movements of the hands is required for vocational activities as well as sports and play. The research of Cratty [4], Kephart [7], and others is cited as a basis for the theoretical constructs of the BOTMP.

Content and Test Administration

Content

The test includes items in the following domains: (1) gross motor ability, (2) gross and fine motor abilities, and (3) fine motor abilities.

GROSS MOTOR ABILITY. Within this area are items measuring running speed and agility (one item), static standing balance (three items), dynamic balance while engaged in various walking movements (five items), bilateral coordination of the arms and legs (eight items), and strength of arms, legs, and abdominals (three items).

GROSS AND FINE MOTOR ABILITIES. Upper-limb coordination items are included under this category. Six items assess visual tracking with arms and hand movements, and three items assess precise movements of the hands.

FINE MOTOR ABILITY. Items in this area include response speed (one item), which is the speed with which the hand stops a moving visual stimulus; visual-motor control in paper and pencil tasks (eight items); and upper-limb speed and dexterity (eight items) (Fig. 6-2).

There are a total of 46 items on the complete battery comprised of eight subtests. The subtests include: Running Speed and Agility, Balance, Bilateral Coordination, Strength, Upper-Limb Coordination, Response Speed, Visual-Motor Control, and Upper-Limb Speed and Dexterity. The Short Form contains 14 items from the entire battery and provides a quick screening of motor proficiency. Table 6-2 presents a list of test items.

Setting and Equipment

The test kit includes an examiner's manual, record forms for the complete battery and short form, the student booklet for the visual-motor items, a balance beam, ball with string, wooden beads, block, two small boxes, masking tape, pegboard and wooden pegs, black and red pencils, pennies, response speed stick, scissors, shape cards, shoelace, standing mat, target, tape measure, tennis ball, and testing pad for the table. The examiner must provide two chairs, a table, stopwatch, mat, and clipboard. Special arrangements for placement of the tape on the wall and floor for the response speed, running speed and agility, and balance items, and for placing

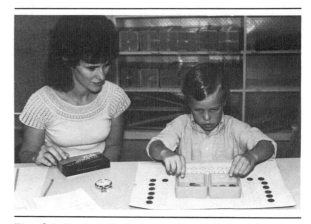

Fig. 6-2. Bruininks-Oseretsky Test of Motor Proficiency. Item from the Upper-Limb Speed and Dexterity Subtest.

Table 6-2. List of test items on the Bruininks-Oseretsky Test of Motor Proficiency

Pretest items: Arm and leg preference are determined prior to testing
  Item 1: Arm preference (throwing tennis ball)
  Item 2: Leg preference (kicking tennis ball)
Subtest 1: Running Speed and Agility
  Item 1: Running speed and agility*
Subtest 2: Balance
  Item 1: Standing on preferred leg on floor
  Item 2: Standing on preferred leg on balance beam*
  Item 3: Standing on preferred leg on balance beam (eyes closed)
  Item 4: Walking forward on walking line
  Item 5: Walking forward on balance beam
  Item 6: Walking forward heel-to-toe on walking line*
  Item 7: Walking forward heel-to-toe on balance beam
  Item 8: Stepping over response speed stick on balance beam
Subtest 3: Bilateral Coordination
  Item 1: Tapping feet alternately while making circles with fingers*
  Item 2: Tapping (foot and finger on same side synchronized)
  Item 3: Tapping (foot and finger on opposite side synchronized)
  Item 4: Jumping in place (leg and arm on same side synchronized)
  Item 5: Jumping in place (leg and arm on opposite side synchronized)
  Item 6: Jumping up and clapping hands*

Table 6-2 (continued)

Item 7: Jumping up and touching heels with hands

Item 8: Drawing lines and crosses simultaneously

Subtest 4: Strength

Item 1: Standing broad jump*

Item 2: Sit-ups

Item 3: Knee push-ups or full push-ups

Subtest 5: Upper-Limb Coordination

Item 1: Bouncing a ball and catching it with both hands·

Item 2: Bouncing a ball and catching it with preferred hand

Item 3: Catching a tossed ball with both hands*

Item 4: Catching a tossed ball with preferred hand

Item 5: Throwing a ball at a target with preferred hand*

Item 6: Touching a swinging ball with preferred hand

Item 7: Touching nose with index fingers (eyes closed)

Item 8: Touching thumb to fingertips (eyes closed)

Item 9: Pivoting thumb and index finger

Subtest 6: Response Speed (one item)*

Subtest 7: Visual-Motor Control

Item 1: Cutting out a circle with preferred hand

Items 2, 3,* 4: Drawing a line through a path with preferred hand

Items 5,* 6, 7, and 8*: Copying a geometric form with preferred hand

Subtest 8: Upper-Limb Speed and Dexterity

Item 1: Placing pennies in a box with preferred hand

Item 2: Placing pennies in two boxes with both hands

Item 3: Sorting shape cards with preferred hand*

Item 4: Stringing beads with preferred hand

Item 5: Displacing pegs with preferred hand

Item 6: Drawing vertical lines with preferred hand

Item 7: Making dots in circles with preferred hand*

Item 8: Making dots with preferred hand

*Items administered on short form.

the target on the wall are described at the beginning of each subtest. These preparations should be made before the testing begins. Children should wear tennis shoes or crepe-soled shoes. The test should be conducted in a distraction-free area. A gymnasium or large room with a space large enough for an 18-yard running course is needed.

Administration Procedures

Each item is administered directly to the child using standardized procedures. The manual is well organized for clinical use. Directions are clear, and verbal directions are printed in bold-face. Scoring for each item is easy to follow and is completed either when the item is administered or when the booklet is scored. In the manual, each item presents a description of what the item is measuring, kit equipment and other equipment needed, general directions for the total subtest, number of trials given, and administering and recording. Although the directions are clear, the examiner must be familiar with how to administer items as some of them require coordinated movement on the part of the examiner.

Scoring

Scores on each test item are expressed as the amount of time taken to complete the task, the number of times performed within a set time interval, the number of errors made, or as a pass/fail by prescribed criteria. A conversion scale is available on the individual record form so that each child's raw score can be converted to the point scores. The child's best performance is selected for items with more than one trial. Appendix A is used to interpret forms drawn on Subtest 7, items 5 through 8.

Part 5 of the test manual is devoted exclusively to scoring procedures. Raw scores are converted to a point scale for each item, which ranges anywhere from 0 to 1 point or from 0 to 15 points. The total point score for each subtest is computed as well as a gross motor composite, fine motor composite, and total battery composite. Subtest scores can be converted into standard scores, percentile ranks, or age equivalents. A set of 20 tables present the standard scores for each 6-month interval for 4½ year olds up through 14½ year olds. Composite standard scores and median age-equivalent scores corresponding to the gross motor, fine motor, and battery composites can be obtained as well. Directions are also provided for the short form, with a corresponding table to interpret scores. Separate norms for boys and girls are provided for the complete battery.

After scoring the test battery, the test user is referred to Part 6 of the manual entitled Interpretation. Since the various derived scores include standard scores, percentile ranks, stanines, and age equivalents, an explanation is given for each on how to interpret these findings. The standard error of measurement is also provided both for gross motor, fine motor, and battery composites and for the short form.

Psychometric Properties

Standardization

A multistage, stratified sampling procedure was used based on the 1970 U.S. census. There was a total of 765 subjects in the final standardization sample, which was relatively equal for males and females. The objective was to have 80 children for each age range of 1 year, although there were more in all age ranges except the 4½ to 5½, 12½ to 13½, and 13½ to 14½ year age groups. The sampling also included a distribution of 84.8 percent white children, 13.7 percent black, and 1.5 percent other races. The community size is also specified to represent children from the central city, suburban area, and rural areas. Children were also tested in the north central, southern, and western regions of the United States as well as in Canada. No children from the northeastern region were included in the sample.

Means and standard deviations were obtained for each age group tested. These point scores were converted to standard scores for each subtest as well as for the three composite scores. Supplementary norms for boys and girls are also given as well as age equivalents for each of the eight subtests.

Reliability

Test-retest reliability was conducted on a sample of 63 second graders and 63 sixth graders within a 7- to 12-day period. Of the subjects, five were mildly retarded or learning disabled. The test-retest reliability coefficients were .77 for gross motor composite and .88 for the fine motor composite for grade 2 and .85 and .68, respectively, for grade 6. The reliability coefficients for the total battery and short form were above .80 for both grades. Test-retest coefficients for the individual subtests ranged from .58 to .89 for grade 2 and from .29 to .89 for grade 6. The lower reliability coefficients for the older subjects may be due to the fact that they achieved maximum or near-maximum point scores. The following subtests achieved a reliability coefficient of .80 or above for grade 2: Bilateral Coordination, Upper-Limb Coordination, Visual-Motor Control, and Upper-Limb Speed and Dexterity. Subtests achieving a reliability coefficient of .80 or above for grade 6 included the following: Running Speed and Agility, Bilateral Coordination, Strength, and Upper-Limb Speed and Dexterity. The individual subtest scores not listed should be interpreted with caution. The standard error of measurement for each subtest and composite by grade is reported as well. Interrater reliability was conducted for the eight items in Subtest 7 (Visual-Motor Control). Five raters independently scored 74 subjects' protocols in one study. In a second study, three raters scored 30 subjects' protocols. Reliability coefficients ranged from .79 to .97 for the first study and from .77 to .97 for the second study for the individual items. The median correlations for the total subtest reached .98 and .90 for the two studies.

Validity

In the validity section of the manual, construct validity of the BOTMP was considered in terms of the relationship of the test content to theories of motor development in research studies, the statistical properties of the test, and comparisons of the performance of groups of handicapped and normal children on the test. In examining the relationship of the test scores to chronological age, correlations ranged from .57 to .86 with a median of .78, which indicates a close relationship between subtest scores and chronological age.

Correlations of item point scores with their subtest and the total test scores were computed to determine whether the subtests measured different functions and whether the subtests are linked together in the same domain of behaviors. Median correlations for the subtests ranged from .65 to .87 for the subtests and from .56 to .86 for the total test. These moderate to high correlations for the subtests indicate that they are somewhat related in their functions. Likewise, the correlations for the total test are quite substantial and indicate that the subtests contribute to overall fine and gross motor development measured by the total test. Factor analysis of the subtest items was completed on the 46 test items to clarify the structure of the test. This analysis gave some support to the grouping of items on the subtests.

Additional construct validity studies were completed to contrast the performance of handicapped subjects with normal age-equivalent subjects. The handicapped subjects included those who were mildly retarded ($n = 72$ in each group with a total n of 144), moderately to severely retarded ($n = 19$ in each group), and learning disabled ($n = 55$ in each group). T test analyses of the three different subgroups revealed that the BOTMP differentiates between normal and handicapped children. These studies also confirm the usefulness of the test with retarded and learning-disabled children.

A study correlating scores on the BOTMP and the Southern California Sensory Integration Tests [1] was conducted [9]. Significant correlations were obtained between the BOTMP composite battery scores and those tests on the

SCSIT with a motor component (Space Visualization, Design Copying, Manual Form Perception, Imitation of Postures, Bilateral Motor Coordination, Standing Balance with Eyes Open and Eyes Closed, and Motor Accuracy). In addition, the fine motor composite on the BOTMP was found to have a significant correlation with 14 of the 18 SCSIT tests. The authors concluded that the BOTMP long form would be useful in screening children who display sensory integrative dysfunction and as a clinical research tool to evaluate the effectiveness of sensory integrative therapy as it affects motor performance [9].

The use of the BOTMP with preschoolers was investigated by Beitel and Mead [2]. The BOTMP was administered to twenty-four 3- to 5-year-old normal children. The short form and the eight different subtests significantly related to age, but no significant sex differences were found. The short form accounted for a large proportion of variance of the complete battery; therefore, it can be used to substitute for the complete test when appropriate. Their study supports the use of the BOTMP with preschoolers; however, further standardization data are needed on 3 and 4 year olds before the test is used for this purpose.

Guidelines for Use in a Clinical Setting

The BOTMP is useful in testing retarded, learning-disabled, and normal children. It can be used as a screening instrument by using the short form or as a clinical diagnostic tool by using the long form. Inspection of individual subtest scores may assist the teacher or therapist in developing appropriate activities to remediate motor delays. Because test-retest reliability was low for many of the individual subtests, results should not be interpreted based on subtest scores alone. The fine motor composite is more reliable for children in grade 2 than grade 6, and the gross motor composite is more reliable for children in grade 6 than grade 2. Since the short form accounts for a large proportion of the variance of the complete battery, it can be administered in place of the complete test when appropriate. The BOTMP may also be useful in measuring progress as a result of educational or therapeutic intervention for motor delays.

A child with learning disabilities or perceptual problems who exhibits delays in fine and/or gross motor skills on the BOTMP may also have sensory integrative problems and should receive further testing. If the BOTMP is being administered as a screening instrument, it may be helpful to administer the Quick Neurological Screening Test as well in order to differentiate those children who may require more in-depth testing.

Review

The BOTMP is a test of fine and gross motor skill development in children ranging in age from 4½ to 14½ years of age who exhibit motor impairments. It can be used with children with mental retardation, learning disabilities, and developmental delays as a screening or diagnostic tool. The BOTMP is useful in determining which children may require developmental or therapeutic motor intervention. The content of test items reflects research regarding components of posture, visual-perceptual skills, and other factors that contribute to fine and gross motor development.

The BOTMP is easy to administer and score and requires no special training, although the examiner must be practiced in the administration of items since coordination is involved on the part of the examiner. The BOTMP is well standardized, and reliability studies indicate fair to good test-retest and interrater reliability for second and sixth graders. Test-retest reliability was better on the fine motor composite for the younger ages and better on the gross motor composite for the older ages. Better reliability was obtained for the total test battery and short form (> .80) than for the individual subtests; therefore, decisions based on the subtests alone are not recommended. Construct and decision validity studies described previously were also conducted with good results.

REFERENCES

1. Ayres, A. J. *Southern California Sensory Integration Tests.* Los Angeles: Western Psychological Services, 1980.
2. Beitel, P. A., and Mead, B. J. Bruininks-Oseretsky Test of Motor Proficiency: A viable measure of 3- to 5-year-old children. *Percept. Mot. Skills* 51 : 919, 1980.
3. Bruininks, R. H. *Bruininks-Oseretsky Test of Motor Proficiency.* Circle Pines, Minn.: American Guidance Service, 1978.
4. Cratty, B. J. *Perceptual and Motor Development in Infants and Young Children.* New York: Macmillan, 1970.
5. Doll, E. A. (ed.). *The Oseretsky Test of Motor Proficiency.* (Translated from the Portuguese Adaptation.) Circle Pines, Minn.: American Guidance Service, 1946a.
6. Doll, E. A. The Oseretsky Test. *Ill. Training Sch. Bull.* 43 : 1, 1946b.
7. Kephart, N. C. *The Slow Learner in the Classroom.* Columbus, Oh.: Merrill, 1971.
8. Stott, D. H. A general test of motor impairment for children. *Dev. Med. Child. Neurol.* 8 : 525, 1966.
9. Ziviani, J., Poulsen, A., and O'Brien, A. Correlation of the Bruininks-Oseretsky Test of Motor Proficiency with the Southern California Sensory Integration Tests. *Am. J. Occup. Ther.* 36 : 519, 1982.

DEGANGI-BERK TEST OF SENSORY INTEGRATION

Descriptive Information

Test Identification

The title of this test is *DeGangi-Berk Test of Sensory Integration* (TSI), 1983. Its authors are Ronald A. Berk, Ph.D., and Georgia DeGangi, M.S., OTR. Berk is an associate professor at Johns Hopkins University in the Division of Education. His specialty is educational measurement. DeGangi is an occupational therapist in private practice and a clinical instructor at Georgetown University, Department of Pediatrics. Western Psychological Services (12031 Wilshire Blvd., Los Angeles, California 90025) publishes the test at a cost of $43–$45 for the test kit and $13–$15 for the manual.

Age and Type of Client

The TSI is constructed as a criterion-referenced test to be administered to children 3 to 5 years of age with delays in sensory, motor, and perceptual skills or to children suspected of having learning problems.

Purpose

The TSI is designed to measure overall sensory integrative dysfunction in preschoolers. It focuses primarily on the vestibular-based functions and includes subtests measuring postural control, bilateral motor integration, and reflex integration. The TSI can be used for diagnosis of sensory motor dysfunction. When used for this purpose, the results of the TSI should be incorporated with other relevant test results to diagnose the problem areas of sensory motor functioning in the preschool child and to devise an appropriate plan of therapy. The TSI can also be used as a screening instrument to determine the child's overall level of functioning. Potential problems that emerge should then be examined using more in-depth assessment techniques.

Time Required to Administer and Score Test

The test is administered individually in about 30 minutes. It takes an additional 5 to 10 minutes to complete scoring and interpret findings using the criteria in the manual.

Evaluator

Although the TSI was devised as a diagnostic tool to be administered by occupational and physical therapists with background and training in the theory of sensory integration and its application to sensory integrative dysfunction, other specialists including special educators, motor development specialists, and occupational and physical therapy assistants trained in the administration of pediatric motor tests can administer the test for screening purposes. In the test's use

as a diagnostic tool, an occupational or physical therapist should interpret the test scores, especially in children with suspected or definite findings that may require intervention. Approximately 2 hours of training using the administration procedures is needed to become familiar with the scoring and administration of the test items.

Historical Perspective of Test Construction

Development and Source of Items

The original set of test items was developed in 1978 [5]. Several psychometric studies were conducted from these test items [3, 6]. After these preliminary studies, the test was revised and a third series of reliability and validity studies were undertaken [7, 8].

Review of Literature in Terms of Test Use

Since the TSI is a new instrument, only studies conducted by the authors are available and are reported in the test manual. A study has been completed, however, on the original version of the test by Harris and colleagues [10]. In this study, the relationship of the Assessment of Sensorimotor Integration in Preschool Children [5], the Peabody Developmental Motor Scales (PDMS) [9], and the Tactile Sensitivity Checklist [2] were investigated on a sample of 61 preschool children (12 normal and 49 with mild developmental delays). A significant correlation was found between the scores on the Assessment of Sensorimotor Integration in Preschool Children and the PDMS, but not between the Assessment of Sensorimotor Integration and the Tactile Sensitivity Checklist. Since the instrument developed by DeGangi and Berk focused on the vestibular-based functions, it is not surprising that there was a high correlation between those functions and fine and gross motor skills but not tactile sensitivity. It is possible that the Assessment of Sensorimotor Integration would correlate with tactile behaviors if an instrument

Table 6-3. Behaviors assessed by the DeGangi-Berk Test of Sensory Integration (TSI) items in three subdomains of sensory integration

Items	Task	Behaviors assessed
Postural Control		
1–2	Monkey task	Ability to assume and maintain an antigravity posture of flexion
3–4	Side-sit cocontraction	Cocontraction of upper extremities and trunk
8	Prone on elbows	Neck cocontraction in the prone position
9–10	Wheelbarrow walk	Stability of the neck, trunk, and upper extremity extensors
11–14	Airplane	Ability to assume and maintain an antigravity posture of extension
18	Scooter board cocontraction	Cocontraction of the upper extremities
Bilateral Motor Integration		
5–7	Rolling pin activity	Bilateral motor coordination, trunk rotation, crossing the midline
15–17	Jump and turn	Bilateral motor coordination of the lower extremities, trunk rotation
25–27	Diadokokinesis	Complete forearm rotation
30	Drumming	Bilateral motor coordination
31–36	Upper extremity control	Motor speed, disassociation of the trunk and arm, crossing the midline
Reflex Integration		
19–22	Asymmetrical tonic neck reflex (ATNR)	Integration of the ATNR in the quadruped position
23–24	Symmetrical tonic neck reflex (STNR)	Integration of the STNR in the quadruped position
28–29	Diadokokinesis	Isolation of forearm rotation, associated reactions

that accounted for tactile functions other than tactile sensitivity were used. Strengths and limitations of the original version of the instrument are presented in the article as well. Strengths included the brevity of administration, its usefulness in screening children, the availability of test materials, and the appeal of the test items for this age group. The limitations described included the failure to discriminate among age levels, failure to include items to test equilibrium reactions, and lack of discrimination in the scoring for failure to perform item because of refusal or inability to perform the item. The first and third limitation have been addressed in the revised version of the instrument.

Theoretical Constructs and Implications for Intervention

The TSI is based on the theory of sensory integrative dysfunction described by A. Jean Ayres [1]. Since preschool children with poor sensory integration typically exhibit delays in fine and gross motor skills as well as visual-spatial perception, poor balance, incoordination, poor motor planning abilities, and lack of an established dominance, the domain of vestibular-based functions was selected from the general domain of sensory integration because of its impact on the development of these skills. The three areas of postural control, bilateral motor integration, and reflex integration were specifically selected because of their clinical significance in the development of sensory integrative functions in the preschool child.

Content and Test Administration

Content

The TSI contains three subtests—postural Control (12 items), Bilateral Motor Integration (20 items), and Reflex Integration (four items)—with a total of 36 test items. The test items and the behaviors they assess are presented in Table 6-3.

Setting and Equipment

A space of at least 10 feet by 15 feet is required to administer the test since several items (e.g., wheelbarrow walk) are completed over a distance. The test equipment should also be set up prior to testing.

The test kit includes a 12-inch circle, 2-foot circle marked in eighths and lettered, colored foam ball, printed clown picture, and printed star design, most of which are needed for several of the test items. Additional test materials (not included in the test kit) are a table and chair suitable for a preschool child, masking tape, pencil, stopwatch, wood dowel, rolling pin, scooter board, hula hoop, and a floor mat. Specifications for the equipment are presented in the chapter on administration and scoring.

Administration Procedures

A set of 36 test items is administered individually to the child. The test items should be administered exactly as described, and the verbal directions given as they are specified for each item. Each item is presented with exact procedures on how to administer the test. Verbal directions appear in boldface in the manual. Directions are clear and simple to administer.

Although the procedures are described in detail, the examiner needs to practice the items, especially those requiring timing while simultaneously lifting the child (e.g., monkey task) (Fig. 6-3). The examiner must also be able to administer varying degrees of resistance on several items and be able to consistently apply a certain amount of force for test items examining cocontraction (i.e., 1 to 1½ pounds of resistance for "slight resistance"). In addition, the test items are sequenced so that the child can move easily from one position to the next. The test manual and scoring sheet are designed to facilitate ease of administration.

Scoring

Most of the test items can be scored easily and objectively. For instance, the item may involve recording the number of seconds that the child performed the task. Thirteen actual tasks are administered; however, 36 items are scored. Each task has anywhere from one to six different items that are scored by observing different components of the task. For instance, on the rolling pin activity, which involves holding the rolling pin and batting a suspended ball held at various positions to the right and left of the child, three items are scored: the ability to maintain grasp on the rolling pin over the various trials and the ability to cross the midline to the right and left sides. Scoring for each item is delineated in considerable detail. Each item is weighted, with point values ranging from 0–1 to 0–4 points. Guidelines are also provided for children who refuse to cooperate or to attempt an item. This problem should not be encountered frequently since the tasks are designed to be fun for the child.

Scores are recorded on the protocol booklet while administering the test. They are added for the three different subtests and for the total test and are then interpreted based on a profile that delineates performance by age range and by level of function. Cutoff scores were used to differentiate the performance of normal and delayed

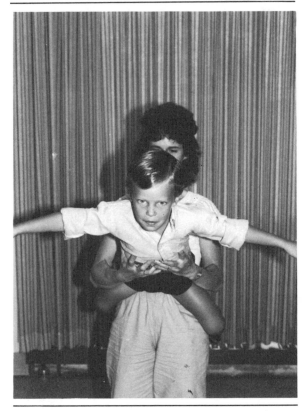

Fig. 6-3. DeGangi-Berk Test of Sensory Integration. Item from the Postural Control Subtest.

children. A child's score is interpreted as normal, at risk, or deficient in postural control, bilateral motor integration, and overall sensory integration function. Since interobserver reliability coefficients were inadequate for the Reflex Integration Subtest, scores for this subtest are not used for decision making, although the results are included in the total test scores. The inclusion of results from the Reflex Integration Subtest into the total test score did not affect the interobserver reliability coefficient for the total test; therefore, results from this subtest can be used only as part of the total test score when making decisions regarding the child's overall sensory integrative functioning.

An entire chapter in the test manual describes how scores should be interpreted for diagnosis and screening. A sample case history includes recommendations for therapy based on test results. An example of how to score the protocol booklet is also provided.

Psychometric Properties

Standardization

The TSI is not a standardized instrument. Rather, it is validated on a sample of 3- to 5-year-old children using the criterion-group's validation model. Because the test is intended for use with children who are suspected of having developmental delays, a sample of children who were found to have a delay of at least 1 year in fine and/or gross motor skills were compared with a sample of normal preschoolers. Selection criteria for the delayed sample are presented in detail in the manual. The samples included 101 normal children from the Washington, D.C., metropolitan area preschools, 30 delayed children enrolled in schools from the same area, and 8 additional delayed children from a child development center in Bristol, Indiana. All three age levels (i.e., 3 through 5 years) and three ethnic groups (i.e., black, Hispanic, and white) were represented in the sample. There was a total of 62 boys and 77 girls in the study. The predominance of 3 and 4 year olds in the sample was expected to lower performance estimates in certain skill areas.

Reliability

Interobserver reliability was completed on 33 children (26 normal and 7 delayed). Three observers, two of whom were occupational therapists and one who was a certified occupational therapy assistant, were the examiners. Two pairs of observers were used. Each child was rated by two examiners within 1 week of the other. Generalizability (interobserver) coefficients were derived from the variance components. The use of generalizability coefficients allows for analysis of observer bias by partitioning out all possible variance components. For both pairs of observers, the coefficients for the dependability of a single observer (i.e., estimates of the average agreement between one observer and another) were .67 and .79 for Postural Control, .76 and .74 for Bilateral Motor Integration, .49 and .14 for Reflex Integration, and .73 and .79 for the total test. The estimates for the case of both observers (i.e., estimates of the average agreement between the sample of observers used in this study and a theoretical set of other samples drawn from the same universe) were .80 to .88 for the three subtests and the total test, except for Reflex Integration which was .66. The coefficients for both observers are generally used when determining if an instrument has acceptable levels of reliability. Since Reflex Integration showed inadequate interobserver reliability, diagnosis based on this subtest alone is discouraged. Although less precise than the generalizability coefficients, *Pearson coefficients* (or interclass correlations) were also reported, with values ranging from .67 to .82 for the total test and Postural Control and Bilateral Motor Integration Subtests.

Decision-consistency reliability was calculated to identify the proportion of children who would be consistently classified as normal and delayed on repeated testings. It furnishes evidence as to the degree of confidence that can be placed in the initial decisions. A sample of 29 children (23 normal and 6 delayed) were tested twice using a 1-week retest interval. The same three observers were used as in the interobserver reliability study. The P_0 estimates for the three subtests and the total test ranged from 79 to 93 percent, with the lowest index for Reflex Integration. The standard errors, however, were found to be quite large, which appears to be due to the small sample size. As a consequence, less weight should be attached to the specific value for the P_0 index, and interpretation should focus instead on a range of values. The accuracy of making a correct decision that the child will be delayed or normal will tend to range from 83 to 100 percent (for the 95 percent confidence interval).

Test-retest reliability was also completed to examine the stability of individual scores. The same subjects and examiners were used in this study as in the decision-consistency reliability study. The stability coefficients for each subtest and the total tests over a period of 1 week ranged from .85 to .96 for the three subtests and the total test.

Validity

To examine domain validity, eight occupational therapists were asked to evaluate whether each item on the test measured the intended specific behavior. Overall, the judges rated the items as having a high degree of congruence with the domain being tested. Twelve judges, including ten occupational therapists, one certified occupational therapy assistant, and one motor development specialist, were asked if the collection of items was representative of their respective subdomain (postural control, bilateral motor integration, and reflex integration). All the ratings of representativeness were high for postural control; 83 percent rated bilateral motor integration and reflex integration as high and 17 percent as moderate.

Construct validity was obtained on three levels: item, subtest, and total test. The effectiveness of each item was determined by comparing the mean scores for the normal and delayed groups, then calculating a discrimination index. The statistical significance (using a *t* test for independent samples) and the magnitude of this discrimination index were evaluated. The 37 items insensitive to the developmental status of normals or not discriminating between the performance of normal and delayed children were discarded. All but three items produced mean differences significant at the .05 level and beyond. In addition, 79 percent of the items displayed a medium or large discrimination index effect, while 21 percent satisfied the criterion for a small effect.

Tasks requiring motor planning, balance, and eye-hand coordination in the Bilateral Motor Integration Subtest exhibited small effects, probably because these functions are emerging and are being refined in the preschool years.

To establish decision validity, optimal cutoff scores were located to determine the best points of each group's discrimination. Correct and incorrect classification probabilities were computed, including the false-normal and false-delayed error rates. Cutoff scores were weighted to minimize the false-normal error rate since it was judged to be the more serious type of error in screening delayed children. This error rate ranged from 4 to 9 percent for the three subtests and 9 percent for the total test. The error rate for false delayed (i.e., classifying a normal child as delayed) ranged from 17 to 26 percent for the three subtests and 10 percent for the total test. The classification accuracy of the total test was 81 percent. In addition, the sensitivity of the cutoff scores (the probability of correctly identifying a delayed child in a sample of actual delayed children) ranged from 66 to 84 percent. Likewise, the specificity of the cutoff scores (the probability of correctly identifying a normal child in a sample of actual normal children) ranged from 64 to 85 percent for the subtests and total test scores.

The structure of the total test and subtests were examined by comparing the relationship of the subtests with each other and the total test. Pearson correlation coefficients were computed with moderately low subtest correlations ranging from .39 to .65. These values indicate that each subtest is measuring different vestibular-based functions from the others, which provides empirical support for the domain structure. The amount of overlap (explained variance) between the subtests ranged from 15 to 42 percent, providing sufficient data to warrant their inclusion in one total score. The correlations of the subtests and the total test were quite substantial (.64–.93). From this analysis it was apparent that the subdomains of postural control and bilateral

motor integration appear to be more vital to overall sensory integration than reflex integration.

Guidelines for Use in a Clinical Setting

The TSI is appropriate for preschool children with developmental delays who exhibit (1) fine and gross motor delays of 1 to 2 years, (2) perceptual problems, (3) mild to moderate mental retardation, or (4) learning disabilities. The child must comprehend both verbal directions requiring him or her to hold various body positions and the notion of continuing a task until completion. Some children with moderate mental retardation are not appropriate for this test. Likewise, the test is not designed for children with orthopedic handicaps or cerebral palsy. The TSI can be used on older children; however, items requiring lifting the child will need to be adapted (e.g., using a bolster for the airplane task). The scores can be interpreted based only on the data presented for preschool children. A school-aged child (over 6 years) who receives a suspect or deficient score would be considered to have a definite deficit in sensory integration; in this case, evaluation using the Southern California Sensory Integration Tests is recommended to determine if the child would benefit from sensory integrative therapy.

Since the TSI is intended as an assessment of overall sensory integrative functioning, other instruments should be used when the TSI is used as a diagnostic instrument. Tests such as the Peabody Developmental Motor Scales, the Miller Assessment for Preschoolers, and the Southern California Postrotary Nystagmus Test may be useful in delineating the child's problem areas.

Review

The TSI is a criterion-referenced test designed to measure overall sensory integration in 3- to 5-year-old children with delays in sensory, motor, and perceptual skills or suspected of being at risk for learning problems. The test focuses primarily on the vestibular-based functions and includes subtests measuring postural control, bilateral motor integration, and reflex integration. The test is useful in screening and in diagnosing (in combination with other instruments) children with sensory integrative dysfunction. In addition, it is useful in delineating areas in need of therapeutic intervention. The test is easy to administer and score; however, it requires practice to administer and interpret findings. Studies of interobserver, test-retest, and decision reliability indicated good reliability for the total test and Bilateral Motor Integration and Postural Control Subtests. Since the Reflex Integration Subtest showed inadequate interobserver reliability, diagnosis based on this subtest alone is discouraged. Studies of validity indicated good domain, construct, and decision validity. Cutoff scores are presented and are used to make decisions regarding the child's level of functioning in the areas tested.

The major limitation of the TSI is the predominance of 3 and 4 year olds in the sample. Further data should be collected to expand the data base, especially on 5 year olds. Statistical studies indicated that the Reflex Integration Subtest was a weak area of the test. Additional items should be added to this subtest in future revisions to include standing balance items as well. Predictive validity studies are needed to determine if children identified in their preschool years as having sensory integrative dysfunction on the TSI demonstrate learning disabilities in the school years. In addition, the relationship of the TSI to other instruments should be examined.

REFERENCES

1. Ayres, A. J. *Sensory Integration and Learning Disorders.* Los Angeles: Western Psychological Services, 1972.
2. Bauer, B. A. Tactile sensitivity: Development of a behavioral responses checklist. *Am. J. Occup. Ther.* 31 : 357, 1977.
3. Berk, R. A., and DeGangi, G. A. Decision reliability of the Assessment of Sensorimotor Integration: Preliminary findings. *Phys. Occup. Ther. Pediatr.* 1 : 53, 1980.
4. Berk, R. A., and DeGangi, G. A. *DeGangi-Berk Test of Sensory Integration.* Los Angeles: Western Psychological Services, 1983.
5. DeGangi, G. *Assessment of Sensorimotor Integration in Preschool Children.* Baltimore: Johns Hopkins University, 1979.
6. DeGangi, G. A., Berk, R. A., and Larsen, L. The measurement of vestibular-based functions in preschool children. *Am. J. Occup. Ther.* 34(7) : 452, 1980.
7. DeGangi, G. A., and Berk, R. A. Psychometric analysis of the Test of Sensory Integration. *Phys. Occup. Ther. Pediatr.* 3 : 43, 1983a.
8. DeGangi, G. A., and Berk, R. A. Assessment of sensory integrative dysfunction in the preschool years. *Learn. Disabil.* 2 : 1, 1983b.
9. Folio, M. R., and Fewell, R. R. *Peabody Developmental Motor Scales* (Revised Experimental Edition). Hingham, Mass.: Teaching Resources Corp., 1974.
10. Harris, S. R., et al. The relationship between tests of sensorimotor integration, tactile sensitivity, and gross motor skills in normal and developmentally delayed preschool children. *Phys. Occup. Ther. Pediatr.* 4 : 5, 1984.

THE MARIANNE FROSTIG DEVELOPMENTAL TEST OF VISUAL PERCEPTION

Descriptive Information

Test Identification

The title of this test is *The Marianne Frostig Developmental Test of Visual Perception* (DTVP), 1966. Its authors are Marianne Frostig, Phyllis Maslow, D. Welty Lefever, and John R. B. Whittlesey. Both Frostig and Maslow were working at the Marianne Frostig School of Educational Therapy in Los Angeles at the time of the printing of the monograph. No other information is given regarding their discipline. In addition to the Frostig Developmental Test of Visual Perception, Frostig has also developed the Frostig Program for Individualized Training and Remediation in Visual Perception and the Frostig Move-Grow-Learn Program, which is a movement education program to improve motor and perceptual skills in young children. Both programs are available through Consulting Psychologists Press and Modern Curriculum Press.

Consulting Psychologists Press (577 College Ave., P.O. Box 60070, Palo Alto, California 94306) publishes the test at a cost of $20–$22 for an examiner's kit containing 10 test booklets, a set of scoring keys, a set of demonstration cards, and the monograph and manual; and $18–$22 for each set of 25 tests.

Age and Type of Client

Although the norms are available for 4 to 8 year olds, the normative curves indicate that there is little change in perceptual development after the age of 7; therefore, the test is designed mainly for use with children from 4 to 7 years of age. It appears that the DTVP is designed for children with learning disabilities, neurological impairments, or general developmental delays that cause the child to exhibit difficulties in visual perception. The test is intended to be used as part of the evaluation of children who need remedial or school readiness programs. The authors state that the DTVP is particularly useful in screening groups of nursery, kindergarten, and first grade children who may require perceptual training. The test may also be administered to older children with severe learning disabilities who exceed the norms for the test.

Purpose

The test is designed to test visual perceptual functions in children from 4 to 8 years of age. It can be administered individually or in groups. The authors suggest that the DTVP may be useful either in screening 4 to 6 year olds or as a diagnostic tool for older children with visual perceptual problems.

Time Required to Administer and Score Test

The time required to administer the test to a group is less than 1 hour. When administering the test to individuals, it takes between 30 and 45 minutes. Scoring takes approximately 5 to 10 minutes.

Evaluator

The DTVP is intended as a screening tool suitable for group or individual administration by professionals who are thoroughly familiar with the instructions, test items, and scoring criteria. The authors recommend that the test not be administered by a regular classroom teacher unless the teacher is trained by a school psychologist and has given practice tests individually and in a small group. Children who are handicapped or severely disturbed should be tested by an experienced psychologist.

Historical Perspective of Test Construction

Development and Source of Items

Preliminary construction of test items began in 1958; the items were field tested in 1959 on several groups of about 100 schoolchildren. The first formal version of the test was developed and standardized in 1961, and the final version was published in 1963, after revisions were made in the items for a third time. The testing materials were not revised; however, the manual was revised in 1966.

Test items selected were based on good age progression in the five areas tested and a low degree of overlap with other abilities. The DTVP was developed because existing tests of visual perception, such as the Bender-Gestalt, required individual administration. Many of the tests available at that time also did not provide normative data.

Review of Literature in Terms of Test Use

Several studies have examined the usefulness of the DTVP with children exhibiting physical handicaps, mental retardation, and learning disabilities. Abercrombie and colleagues [1] used the DTVP as part of the assessment of physically handicapped children and found that disturbances in visual-motor skills were associated with spasticity and not athetosis. They found the DTVP to be useful in examining disorders of visual-motor rather than visual-perceptual skills. Frostig has stated that the DTVP can be used with cerebral-palsied children; however, the examiner must use clinical judgment in giving Subtest 1 (Eye-Hand Coordination). When administering the DTVP to mentally retarded children, Frostig recommends that the scale scores and perceptual quotients be compared with the child's mental age since the tests are too difficult for this population. In another study, Frostig and colleagues [9] found that 71 children with learning disabilities demonstrated a high percentage of scatter in their subtest scores, with a lower total test score compared with normal children. A high percent of children in their sample were diagnosed as neurologically handicapped.

In a review of the DTVP, Chissom [4] views the test as useful for a variety of populations, but stresses that further research is needed on the instrument before it can be considered more than just an adequate visual perception instrument. Kephart [11] also views the DTVP favorably when used as Frostig intended (i.e., as part of a total diagnostic procedure). He states that the DTVP contributes valuable information regarding the child's visual perception skills. Concerns regarding the validity of the DTVP have been expressed by Rosen [14], who reports that none of the studies provided predictive or concurrent validity. Rosen also criticizes the fact that not enough attention is provided toward recommended uses of the test, and he cautions against misuse of the instrument as an evaluative tool. Mann [12] also adds that the DTVP does not seem to assess five different areas of visual perception, and that low scores on the DTVP may not actually imply visual perception problems.

Theoretical Constructs and Implications for Intervention

The development of the DTVP is based on the premise that visual perceptual disturbances are more prevalent in learning-disabled children than other symptoms that contribute to learning difficulties and that disturbances in visual perception are likely to affect reading abilities. The authors' clinical observations were used to select five visual perceptual areas relevant to school performance. Children with difficulties in handwriting appeared to have disturbances in eye-hand coordination, and children with difficulties recognizing words seemed to have poor figure-ground perception. Those children who could not recognize letters or words presented in lower- or uppercase were expected to have poor form constancy. Reversals in writing were thought to reflect difficulties in position in space, and interchanging of letter order appeared to suggest poor spatial relations. Based on the observations of Frostig and Maslow, the DTVP was constructed to explore these five areas of visual perception. These five areas were hypothesized to be most relevant to school performance, although they may not be the only factors contributing to visual perception. Recognition skills (Subtests 2, 3, and 4) were separated from copying skills (Subtest 5) in order to differentiate visual perception from visual-motor integration. Subtest 1 taps simple motor skills so that the effects of poor eye-hand coordination can be examined as it affects handwriting and visual-motor integration.

Content and Test Administration

Content

Five visual perception areas are tested by the DTVP.

Test 1: Eye-Motor Coordination. Sixteen items measure the child's ability to draw within a straight, curved, or angular pathway of decreasing size, to draw on a line, and connect dots between two points.

Test 2: Figure-Ground. The eight test items within this subtest involve finding an intersecting or hidden geometric form against increasingly complex backgrounds.

Test 3: Constancy of Shape. The four items on this subtest involve recognizing circles and squares presented in a variety of sizes, shadings, textures, and positions in space as well as discriminating them from similar geometric forms.

Test 4: Position in Space. This subtest includes four items requiring the child to distinguish which line drawing differs in position from the others and four items requiring the child to match a stimulus figure with one of four line drawings presented in different orientations (Fig. 6-4).

Test 5: Spatial relationships. This subtest includes eight items that involve copying simple forms and patterns on a dot grid.

Setting and Equipment

The DTVP can be administered individually or in groups; therefore, the setting is usually a classroom or small room. The test materials include a 35-page booklet, eleven demonstration cards showing various shapes such as the "kite" for the items used in the Subtests 2 and 3, and three transparent scoring tissues for items 10 through 16 on the first subtest. The examiner must also provide four sharp-colored pencils of contrasting color and a regular lead pencil. A blackboard is needed for group administration. If the test is administered individually, paper or a slate is needed for demonstration.

Administration Procedures

There are verbal directions and procedures for administering each subtest and item or set of

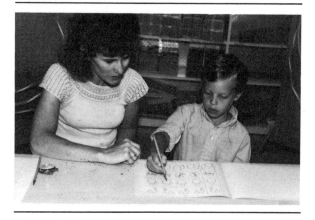

Fig. 6-4. The Marianne Frostig Developmental Test of Visual Perception. Item from the Position in Space Subtest.

items. The procedures are simple and easy to administer.

Scoring

Scoring of items is performed by using the criteria in the administration and scoring manual. Specific guidelines are given for scoring items, with criteria delineating the different point counts that can be assigned. Some items range from 0 to 2 points while others are 0 or 1 point. After scoring all items, the total raw score is obtained for each subtest. Table 1 is used to convert raw scores to perceptual age equivalents. Table 2 is used to find the child's scale score corresponding to his or her chronological age. A perceptual quotient is attained from which a percentile rank is recorded from Table 2 as well. Scale scores are provided for children ranging in age from 4 years to 7 years 11 months in 3-month intervals. Suggestions for interpreting scores of children who are 3 or 8 to 10 years of age are provided in the manual. Frostig recommends that when interpreting results on 3 and 4 year olds and 8 to 10 year olds that Table 1 be used for the perceptual age equivalent. For children ranging in age from 4 to 8, the conversion scores in Table 2 are suggested. Results on children over 10 years of age can be interpreted by examining whether the child reaches the maximum perceptual age equivalent.

Test scores can be converted from a raw score on each subtest to perceptual age equivalents, which are available in Table 2 of the monograph. Sixteen tables are divided for each 3-month increment of age in order to convert raw scores of individual subtests and total test scores to scale scores and perceptual quotients for below and above average performance. *Scale scores* are the perceptual ages divided by the chronological age and multiplied by 10 and are defined in terms of a ratio. The *perceptual quotient* is a deviation score expressed in percentiles and is based on the summation of the subtest scores, which corrects for age variation. The perceptual quotient was found to be a better indicator of prognosis than the perceptual age. A perceptual quotient of 90 is recommended as a cutoff point in scores in kindergarten children. Children falling below this cutoff score should receive special training. No other cutoff scores are given, and how the cutoff score of 90 is derived is questionable. It is based on results of 25 children, ranging in age from 4½ to 6½ years, who later developed reading problems. Scores for children over 10 years of age should be interpreted in terms of their subtest perceptual age equivalents.

Psychometric Properties

Standardization

In the 1963 standardization of the DTVP, there were a total of 2116 children ranging in age from 3 to 9 years. The children were grouped in half-year increments, with anywhere from 107 to 240 children in each group. All children lived in Southern California and were predominantly white, middle-class. Exact information on socioeconomic status and race of the children is not available. Poor geographic distribution and poor representation across low socioeconomic groups and minority groups is a major criticism of the DTVP [4, 12].

Reliability

Test-retest reliability conducted on 50 children with learning difficulties at all ages with a 3-week interval between tests yielded a coefficient of .98. Interobserver reliability between two administrators, both psychologists, on a sample of 35 first graders and 37 second graders was .80 for the entire test. Subtest scale score test-retest correlations ranged from .42 (Subtest 2) to .80 (Subtest 3). Another study of interobserver reliability using persons who were trained in the administration of the test but who were not psychologists on 55 kindergartners and 72 first graders yielded reliability quotients of .69 for the total test for both groups. Product-moment coefficients ranged from .29 to .74 on the subtest scale scores for the kindergartners and from .39 to .67 for the first graders. Subtest 1 had the lowest correlation in both samples. Low test-retest reliability on the subtest scale scores, with correlations ranging from .29 to .74, was also found by Hammill, Colarusso, and Wiederholt [10] for kindergarten and first grade children. Split-half reliability correlation coefficients yielded coefficients ranging from .78 to .89 for large groups of 5 to 9 year olds for total test scores. Correlation coefficients for split-half reliability ranged from .35 on Subtest 4 to .96 on Subtest 2.

Validity

Several studies have examined the validity of the DTVP. A major premise held by Frostig is that problems in visual perception will affect academic skills. To investigate the ability of the DTVP to detect children with academic problems, Frostig correlated teacher ratings of classroom adjustment with the DTVP. A correlation of .44 was obtained, which Frostig interpreted as suggestive that disturbances in visual perception may be reflected in problematic classroom behavior. Correlations between scores on the DTVP and the Goodenough test, a test of body image, yielded correlation coefficients ranging from .318 to .466 for kindergartners and first and second graders. These coefficients suggest that the two tests measure relatively different functions but that there is some overlap. Olson and Johnson [13] compared the DTVP to the Gates Reading Readiness Test, the Metropolitan Reading Test, and the Olson Reading Readiness Test and found the DTVP to be the least useful in predicting reading readiness.

The only study of predictive validity reported by Frostig is one in which 25 children ranging from 4½ to 6½ years of age were tested, then scores compared to later reading achievement. It was predicted that the eight children who had perceptual quotients of 90 or below would not attempt to learn to read. Later ratings of reading achievement revealed that none of these children had begun to read, while only one child with a perceptual quotient of over 90 had reading difficulties. The method by which Frostig selected the cutoff score of 90 is not described, nor is the accuracy of this cutoff score in classifying children as delayed versus normal in visual perception skills examined.

Several factor analytic studies have been conducted regarding the validity of the subtests in measuring five distinct areas of visual perception. In establishing these five areas, Frostig relied on clinical judgment and had not completed any factor analytic studies. Of the studies that have been completed, conflicting results are present. Several investigators found the DTVP to measure only one central factor identified as perceptual development or intelligence [2, 3]. Corah and Powell [5] compared the results of other factor analytic studies and arrived at two major factors accounting for the majority of variance: general intelligence and developmental changes in perception. A study by Sabatino and colleagues [15] determined that the DTVP measures two specific components: visual perception and manual motor coordination. This study

and several others [7, 8] found that the DTVP is not a significant predictor of reading abilities. One study [6] compared the DTVP and Bender-Gestalt and concluded that the DTVP is not a pure measure of visual perception, and that nonperceptual cognitive skills appear to influence performance on the test. In the study by DuBois and Brown [8], correlations between the DTVP and Slosson Intelligence Test showed that there was significant overlap. The authors concluded that the DTVP measures very little different from a language-based intelligence test, and it does not measure any additional specific skills related to reading when compared with the Bates-MacGinitie Reading Survey. Likewise, Smith and Marx [16] found that the DTVP was weakly associated with intelligence and unrelated to reading ability. They also criticized the scaling used to derive scores, since a poorer raw score would yield a higher scaled score for normal children over 8 years. Overall, the studies view the DTVP as having limited value as a test of visual perception and stress that it should not be used to predict reading ability.

Guidelines for Use in a Clinical Setting

Because of research cited in the review of the literature that the DTVP does not necessarily measure visual perception and does not correlate with later reading abilities, the test is not recommended for screening or diagnosis of visual perception skills. Since Subtest 3 (Constancy of Shape) was the most reliable of the subtests, it may be useful in making clinical observations. Since the instrument was most reliable for first and second graders, observations using the DTVP should be on this age group.

Review

The DTVP is a test of visual perception developed for use with 4 to 8 year olds with learning disabilities, particularly children with reading disorders. It was initially developed as a screening instrument for individual or group administration. The test includes five areas of visual perception; however, research on the instrument suggests that it does not necessarily measure visual perception and does not correlate with later reading performance. Only one cutoff score is given, based on the performance of only 25 children, and is to be used in making diagnostic decisions regarding children who may require intervention. Since visual perception should improve with age, the use of this cutoff score is questionable. Likewise, scaling of scores for children over 8 years is problematic. Interobserver reliability (r) was only fair ($r = .69$) for persons trained in the use of the test but who were not psychologists for kindergartners and first graders. Interobserver reliability was good ($r = .80$) for a small sample of first and second graders tested by psychologists. Test-retest reliability was .98 for the total test; however, only subtest 3 yielded fair ($r = .74$) to good ($r = .80$) correlation coefficients, while the other subtests were poor in their stability. In light of the poor construct validity, fair interobserver reliability, and poor decision validity, the DTVP is not recommended as a test to measure visual perception. Other instruments should be selected in its place.

REFERENCES

1. Abercrombie, M. L. J., et al. Visual, perceptual, and visuo-motor impairment in physically handicapped children. *Percept. Mot. Skills* 18 : 561, 1964. (Monogr. Suppl. 3-V18)
2. Boyd, L., and Randle, K. Factor analysis of the Frostig Developmental Test of Visual Perception. *J. Learn. Disabil.* 3 : 253, 1970.
3. Chissom, B. S., and Thomas, B. J. Comparison of factor structures for the Frostig Developmental Test of Visual Perception. *Percept. Mot. Skills* 33 : 1015, 1971.
4. Chissom, B. S. Review of the DTVP. In O. K. Buros (ed.), *The Seventh Mental Measurements Yearbook (Vol. 2)*. Highland Park, N.J.: Gryphon Press, 1972. P. 871.
5. Corah, N. L., and Powell, B. J. A factor analytic study of the Frostig Developmental Test of Visual Perception. *Percept. Mot. Skills* 16 : 59, 1963.
6. Culbertson, F. M., and Gunn, R. C. Comparison of the Bender-Gestalt Test and the Frostig Test in several clinical groups of children. *J. Clin. Psychol.* 22 : 439, 1966.
7. DuBois, N. F. Selected correlations between reading achievement and various visual abilities of children in grades 2 and 4. *Percept. Mot. Skills* 37 : 45, 1973.
8. DuBois, N. F., and Brown, F. L. Selected relationships between Frostig scores and reading achievement in a first grade population. *Percept. Mot. Skills* 37 : 515, 1973.
9. Frostig, M., Lefever, D. V., and Whittlesey, J. R. B. A developmental test of visual perception for evaluating normal and neurologically handicapped children. *Percept. Mot. Skills* 12 : 383, 1961.
10. Hammill, D. D., Colarusso, R. P., and Wiederholt, J. L. Diagnostic value of the Frostig test: A factor analytic approach. *J. Spec. Ed.* 4 : 279, 1970.
11. Kephart, N. C. Review of the DTVP. In O. K. Buros (ed.), *The Seventh Mental Measurements Yearbook (Vol. 2)*. Highland Park, N.J.: Gryphon Press, 1972. P. 871.
12. Mann, L. Review of the DTVP. In O. K. Buros (ed.), *The Seventh Mental Measurements Yearbook (Vol. 2)*. Highland Park, N.J.: Gryphon Press, 1972. P. 871.
13. Olson, A. V., and Johnson, S. Structure and predictive validity of the Frostig Developmental Test of Visual Perception in grades one and three. *J. Spec. Ed.* 4 : 49, 1970.
14. Rosen, C. L. Review of the DTVP. In O. K. Buros (ed.), *The Eighth Mental Measurements Yearbook (Vol. 2)*. Highland Park, N.J.: Gryphon Press, 1978. P. 871.
15. Sabatino, D. A., Abbott, J. C., and Becker, J. T. What does the Frostig DTVP measure? *Excep. Child.* 40 : 453, 1974.
16. Smith, P. A., and Marx, R. W. Some cautions on the use of the Frostig test: A factor analytic study. *J. Learn. Dis.* 5 : 357, 1972.

A GUIDE TO TESTING CLINICAL OBSERVATIONS IN KINDERGARTNERS

Descriptive Information

Test Identification

The title of this guide is *A Guide to Testing Clinical Observations in Kindergartners,* 1981. Its author is Winnie Dunn, M.Ed., OTR. Dunn is an occupational therapist with expertise in the theory of sensory integrative dysfunction and test administration. American Occupational Therapy Association, Inc. (1381 Piccard Dr., Rockville, Maryland 20850) publishes the test at a cost of $7–$9 for members of the association and $10–$12 for nonmembers.

Age and Type of Client

This set of clinical observations is designed for 5 to 6½ year olds. Although the data are presented only for children with normal functioning, they may be useful as a guide in identifying children with suspected sensory integrative deficits.

Purpose

The purpose of the guide is to provide standardized procedures for clinical observations of ocular-motor, postural mechanisms, reflex integration, muscle tone, and vestibular functioning and a scoring procedure to quantify the observations.

Time Required to Administer and Score Test

Although it is not stated in the manual, it should take approximately 30 minutes to administer and score the observations.

Evaluator

The observations would most likely be administered by an occupational or physical therapist familiar with sensory integration theory and testing. No special training is indicated to use the guide.

Historical Perspective of Test Construction

Development and Source of Items

The items presented in this guide were initially described by A. Jean Ayres in her book, *Sensory*

Integration and Learning Disorders (1972). The observations described by Ayres, however, were not presented in a standardized format with specific procedures and scoring criteria. Dunn has made these improvements in this guide. These clinical observations were initially designed to be administered in conjunction with the Southern California Sensory Integration Tests [2].

Review of Literature in Terms of Test Use

Ayres [1] has described the clinical significance of observations of the qualitative performance of vestibular and/or proprioceptive tasks. Children exhibiting sensory integrative dysfunction may demonstrate problems in some or all of the following areas: low muscle tone, poor ocular-motor control, presence of primitive reflexes with poor balance functions, poor flexion and extension against gravity, poor shoulder and neck cocontraction, postural insecurity, and poor integration of the two body sides. Children with problems in these functions typically have vestibular and/or proprioceptive processing problems. Ayres [3] has found that 50 percent of children identified as learning disabled also demonstrated inadequate vestibular functioning. Steinberg and Rendle-Short [15] reported that children with minor neurological dysfunction have a high proportion of deficits in postural reactions (particularly in the prone position), vestibular functions, and visual-spatial skills. Rider [12, 13] reported that both children with learning disabilities and children with dysphasia had significantly more abnormal postural reflexes than their normal counterparts.

Research on this particular set of clinical observations first described by Ayres is very limited. Harris [8] found a significant difference between 4 and 8 year olds in their ability to hold a prone extension posture against gravity, which supports the notion of developmental differences in postural stability. Gregory-Flock and Yerxa [7] recently standardized the prone extension postural test on 4 to 8 year olds. They assessed prone extension through a quality rating scale that accounted for the degree to which the child could assume and maintain the posture as well as head, trunk, and leg posture. Their data indicated that 4 and 5 year olds performed similarly but differed significantly from 6 to 8 year olds. The authors also found that the test differentiated the performance of 10 learning-disabled children from that of the normal sample, with the exception of the 4 year olds.

Ottenbacher [9] compared the supine flexion and prone extension postures and found a significant relationship between them; however, there was a high correlation between vestibular function and the prone extension posture only. In a study examining the relationship of prone extension to other vestibular functions, Bundy and Fisher [4] found that equilibrium reactions in sitting and kneeling, crossing midline of the eyes, and below-average academic performance were related to prone extension abilities. They also found that poor performance on one vestibular measure does not necessarily mean that performance is poor on other vestibular functions, a finding that reflects the need to delineate which type of vestibular function (i.e., otolithic versus semi-circular canal) a task is actually testing.

Several investigators have examined the prevalence of the asymmetrical tonic neck reflex in children and have devised rating scales to assess this reflex in a clinical setting. Since the ATNR has been shown to be less suppressed in children with learning disabilities than in normal children [1, 12], its assessment may be valuable in determining the degree of integration of brain stem level functions. Parmenter [11] has developed a quantitative rating scale for evaluation of the reflex in the quadruped position with four sequences of lateral head rotation. A four-point rating scale was developed, which Parmenter used in evaluating the performance of first and third graders. In an earlier study by Parmenter [10], she found that elbow flexion of more than 30 degrees on the skull-side arm in first and third graders may indicate poor inhibition of the reflex.

Sieg and Shuster [14] examined the asymmetrical tonic-neck reflex (ATNR) in three different positions including quadruped, the quadruped-reflex inhibiting posture, and standing, and found that the quadruped position was the most reliable. Both Parmenter and Sieg and Shuster used four or more slow rotations of the head in evaluating the position. Zemke [16] examined the incidence of the ATNR in normal preschool children and found that its prevalence was very high in both 3 and 5 year olds when tested in both the supine and quadruped position using electrogoniometry of elbow flexion and head rotation. Zemke concluded that the presence of the ATNR in preschool children may not be indicative of an abnormality, and she stressed that more precise examination of the reflex is needed.

Theoretical Constructs and Implications for Intervention

Since the literature cited thus far indicates a prevalence of poor postural mechanisms as well as other vestibular-based, tactile, and proprioceptive functions in learning-disabled children, intervention should be directed toward integrating these underlying sensorimotor functions when deficits are identified.

Content and Test Administration

Content

The guide contains test items in the following areas:

Eye preference, independent eye closure
Eye movements
Muscle tone
Cocontraction
Slow motions of the upper extremities
Finger-to-nose test
Schilder's arm extension test
Flexion in supine
Prone extension
Symmetrical and assymmetrical tonic neck
  reflex

Diadokokinesis
Mouth motor planning
Postural security
Rising to stand with symmetry
Protective extension in kneeling
Equilibrium reactions in four positions
Postrotary nystagmus

Setting and Equipment

There is no test kit; however, a tiltboard is required, and a Dunnometer (purchased from Be O. K. Fred Sammons, Inc.) is used to calibrate the number of degrees tilted by the tiltboard for equilibrium reactions. A pencil, goniometer, centimeter ruler, stopwatch, and rotation board used in the Southern California Postrotary Nystagmus Test [3] are also needed. A recording form is presented in the back of the manual.

Administration Procedures

A set of clearly presented standardized procedures accompanies each observation. Diagrams or drawings are given for some items. Criteria for scoring are presented in detail. Although the procedures are not highly complex, practice in administering and scoring the items is needed in order to devote attention to observing the quality of the performance.

Scoring

The scoring criteria are clearly presented for each observation. The recording form presented can be easily used while administering the items. Scores are not computed as a total test but rather are interpreted as individual test scores. Data are presented in standard scores for each item. An interpretation of the scores or range of expected responses is given at the end of each item's description. Dunn stresses that the standard scores presented are to be used in characterizing trends and are not to be used as norms.

Psychometric Properties

Standardization

Data were collected on 263 children ranging in age from 5 to 6½ years. The mean age was 5 years 7 months; and all children were described by Dunn as functioning as normal. Dunn reports that the children in the sample were not at the top of the scales in performance so that results were not distorted. No intelligence scale scores are reported on the subjects. In addition, no additional data are given regarding race, cultural or socioeconomic background, sex distribution, or geographic location of the sample.

Reliability

No reliability studies were conducted on the guide; therefore, much reservation is needed when interpreting the results.

Validity

Construct validity was the only type of validity examined on the guide. The percent of children performing at each level of performance for each item was reported and interpreted for discriminative ability for the kindergarten population. In addition, Pearson r correlations were computed to determine the relationship among test items as well as the relationship within an item for the various components scored. Although Dunn describes aspects of a particular item that discriminate well for the sample, adjustments were not made in the scoring criteria to aid the user in interpretation of the items. For instance, scoring for head position on prone extension was the only valid measure for this item, as the other three parts of the item (legs only, together straight, together bent) were too difficult for the majority of children in the sample. Inspection of the data reveals that the only items that should be deleted include independent eye closure and prone extension (leg items only). Although some items appeared to discriminate among the normal subjects, caution should be taken when interpreting results. Research by Bundy and Fisher [4] found that children who score poorly on one measure of vestibular function will not necessarily perform poorly on other measures of vestibular function. In research conducted by DeGangi and colleagues [5], the authors found that some items measuring postural control and reflex integration had a high overlap in performance between delayed and normal subjects. This was true of the Schilder arm extension test (degree of trunk rotation), eye-hand dominance, and ocular-motor control in horizontal eye movements. Since data were collected on 3 to 5 year olds in their sample, conclusions from this study cannot necessarily be correlated with Dunn's findings. The importance of comparing the results of normal and learning-disabled subjects should not be overlooked, however.

Guidelines for Use in a Clinical Setting

The clinical observations described by Dunn are intended as a guide for interpreting responses in normal kindergarten children. These observations can be used as a gross screening tool. Children who perform poorly can be referred for further testing using the Southern California Sensory Integration Tests or other standardized instruments. Since no data were collected on children with developmental delays or learning disabilities, it is difficult to determine if all items in the set of observations would discriminate children with deficits from age-matched normal children. In addition, data were collected only on kindergartners; therefore, judgments regarding the performance of 3 and 4 year olds and children over 6 years should not be made using the data presented by Dunn. Older children who perform considerably below the expected performance of a kindergartner should definitely be referred for additional testing. Three and four year olds may be more accurately screened with the DeGangi-Berk Test of Sensory Integration. The major advantage of this guide developed by Dunn is

that it presents a written, formalized procedure for clinical observations commonly examined by physical and occupational therapists.

Review

A Guide to Testing Clinical Observations in Kindergartners provides a formalized set of procedures that should prove useful to occupational and physical therapists. Because data were collected only on normal subjects, the guide is primarily helpful when administered to normal children. Five- and six-year-old children falling well below the guidelines set forth for normal performance should be tested with standardized instruments to determine if a delay indeed exists. Since the standard scores presented in the guide are used only to characterize trends, caution should be taken when interpreting results from the guide. Data on older children and on children with learning problems need to be collected in order to validate the usefulness of the items in detecting children with sensory integrative dysfunction. More extensive data collection and validity and reliability studies are also needed before this set of clinical observations can be used as a sound clinical instrument.

REFERENCES

1. Ayres, A. J. *Sensory Integration and Learning Disorders.* Los Angeles: Western Psychological Services, 1972.
2. Ayres, A. J. *Southern California Sensory Integration Tests (Revised).* Los Angeles: Western Psychological Services, 1980.
3. Ayres, A. J. *Southern California Postrotary Nystagmus Test.* Los Angeles: Western Psychological Services, 1975.
4. Bundy, A. C., and Fisher, A. G. The relationship of prone extension to other vestibular functions. *Am. J. Occup. Ther.* 35 : 782, 1981.
5. DeGangi, G. A., Berk, R. A., and Larsen, L. The measurement of vestibular-based functions in preschool children. *Am. J. Occup. Ther.* 34(7) : 452, 1980.
6. Dunn, W. *A Guide to Testing Clinical Observa-*

tions in Kindergartners. Rockville, Md.: American Occupational Therapy Association, 1981.

7. Gregory-Flock, J. L., and Yerxa, E. J. Standardization of the prone extension postural test on children ages 4 through 8. *Am. J. Occup. Ther.* 38(3) : 187, 1984.

8. Harris, N. P. Duration and quality of the prone extension position in four-, six-, and eight-year-old normal children. *Am. J. Occup. Ther.* 35 : 26, 1981.

9. Ottenbacher, K. Identifying vestibular processing dysfunction in learning-disabled children. *Am. J. Occup. Ther.* 32 : 217, 1978.

10. Parmenter, C. The asymmetrical tonic neck reflex in normal first and third grade children. *Am. J. Occup. Ther.* 29 : 462, 1975.

11. Parmenter, C. L. An asymmetrical tonic neck reflex rating scale. *Am. J. Occup. Ther.* 37(7) : 462, 1983.

12. Rider, B. A. Relationship of postural reflexes to learning disabilities. *Am. J. Occup. Ther.* 26 : 239, 1972.

13. Rider, B. A. Abnormal postural reflexes in dysphasic children. *Am. J. Occup. Ther.* 28 : 351, 1974.

14. Sieg, K. W., and Shuster, J. J. Comparison of three positions for evaluating the asymmetrical tonic neck reflex. *Am. J. Occup. Ther.* 33 : 311, 1979.

15. Steinberg, M., and Rendle-Short, J. Vestibular dysfunction in young children with minor neurological impairment. *Dev. Med. Child Neurol.* 19 : 639, 1977.

16. Zemke, R. Incidence of ATNR response in normal preschool children. *Phys. Occup. Ther. Pediatr.* 1(2) : 31, 1980.

THE IMITATION OF GESTURES

Descriptive Information

Test Identification

The title of this test is *The Imitation of Gestures,* 1965. Its authors are Jean Bergès, M.D., and Irène Lézine, M.D. Both Bergès and Lézine are physicians, although it is not presented in the book whether they are pediatricians or neurologists. The test first appeared in *Clinics in Developmental Medicine* (No. 18), 1965, published by the Spastics Society Medical Education and Information Unit (London, England). The Imitation of Gestures is currently out of print; however, it is included in this chapter because it measures a domain of behaviors not included in many of the scales currently available, and it is available in medical libraries.

Age and Type of Client

The Imitation of Gestures was developed for 3 to 6 year olds. Although the type of client is not described in the book, it appears that children with learning disabilities or mild neurological deficits or slow learners may be most appropriate for the test.

Purpose

The test was developed for the purpose of examining body scheme and motor planning (praxis).

Time Required to Administer and Score Test

It takes approximately 20 minutes to administer and score the test.

Evaluator

Pediatricians, neurologists, clinical psychologists, and occupational therapists are most likely to administer The Imitation of Gestures.

Historical Perspective of Test Construction

Development and Source of Items

The test items were developed out of a need for a test of body scheme and praxis. The items were based on the clinical experience of the authors.

Review of Literature in Terms of Test Use

There is little in the literature regarding the use of The Imitation of Gestures test. Other than selected tests from the Southern California Sensory Integration Tests, the revised Sensory Integration Praxis Test, and the Short Screening Test for Clumsy Children by Gubbay [5], no other instruments are commercially available to detect motor planning problems in children. The Praxis Test for Children developed by Conrad, Cermak, and Drake [4] for a research study is based on the classification of types of praxis developed by Luria [3] for brain-damaged adults. The test items are drawn from several instruments including the Imitation of Gestures. The authors found that the types of praxis that differentiated learning-disabled and normal school-aged children were dynamic (e.g., movement pattern of arm) and optic-spatial (i.e., nonmeaningful gestures of hands and arms). The Optic-Spatial Subtest was most like the postures on The Imitation of Gestures test.

Theoretical Constructs and Implications for Interventions

Ayres [1, 2] has described *dyspraxia* as a disorder of sensory integration that interferes with the ability to plan and execute skilled, nonhabitual motor tasks. It is often associated with inefficient processing of tactile and/or vestibular input. Establishment of a good body schema is felt to be a necessary foundation for the presence of good motor planning skills. Bergès and Lézine view *praxis* as the ability to efficiently assume and control body postures and movements in space. They also interpret the ability to imitate another person's actions as demonstrating an awareness of another person's body. Since body schema is the perceptual component underlying praxis, observations of body schema are also included in the test.

Content and Test Administration

Content

There are two parts to the praxis part of the test:

1. Simple Gestures
   a. The child stands in front of the examiner who is seated and imitates a series of hand movements (10 items).

b. This is similar to a but in this section the child imitates arm movements in a series of 10 items.
2. Complex Gestures
   a. Complex hand and finger movements are imitated (16 items).
   b. In this part of the test, the child must reverse the examiner's gestures, which are those presented in 1.b.

In addition to the praxis items described above, the children who receive The Imitation of Gestures test also completed the Goodenough Draw-a-Man Test and the Grace Arthur Mannequin Puzzle.

Setting and Equipment

No equipment is needed except recording sheets. Enough space is needed to perform the arm movements.

Administration Procedures

The directions for administering the items are clear and simple. The child is simply asked to do what the examiner did. The test manual presents drawings for each test item illustrating the examiner's position. Although the different arm and hand positions are very clear, the examiner should have practiced these movements previously, so that the child does not see the method of assuming the position but only the final posture or gesture.

Scoring

Each response is recorded as a pass, a fail, or an incomplete. Criteria for scoring are presented in detail for each item. A success is considered an immediate or hesitant form, mirror or nonmirror versions of the posture (except for part 2. b.), and a final correct position of the body. A failure is any alteration in the test body position. An incomplete may be that only one side of the body was accurate. The items are not timed; therefore, a child who is hesitant or takes time to motor plan the position is not penalized. This factor may not be important given the age of the children being tested (3 to 6 year olds) by this instrument.

The number of successes are added for each part of the test, then compared with tables of percentages of passes in the normative sample. These percentages are presented by each age level and by item. A motor age can be obtained as well.

Psychometric Properties

Standardization

The normative sample includes 489 children from Paris and Sceaux public schools. The data were collected from 1959 to 1961. There were between 86 and 146 children in each age group (1-year intervals) from 3 to 6 years of age. There were also twenty-nine 7 year olds and twenty-one 8 year olds. There is no information presented regarding sex, race, or socioeconomic breakdown. In addition, there were 100 children ranging in age from 30 months to 9 years who were from the premature follow-up clinic. These children were used to validate the instrument; however, no information is presented regarding their eventual outcome (i.e., learning disabled, physically handicapped, or normal). The breakdown by age is also not given on the sample population; therefore, differentiation of performance by age cannot be done.

Reliability

No reliability studies were completed on *The Imitation of Gestures* test.

Validity

Unfortunately, validity studies are not well controlled or systematic in validating the domain of behaviors assessed and the usefulness of the instrument in identifying children with motor planning problems. Construct validity was examined in several ways, although the statistical procedures used were inadequate in the analyses. The total number of successes for the test differentiated performance across ages for the 3- to 5-year age group. The imitation of simple gestures was too easy for 6 year olds, however, causing a leveling off in the number of successes. Item difficulty was evaluated by age as well, but there was no comparison with a criterion-group to determine if children with dyspraxia would perform differently. Several items in Part 2 of the test were found to be too difficult for the 7 and 8 year olds; however, these items were not discarded from the sample. The only criterion group examined included a sample of 100 children ranging in age from 30 months to 9 years who were premature at birth. This sample was not well-defined, and it is not known if these children exhibited learning disabilities or other types of deficits. The authors report a significant difference between the results of the normal and "premature" sample. None of the premature children had scores above the median of the normal sample. The various types of aberrant responses also appeared frequently in the children with neurological disturbances.

The relation between The Imitation of Gestures test and other tests of body image was examined. The findings are presented in a supplemental section of the test manual. Other observations examined included right-left orientation on oneself and others, knowledge of body parts named and pointed to on verbal command, the Goodenough Draw-a-Man Test, and the Grace Arthur Mannequin Puzzle. The percentage of successes for performance on these measures is presented by age level in the manual. The results from the Draw-a-Man Test differed very little from norms established from Goodenough. Intercorrelations between the various tests were also completed on 3 to 5 year olds. The tests of imitation of simple gestures and imitation of complex gestures yielded a high correlation of .81. The correlation between Imitation of Simple Gestures and Draw-a-Man was significant but weak (.33). The correlation between simple gestures and the mannequin puzzle was moderate (.49). The lowest correlation was found for verbal naming and point of body parts and the imitation of simple gestures ($r = .31$). The imitation of complex gestures shows no significant correlations with the other tests. This finding may reflect the fact that imitation of complex gestures is just emerging in the 5 year old and was not an age-appropriate measure for the sample studied for intercorrelations.

Guidelines for Use in a Clinical Setting

The Imitation of Gestures test can be administered to preschool and young school-aged children suspected of having motor planning problems. It is most appropriate for children with learning disabilities and children experiencing difficulties in motor skills, particularly skills involving sequencing and imitation (e.g., skipping, lacing). It is necessary that the child understand the instructions to imitate the examiner's position exactly. Three to five year olds who are unable to complete the imitation of simple gesturs and who exhibit other signs of dyspraxia (i.e., difficulty sequencing, poor body scheme) should be referred for further testing to determine if a motor planning deficit is present. Results should be interpreted with caution because of the lack of reliability studies and the limited validity presented on the instrument. Although criteria are presented for scoring responses, they are ambiguous and difficult, which may affect the reliability of the instrument.

Review

The Imitation of Gestures test was developed for use with 3 to 6 year olds in evaluating body scheme and praxis. The test is quick and easy to administer, although the examiner must be practiced in assuming the different arm and hand positions and in scoring the various responses. It is questionable whether the scoring criteria are sensitive to differentiating children with dyspraxia and those without. For instance, a hesitant response is scored as a success; however, a child who takes time to motor plan a posture may indeed have dyspraxia. Since no reliability studies were conducted on the test and validation studies were poorly controlled, the test should not be used for any type of diagnostic decision making. Because recent research [2, 4] supports the notion that dyspraxia is not solely limited to the imitation of gestures, but also includes sequencing of movements over time and space, a test for diagnosing dyspraxia should also examine these components.

The Imitation of Gestures test can be administered as an observational tool in determining if a child (ages 3 to 5 years) may have motor planning problems and should be referred for additional testing. It should be kept in mind that a child with dyspraxia may be able to imitate gestures with no difficulty because of cognitive compensation; therefore, additional observations should be made on children suspected of learning problems involving praxis. The model presented by Bergès and Lézine in testing body scheme in addition to praxis appears to be a valid one and may prove useful to the children in documenting the problem. Additional tests of body scheme should supplement a test of praxis. Although dyspraxia is not treated by simply practicing the imitation of simple or complex gestures, results from the test may prove useful in determining at what level activities should be geared.

REFERENCES

1. Ayres, A. J. *Sensory Integration and Learning Disorders*. Los Angeles: Western Psychological Services, 1972.
2. Ayres, A. J. *Developmental Dyspraxia and Adult Onset Apraxia*. Torrance, Calif.: Sensory Integration International, 1985.
3. Luria, A. R. *The Working Brain*. New York: Basic Books, 1973.
4. Conrad, K. E., Cermak, S. A., and Drake, C. Differentiation of praxis among children. *Am. J. Occup. Ther.* 37 : 466, 1983.
5. Gubbay, S. *The Clumsy Child*. Philadelphia: Saunders, 1975.

JORDAN LEFT-RIGHT REVERSAL TEST

Descriptive Information

Test Identification

The title of this test is the *Jordan Left-Right Reversal Test,* Revised Edition, 1974. Its author is Brian T. Jordan, Ph.D. Jordan is a clinical psychologist and has worked extensively in the diagnosis of learning-disabled children. Academic Therapy Publications (20 Commercial Blvd., Novato, California 94947-6191) publishes the test at a cost of $10–$12 for the manual, and approximately $6–$8 for a set of 25 test sheets.

Age and Type of Client

The Jordan Left-Right Reversal Test (Jordan) is designed for 5- to 12-year-old children with minimal neurological impairment.

Purpose

The test is intended as a screening instrument for children with reading problems and learning disabilities involving reversals.

Time Required to Administer and Score Test

The Jordan can be administered individually or in groups. It takes 20 minutes to administer level 1 to an entire class of 6 through 8 year olds, although there is no time limit on the test. For children 9 through 12, the entire test can be administered to a group in about 25 minutes.

Evaluator

Teachers and other professionals qualified to test learning-disabled children can administer the Jordan. A classroom teacher may find the test useful in screening children with reversal problems. No special training is required to give the test.

Historical Perspective of Test Construction

Development and Source of Test Items

The initial version of the Jordan was published in 1972. This version focused on children from 5 through 8 years of age. The revised test extended the norms for children up through 12 years of age. The initial test measured reversals by identifying letters and numbers. Actual reading texts for use by older children were added in the revision.

Review of Literature in Terms of Test Use

Little research has been conducted on the use of the Jordan as a clinical instrument. Strichart [4] tested 91 learning-disabled children, ranging in age from 5 to 12 years, using the Jordan. The learning-disabled children were found to make more errors than all normal children in Jordan's normative sample. It was concluded that the Jordan is effective in measuring the overall tendency to make visual reversal errors and that it is an appropriate diagnostic tool. Test-retest reliability on the learning-disabled sample was .89 to .92.

A test review by Krichev [3] reported that the Jordan should be useful in diagnosis and that the test has sufficient reliability and validity, but there was limited information presented on the normative sample. Bannatyne [1] also reviewed the Jordan and felt that it was a useful diagnostic tool for learning-disabled children. Significant age and sex differences, as well as significant differences between the performance of learning-disabled and normal children, support the use of the Jordan as a valid tool.

Theoretical Constructs and Implications for Intervention

The Jordan was developed because of the prevalence of reversal problems in children with reading disabilities. The occurrence of reversals may be a result of competition between the two hemispheres without adequate suppression of the right hemisphere. Compared with normal children, visual reversals occur more frequently in children diagnosed as having reading disabilities.

Content and Test Administration

Content

Level 1 items were selected for children ranging in age from 5 through 8 years. Large-sized letters and numbers are presented in either a correct or reversed orientation. Only letters that were considered clear-cut reversals (e.g., b and d) by a panel of judges were selected. The letters and numbers are presented in large bold-faced print for easy reading. Twenty-seven letters are printed on the booklet page along with 14 numbers. Level 2 is more advanced and is intended for 9 to 12 year olds. One page lists 20 sets of five words, including some with individually reversed letters, making the word incorrect. Page 2 of Level 2 includes 20 sentences with either a noun or verb printed in reversed form (e.g., "was" instead of "saw"). The sentences are simple and are presented at a third grade reading level.

Setting and Equipment

Any classroom or office setting can be used for administering the test. Care should be taken that the alphabet or numbers are not exposed. The only materials needed are the test booklet and a pencil.

Administration Procedures

Different verbal instructions are given for ages 5, 6 through 8, and 9 through 12. Five to eight year olds should be given only level 1, while older children are given both levels 1 and 2. Verbal directions are given for each part of the test. Each child fills out the worksheet, although the test examiner may fill out the identifying information on the cover sheet for young children. The procedures are very simple.

Scoring

Guidelines for scoring are given for levels 1 and 2. The number of errors are added to obtain a total raw error score. This score is converted to a percentile score for boys and girls using Tables 8 to 11. These tables present norms for 5 through 12 year olds in 6-month intervals. Scores interpreted as abnormal fall beneath the heavy black line on the chart. The median average percentile score is marked with an asterisk.

Psychometric Properties

Standardization

The Jordan was administered within the classroom setting to over 4350 normal children ranging in age from 5 to 12 years. Children in the sample came from rural and urban areas, all socioeconomic levels, and included a 10 percent sample of nonwhite racial background. No charts are presented giving specific numbers of children in each group, and no information is given regarding the number of girls and boys in the sample. The schools were located in eight different states across the United States.

A significant correlation was found between age level and test error scores. An analysis of variance revealed that the younger children through 8 years made more number errors than letter reversals. Boys made more errors than girls. These data support the notion that girls mature faster in directionality than boys.

Reliability

A test-retest sample was completed for level 1, with 1 month between tests and equal distributions of 5 through 10 year olds. Two hundred and thirty children were retested for level 2 for ages 8 through 12, with a retest period of 2 weeks. Test-retest coefficients ranged from .87 to .98 for level 1 and from .83 to .91 for level 2.

Validity

To determine content validity, a panel of three judges selected items showing a clear reversal. To investigate whether the Jordan could discriminate between normal children and those with minimal neurological impairments, a sample of 325 children ranging in age from 6 to 12 years were selected and compared with age-matched normal children. T tests of the mean test error scores were significant between the groups at all age levels. Another sample was selected to investigate if the Jordan could discriminate between children who were below average in their grade achievement. A sample of 60 children was chosen; the children ranged in age from 9 to 12 years, with about half classified as average and the other half as below-average achievers. No criteria were presented regarding how the children received these classifications as low or average achievers. Using a Pearson product moment correlation, it was found that the Jordan scores correlated negatively with reading achievement on the Wide Range Achievement Test, while there was a positive correlation with error scores on the Bender-Gestalt [2]. As reading achievement decreases, the number of errors on the Jordan increases. Likewise, as perceptual-motor errors increase on the Bender-Gestalt, errors on the Jordan also increase. High correlations were found with reading achievement and perceptual-motor problems reaching the level of significance for all correlations except between the Bender-Gestalt and children classified as average achievers.

Guidelines for Use in a Clinical Setting

The Jordan is a quick and easy test to administer, score, and interpret. It can be administered individually and in groups to screen children ranging in age from 5 to 12 years with reversal problems.

It should be particularly useful to classroom teachers. A child who is detected as having reversal problems on the Jordan should be further tested to determine the effect of the reversals on reading ability. Since the reversals may be attributable to more underlying processing problems, a test such as the Quick Neurological Screening Test may also be administered to determine if problems in bilateral integration and other neurophysiological functions related to learning may be present. Children with positive findings on these screening instruments require more extensive diagnostic procedures to determine the nature of the learning problem and the appropriate method of remediation.

Review

The Jordan is a screening instrument designed to detect mirror image and reversal problems in children with learning disabilities and reading problems. It is useful with children ranging in age from 5 to 12 years. The test can be given individually or in groups and is quick and easy to administer. Good test-retest reliability was obtained; however, no interobserver reliability studies were conducted. There was a large normative sample, although the sample should have been further defined in terms of age, sex, race, and other factors. Likewise, subjects in the validity studies are not well-defined regarding criteria for classification as low or average achievers. The validity studies demonstrated good discrimination of performance by age and sex in the normative sample. Learning-disabled children were found to perform well below the normative sample.

The Jordan is intended to be administered in conjunction with other tests. It is primarily a reading test; therefore, results from the Jordan can assist the examiner only in determining if reversals are related to reading problems. Further assessment of other types of reversals (e.g., reversing directions or imitating postures in a mirror-image) should be completed to determine the extent and type of the reversal problem. Further research is needed in this area since none of the available tests measure reversals in other contexts. Therefore, only clinical observation can be used at this time in measures of this type. Since sensory integrative problems (i.e., poor bilateral integration and laterality) may underlie the cause of the reversals, further assessment in these areas may be needed especially if observations indicate additional laterality and directionality problems.

REFERENCES

1. Bannatyne, A. Review of the Jordan Left-Right Reversal Test. *J. Learn. Disabil.* 8 : 4, 1975.
2. Koppitz, E. M. *The Bender-Gestalt Test for Young Children.* New York: Grune & Stratton, 1964.
3. Krichev, A. Review of the Jordan Left-Right Reversal Test. *Psychol. Sch.* 13 : 240, 1976.
4. Strichart, S. S. Use of the Jordan Left-Right Reversal Test with learning disabled children. *Percept. Mot. Skills* 47 : 1291, 1978.

MOTOR-FREE VISUAL PERCEPTION TEST

Descriptive Information

Test Identification

The title of this test is *Motor-Free Perception Test* (MVPT), 1972. Its authors are Ronald P. Colarusso, Ed.D., and Donald D. Hammill, Ed.D. Both authors have doctoral degrees in education. No other background information is provided in the test manual. Academic Therapy Publications (20 Commercial Blvd., Novato, California 94947-6191) publishes this test at a cost of $8–$10 for the manual, $20–$22 for a set of test plates and $5–$7 for a set of 50 recording forms.

Age and Type of Client

The MVPT is designed for use with 4- to 8-year old children. Since the test focuses on visual perception without requiring the child to engage in a motor response, it is very useful as a screening

and diagnostic tool for children with motor impairments such as cerebral palsy. The test, of course, can be used with children with a wide variety of developmental disabilities.

Purpose

The MVPT is designed as a test of visual perceptual processing ability in children and can be used for screening, diagnostic, or research purposes.

Time Required to Administer and Score Test

The MVPT takes less than 10 minutes to administer, but it is not a timed test. The manual does not describe how much time it takes to score the test. Scoring is simple, however, and can probably be accomplished within a few minutes.

Evaluator

The MVPT was developed for use by teachers, psychologists, educators, and other professionals. No special training is required; however, when interpreting the test results, it is recommended that poor performance on the MVPT be compared with the teacher's reports of classroom performance. Although the MVPT can be administered by a nonprofessional, it is apparent that interpretation of the results must be done by a trained professional who can determine what types of remediation are required.

Historical Perspective of Test Construction

Development and Source of Items

A total of 150 test items were originally developed to test visual perception in 5, 6, and 7 year olds. Forty-five items were discarded because they were either too easy or too difficult. The preliminary form of 105 test items was then administered to 119 normal children ranging in age from 5 to 7 years. A final form of the MVPT was compiled. The 36 items on this version reflected acceptable validity and levels of difficulty. Point biserial correlation was used to identify which items correlated with the total test score. Items that had a correlation coefficient between .30 and .80 and that were statistically significant were included in the final form. In addition, items with a 15 to 90 percent level of difficulty at different age levels were considered for the final test version. A table is presented in the manual displaying the final 36 test items, their level of difficulty, and the item validity according to chronological age levels.

Review of Literature in Terms of Test Use

There have been numerous studies on the use of the MVPT with different populations. Studies have supported its use with mentally retarded children [5] and with physically handicapped children [9]. When the MVPT was correlated to findings on the Beery-Buktenica Developmental Test of Visual-Motor Integration (VMI) and The Marianne Frostig Developmental Test of Visual Perception (Frostig) with physically handicapped children, it was found that as the degree of physical handicap increased, the correlation between the MVPT and the Frostig decreased since the Frostig relies heavily on motor output. The authors found a significant difference in the motor and nonmotor perceptual ages on the normal group of children. They concluded that the MVPT was more accurate in assessing visual perception for both motorically handicapped children as well as normal children than the other two instruments.

In a study to determine if the MVPT can predict later academic performance, it was found that the MVPT significantly correlated with the composite achievement score on the Iowa Test of Basic Skills when kindergartners were tested again at the end of first grade [1]. The authors viewed this finding as indicative of the child's ability to attend, follow a progression in task approach, and organize visual and auditory information rather than a function of visual perceptual skills as tested on the MVPT. Donovan and

Mitchell [2] used the MVPT in assessing subtle deficits in kindergartners but questioned the accuracy of the decisions. They compared the MVPT with the Frostig and found both instruments to be comparable in their ability to screen problems in visual perception. A study of Hudgins [4] reports that the MVPT should be used in conjunction with other assessments, particularly the Bender Visual-Motor Gestalt Test (BVMGT) and Southern California Motor Accuracy Test when differentiating the type of visual perception or visual-motor integration problem in 6 and 7 year olds.

In a review of the MVPT, Krichev [6] supports the use of the test as a quick, reliable, and valid instrument of overall visual processing functions. Rosen [8], on the other hand, criticizes the MVPT because of inadequate evidence substantiating its validity. He states that no clear rationale is presented for why a "motor-free" test of visual perception is needed. Correlational studies of the MVPT and tests of visual-motor functions cannot be supported because of lack of comparability between samples in the studies. He also points out that errors of classification are probable using the authors' recommendation for the perceptual quotient of 85 or less since this criterion is not substantiated by the data. He concludes that the MVPT should not be used in its current form because of inadequate validity.

Theoretical Constructs and Implications for Intervention

The authors categorized visual perception into five types—spatial relationships, visual discrimination, figure-ground, visual closure, and visual memory—based on a review of the literature. Each of these types of visual perception is defined in the introduction, and other researchers examining those particular areas are cited. The rationale for the development of the MVPT is described as attempting to isolate visual perception as a discrete skill. Most tests purported to measure visual perception typically require the child to engage in a motor response such as drawing a circle, consequently confounding visual perception with visual-motor integration. A child with a motor handicap would be penalized in visual perception because of poor performance in the motor domain. Another rationale for development of the MVPT is that many of the instruments available are costly, have poor reliability, lack adequate standardization, and take a long time to administer and are therefore not good instruments for use in research.

Content and Test Administration

Content

The test contains items that measure the areas of spatial relationships, visual discrimination, figure-ground, visual closure, and visual memory. The first eight items are designed to measure visual discrimination. In these items the child points to one of four figures to match or find the stimulus figure among the four options. Items nine through thirteen measure form constancy, which is measured by having the child find the stimulus figure among the four options. The stimulus figure is presented in the choices as a different size, rotated in space with a different spatial orientation, or presented darker in outline or embedded in a design. For items 14 to 21, the child sees the stimulus figure for 5 seconds; then the page is turned and the child finds it on the next page to test visual memory. Items 22 to 32 test visual closure by presenting a complete figure, then requiring the child to find which one of the figures composed of dashed lines would make the completed figure if filled in. The last four items measure spatial relationships and require the child to find the one figure that is different from the others. All of the test items are presented in a separate booklet.

Setting and Equipment

No information is offered in the manual regarding physical setting for the test. No equipment is needed except the booklet of test plates, a score sheet, and the test manual.

Administration Procedures

Standardized verbal directions are given along with procedures for each section of items. The examiner scores the subject's responses by checking the appropriate space on the score sheet. The directions for the MVPT are easy to follow.

Scoring

Scores are recorded on the score sheet by marking the child's choice in the appropriate box. A total score is obtained by adding all of the raw scores for each section. Table 7 in the manual presents the perceptual age for each accompanying raw score. Scores of greater than 10 may be interpreted with confidence, whereas a score lower than 10 may be due to chance or other factors affecting performance such as mental retardation. Children with perceptual quotients of less than 85 are considered to have a significant visual perceptual problem.

Psychometric Properties

Standardization

The MVPT was standardized on 881 normal children ranging in age from 4 through 8 years of age in a sample across 22 states. Children with handicaps were excluded from the norming sample. No demographic data are given regarding breakdowns by age, sex, geographic location, race or socioeconomic levels. The manual states that the data pool included samples from all races and socioeconomic levels.

No differences were found between sexes and geographic areas; therefore, data are presented according to age level only. Normative information is provided in terms of perceptual ages and perceptual quotients.

Reliability

Test-retest, split-half, and Kuder-Richardson reliability procedures were performed on the MVPT. For the test-retest reliability, 162 children were retested 20 days after the first test. Coefficients ranged from .77 to .83 across the different age levels with an overall reliability of .81 for the total sample. Split-half reliability coefficients ranged from .81 to .84 at various age levels with .88 for the total sample. Interitem consistency of the test was examined using the Kuder-Richardson formula. Correlation coefficients were .71 to .82, with a total value of .86. The authors state that there were comparatively few 4 year olds in the sample; therefore, they urge that caution be used when interpreting results of 4 year olds.

Validity

Construct validity was examined in several ways. Forty subjects were randomly selected from the 5, 6, and 7 year age levels, and their scores were subjected to an analysis of variance procedure. *F* scores were significant at the .01 level. The authors report that "moderately high" correlations ranging from .31 to .73, with a median of .49, were obtained between the MVPT and the Frostig Developmental Test of Visual Perception and the Copying and Matching Subtests from the Metropolitan Readiness Tests [3]. A median of .49, however, implies that the tests are not measuring the same construct. Lower correlations with medians of .38 and .31 were found between the MVPT and various achievement and intelligence tests, which would support the fact that the MVPT is measuring a different function. One problem is that in comparing these different studies, the subjects are not comparable, which must be kept in mind when interpreting these findings. The internal consistency of the MVPT was ensured through item analysis and selection of items based on item difficulty and biserial correlations between items and total test scores.

Newcomer and Hammill [7] administered the MVPT and the BVMGT to 85 motor-impaired children. They found that the performance on the MVPT was independent of the degree of motor involvement, whereas performance on the BVMGT reflected the degree of motor involvement.

Guidelines for Use in a Clinical Setting

The MVPT is a test of visual perception that should prove useful in the assessment of both motor-impaired children who exhibit visual perception problems and learning-disabled children. The test directions require only that the child point. If a child is unable to point, as in the case of a severely handicapped cerebral-palsied child, further adaptations may be possible with a head pointer, mouth stick, eye gaze, or by having the examiner point and the child respond with a consistent "yes" or "no" gesture (e.g., eye blink). Scores of 10 or greater can be interpreted with confidence. Scores lower than 10 may be due to chance or other factors (e.g., mental retardation). In such a case, further testing may be needed to determine if a visual perceptual problem is present. It is also important to delineate whether the child has a deficit in visual perception alone or if it is coupled with a visual-motor integration problem. This distinction is particularly useful with learning-disabled children; however, motor-impaired children will score low on a visual-motor integration test due to the nature of their handicap. Therefore, it may not be possible to identify a visual-motor integration problem with the cerebral palsy population because of this factor.

Review

The MVPT is a test of visual perception for 4 to 8 year olds that can be used for either screening or diagnosis. It is very simple to administer and score and is a practical instrument for use in schools. The test is well standardized, and test-retest reliability studies are good although there were few 4 year olds in the authors' sample. The authors stress that caution should be taken when interpreting the scores of 4 year olds. Further studies are required to determine interobserver reliability and decision-consistency reliability. Several validity studies have demonstrated the usefulness of the MVPT with mentally retarded and physically handicapped children, although children with subtle visual perceptual deficits may not necessarily be accurately detected. It appears that a child may be more accurately classified as normal on the MVPT than as delayed; therefore, other instruments of visual perception should be used to substantiate and delineate the type of visual perception problem if one is suspected in a child, especially if the child is learning disabled.

REFERENCES

1. Colarusso, R., et al. Predicting first-grade achievement through formal testing of 5-year-old high-risk children. *J. Spec. Ed.* 14 : 355, 1980.
2. Donovan, G., and Mitchell, M. M. Analysis of the Developmental Test of Visual Perception and the Motor-Free Visual Perception Test. *Percept. Mot. Skills* 46 : 1284, 1978.
3. Hildreth, G. H., Griffiths, N. L., and McGauvran, M. E. *Metropolitan Readiness Tests (Revised Edition).* New York: Harcourt, Brace & World, 1965.
4. Hudgins, A. L. Assessment of visual-motor disabilities in young children: Toward differential diagnosis. *Psychol. Sch.* 14 : 252, 1977.
5. Johnson, D. L., Brekke, B., and Harlow, S. Appropriateness of the Motor-Free Visual Perception Test when used with the mentally retarded. *Ed. Training Ment. Retard.* 12 : 312, 1977.
6. Krichev, A. Review of the Motor-Free Visual Perception Test. *Psych. Sch.* 13 : 365, 1976.
7. Newcomer, P., and Hammill, D. Visual perception of motor-impaired children: Implications for assessment. *Except. Child.* 39 : 335, 1973.
8. Rosen, C. L. Review of the Motor-Free Visual Perception Test. In O. K. Buros (ed.), *The Eighth Mental Measurements Yearbook (Vol. 2).* Highland Park, N.J.: Gryphon Press, 1978. P. 883.
9. Zeitschel, K. A., Kalish, R. A., and Colarusso, R. Visual perception tests used with physically handicapped children. *Acad. Ther.* 14 : 565, 1979.

PEABODY DEVELOPMENTAL MOTOR SCALES

Descriptive Information

Test Identification

The title of this test is *Peabody Developmental Motor Scales (Revised Experimental Edition)*, 1983. Its authors are M. Rhonda Folio, Ed.D., and Rebecca R. Fewell, Ph.D. Both authors' backgrounds are in education and physical education of children with special needs.

DLM Teaching Resources (P.O. Box 4000, One DLM Park, Allen, Texas 75002) publishes this test. The test kit costs $175–$200 and includes 15 copies of the Response/Scoring Booklet. The package includes activity cards designed to be used in programming of motor skills measured by the scales. Additional booklets are available at $20–$25 per package of 15.

Age and Type of Client

The Peabody Developmental Motor Scales (PDMS) is intended to be used with children ranging in age from birth to 7 years who are delayed in motor abilities or who exhibit motor handicaps.

Purpose

The PDMS was designed to measure gross and fine motor skills in infants and children with motor delays. The test items are designed in such a way that fine and gross motor skills that the child has mastered, that are emerging, and that are not in his or her repertoire can be evaluated. A program of activities for use in teaching each skill is included in the PDMS.

Time Required to Administer and Score Test

The fine and gross motor scales can each be administered in 20 to 30 minutes, with a total time of 40 to 60 minutes for both scales. The test can be administered in a group for children over 4 years of age.

Evaluator

No special training or background is required to administer the Peabody Scales; however, the authors recommend familiarity with the administration and scoring of the items and practice on at least three children. Occupational and physical therapists, special educators, motor development specialists, adaptive physical education teachers, and teachers are professionals who would most likely use the PDMS.

Historical Perspective of Test Construction

Development and Source of Test Items

The Peabody Scales were developed based on the Revised Experimental Edition of the PDMS [3]. Many of the items from the original test remained the same, although some were modified and new items were included. Test items on the PDMS were developed based on a number of infant intelligence tests and developmental scales. Some of the tests used to develop scale items include the Bayley Scales of Infant Development, The Measurement of Intelligence of Infants and Young Children (Cattell), the Denver Developmental Screening Test, and the Lincoln-Oseretsky Motor Development Scale. Other reference books on development that were also used to develop test items are cited.

Review of Literature in Terms of Test Use

The PDMS is useful in evaluating children up through 7 years of age in gross and fine motor skills. The authors state that the PDMS is appropriate for both normal and handicapped children. Because scores are interpreted in a number of ways, the PDMS is useful in screening children, evaluating fine and gross motor abilities,

reevaluating children to determine progress or to measure progress as a result of specific treatment interventions, and also for research such as comparing performance in motor development to other skill areas. Palisano and Lydic [6] in their review of the PDMS state that the PDMS seems particularly useful for older infants and children suspected of having motor delays and those with known motor impairments.

Theoretical Constructs and Implications for Intervention

Test items that focused on the child's ability to adapt to various situations were selected. Some of the items for older children emphasize body image, since this is reported by the authors to be an important factor in movement efficiency. The test items are designed to measure the degree to which a skill has been developed. Developmental activities can be prescribed using the PDMS based on performance on the test items.

Content and Test Administration

Content

The PDMS contains a test manual, response and scoring booklets, and a package of activity cards that can be used to program motor behaviors measured by the scales. Test items are listed by age levels and represent behaviors common to other motor development scales. There are 170 test items for the Gross Motor Scale, with 10 different skills for each age range. The age levels are at 2-month intervals up to 1 year of age, 3-month intervals up to 17 months, 6-month intervals up to 59 months, and 12-month intervals up to 83 months (7 years). The Gross Motor Scale measures skills in the areas of reflexes, balance, non-locomotion, locomotion, and receipt and propulsion of objects (ball skills).

The Fine Motor Scale includes 112 test items with six to eight test items for every age range. Intervals for the different age ranges correspond to those on the Gross Motor Scale. The Fine Motor

Scale consists of four areas: grasping, hand use, eye-hand coordination, and manual dexterity.

All test items are presented in a chart format. Items are arranged sequentially by age interval. Directions and scoring are presented next to the items in the manual.

Setting and Equipment

The PDMS should be administered in a distraction-free room. A space large enough for gross motor activities such as riding a tricycle and running is needed as well as a set of stairs. The test kit includes about half of the materials needed. The examiner must provide a stopwatch, balance beam, balls, tricycle, markers, scissors, paper, and several other specified toys.

Administration Procedures

Administration procedures are given for each test item, including the child's body position, materials needed, directions for administering the item, and scoring criteria. Some items account for quality of performance such as in the item "copies triangle," the child must use "good form, sides closed, lines straight." Other items, however, do not differentiate varying degrees of performance in what constitutes a pass. For instance, for "ties shoelaces," the child must tie them correctly but there is no mention of the quality of the execution of the skill. This particular item might be measuring motor planning rather than the ability to combine motor planning with fine dexterity control and strength. In the gross motor items, scoring for qualitative performance is not well-defined on many items. For instance, for the item "hops on one foot," it is not described whether the child should hop across the room or remain in the same place. The child passes this item if he or she completes 10 to 12 steps (4½ to 5 year item). A child may pass the item but display excessive movement of the trunk and arms, performance which would differ considerably from the child who keeps the

trunk and arms fairly quiet while hopping either in a small boxed area or along a straight line.

The test items are administered either by observing the child or by directly administering the test items to the child. Items may be scored by parental or teacher report. The test items are easy to administer, and directions and scoring criteria are presented in one sentence in most cases. It is recommended that items be administered at a level slightly below the child's expected motor level in order to instill confidence in the child. Demonstration is not permitted for some items (e.g., placing shapes in formboard); thus, the child must be able to understand simple directions or understand the perceptual process underlying the task. Suggestions are given on how to modify the administration procedure for handicapped children who cannot be given the standardized version.

Scoring

Each item is scored according to a 3-point scale which reflects the degree to which the skill has developed. For instance, a score of 0 is given for unsuccessful performance; 1 for clear resemblance to item criterion but criterion not fully met; and 2 for successful performance, criterion met. Scoring criteria are presented in a behavioral objective format. The scoring criteria, however, do not account for quality of performance. A child may receive a score of 2 but perform the task abnormally. There may also be wide variation in how two examiners would score a "1" performance.

A basal and ceiling are obtained for the fine motor and gross motor scales and for each skill category within the scale. The raw score can be converted into an age-equivalent score, a developmental motor quotient, a percentile ranking, or a standardized Z or T score. Raw scores can also be converted into scaled scores, which are useful for handicapped children in detecting small changes in progress rather than using an age-equivalent score.

Psychometric Properties

Standardization

The PDMS was standardized using a stratified quota sampling procedure, which was used to select a representative sample of the United States population. The sample included children from 20 states (representing the different geographic regions) and was stratified for age and sex. The racial distribution was 85.1 percent Caucasian, 7.3 percent black, and 7.6 percent Hispanic. The majority of children came from middle socioeconomic status (SES), but the sample also included subjects from high and low SES. In addition, the communities were selected to reflect rural-urban characteristics necessary for stratified sampling.

The PDMS was administered to 617 children ranging in age from 0 to 83 months. There were 27 to 33 children in each age group up to 23 months, 46 to 55 children from 24 to 48 months and 60 to 83 months, and 25 children for the 48 to 59 month age groups. Most children were tested in their homes. Thirty-three examiners participated in the data collection.

Reliability

Test-retest reliability studies were conducted on 38 children who were tested twice within a 1-week span. The reliability coefficient for the Gross Motor Scale was .95, and for the Fine Motor Scale, .80. Interrater reliability was obtained on 36 children by having one tester score and administer the test while another person simultaneously scored the items. Interrater reliability was .97 for the Gross Motor Scale and .94 for the Fine Motor Scale. This latter type of reliability indicates that the PDMS can be scored with high reliability by two examiners observing the same child and reflects agreement. However, it does not tell us that two examiners will administer the PDMS on two different occasions in the same manner and obtain the same results. Therefore, interobserver reliability studies are needed.

Validity

Three types of validity were examined on the PDMS: content, construct, and concurrent. Content validity was established by selecting test items from research on normal motor development and from validated motor development tests. Construct validity was determined by testing the significance of improvement in scores as a function of age. Statistically significant gains were obtained for all age levels for both Fine Motor and Gross Motor Scales, except for the 54 to 59 month age level on the Gross Motor Scale. This supports the theory of increasing refinements in motor development as one gets older.

To examine concurrent validity, 104 children with developmental motor problems were tested and their mean standardized scores compared with their normal counterparts. The standardized scores were significantly lower than scores obtained on normal subjects except for the 0 to 5 month age group. Forty-three children were tested on both the PDMS and the Bayley Motor and Mental Scales. The Gross Motor Scale scores and the scores on the balance, nonlocomotion, and locomotion skill categories on the Gross Motor Scale significantly correlated with the Bayley Motor Scale scores. The correlation between the Bayley Mental Scale and the PDMS Gross Motor Scale was nonsignificant; however, significant correlations were obtained between the Bayley Mental and Motor Scale and the PDMS Fine Motor Scale. Also, all four of the Fine Motor Scale categories showed a high correlation with the Bayley Motor and Mental Scales. These high correlations validate the content of the test items on the PDMS.

In addition to the validity studies described in the manual, a study was conducted by Harris and colleagues [4] examining the relationship between the PDMS (1974 version), the Assessment of Sensorimotor Integration in Preschool Children [2] and the Tactile Sensitivity Checklist developed by Bauer [1]. They found a significant correlation between scores on the sensorimotor integration assessment and the PDMS for the sample of 61 preschool children (12 normal and 49 with mild developmental delays). Correlations were not conducted between the PDMS and the Tactile Sensitivity Checklist. Since DeGangi's assessment was designed to assess vestibular-based functions, the results of this study suggest a relationship between fine and gross motor skills and this particular domain of sensory integration behaviors.

Guidelines for Use in a Clinical Setting

Not only can the PDMS be used in assessing fine and gross motor skills, but the test is useful as well in reevaluation of skills, in determining progress in motor behaviors, and as a research instrument. The authors of the PDMS also attempt to bridge the gap between assessment and intervention by providing a set of activity cards to accompany the manual. For every item tested in the motor scales, there are several developmental activities presented that can be used to facilitate the development of that particular skill. The activities are geared toward improving perceptual-motor performance and are presented in such a way that a parent or teacher could understand the various developmental activities. A major problem with the activity cards is that they do not account for the various types of motor handicaps. In addition, the rationale for the intervention strategies developed are not described. Palisano and Lydic [6] in their critique of the PDMS state that the activity cards may promote the use of teaching specific motor skills rather than the skills underlying their development. Montgomery and Richter [5] in their study have documented the importance of focusing on sensory integrative skills underlying the development of fine and gross motor skills rather than the specific skill itself.

Review

The PDMS provides a standardized format for testing fine and gross motor skills in children up to 7 years of age. It can be used for screening children and for testing children with a variety of developmental disabilities who fall developmentally between 0 and 7 years of age in their motor skills. The scoring criteria account for the emergence of skills; however, they do not allow for scoring of qualitative performance in many items. Some children may pass the various items, testing as normal in their fine and gross motor skills. They may demonstrate many qualitative findings, however, that would alert a trained occupational or physical therapist that the child may be at risk for perceptual and/or motor dysfunction. The PDMS, therefore, should be administered in conjunction with other instruments designed to detect qualitative performance (e.g., the DeGangi-Berk Test of Sensory Integration, the Miller Assessment for Preschoolers, or the Quick Neurological Screening Test). Test-retest reliability and interrater agreement correlations were good on the studies conducted on normal children only. They also did not include interobserver reliability studies (two different examiners administering the test on two different occasions). These studies are important since interpretation of what constitutes a score of "1" may vary among examiners. Interobserver and test-retest reliability studies are also needed on children with motor impairments. The validity studies with the Bayley Scales and the Assessment of Sensorimotor Integration in Preschool Children show significant correlations with the PDMS. Additional validity studies should be conducted on how children with various handicaps perform on the PDMS in comparison to normals. Since few motor development tests have been normed for 3 to 7 year olds, the PDMS provides a unique contribution to motor assessments. Caution should be placed on the exclusive use of the developmental activity cards, since they may promote the development of splinter motor skills.

REFERENCES

1. Bauer, B. A. Tactile sensitivity: Development of a behavioral responses checklist. *Am. J. Occup. Ther.* 31 : 357, 1977.

2. DeGangi, D. *Assessment of Sensorimotor Integration in Preschool Children*. Baltimore: Johns Hopkins University, 1979.

3. Folio, R., and Dubose, R. F. *Peabody Developmental Motor Scales (Revised Experimental Edition)*. Nashville, Tenn.: George Peabody College for Teachers, 1974.

4. Harris, S. R., et al. The relationship between tests of sensorimotor integration, tactile sensitivity, and gross motor skills in normal and developmentally delayed preschool children. *Phys. Occup. Ther. Pediatr.* 4 : 5, 1984.

5. Montgomery, P., and Richter, E. Effect of sensory integrative therapy on the neuromotor development of retarded children. *Phys. Ther.* 57 : 799, 1977.

6. Palisano, R. J., and Lydic, J. S. The Peabody Developmental Motor Scales: An analysis. *Phys. Occup. Ther. Pediatr.* 4 : 69, 1984.

THE PURDUE PERCEPTUAL-MOTOR SURVEY

Descriptive Information

Test Identification

The title of this test is *The Purdue Perceptual-Motor Survey* (PPMS), 1966. Its authors are Eugene G. Roach, M.D., and Newell C. Kephart, Ph.D. Kephart has worked extensively in the field of learning disabilities, with particular emphasis on perceptual-motor functions. He was on the faculty at Purdue University, Department of Psychology, at the time the PPMS was developed. Roach is on the faculty in the Department of Psychiatry and Medical Genetics at Indiana University and at Purdue University. Charles E. Merrill Publishing Co. (1300 Alum Creek Dr., Columbus, Ohio 43216) publishes the survey at a cost of $15–$17 per manual and set of cards; and $17–$19 per 25 score forms.

Age and Type of Client

The items in the test are designed primarily for 6 to 10 year olds and are meant to be used with children exhibiting perceptual-motor delays, slow learning, or learning disabilities. The authors stress that the PPMS is not designed for

children who have specific sensory and motor deficits such as cerebral palsy or blindness.

Purpose

The PPMS is not an assessment tool but rather a survey that can be used to make qualitative observations about a child's performance on perceptual-motor tasks and that can be helpful in designing remediation activities.

Time Required to Administer and Score Test

The time required to administer and score the PPMS is not given in the manual, but it probably would take about 30 to 45 minutes to administer and score the observations.

Evaluator

The PPMS is designed for use by classroom teachers and special educators. The scoring criteria are purposely simple so that only a minimum of training using the test manual is necessary to use the survey.

Historical Perspective of Test Construction

Development and Source of Items

Many of the test items were developed as the result of experiences of the authors with retarded children and slow learners and are similar to tasks presented in *The Slow Learner in the Classroom* [3]. No other information about development of the survey was available.

Review of Literature in Terms of Test Use

Several factor analytic studies have been conducted on the Purdue. Both Neeman [6] and Geddes [1] identified nine factors measured by the PPMS. Geddes compared the PPMS with the Perceptual-Motor Attributes of Mentally Retarded Children and Youth Battery developed by

Cratty in 1966 on 80 first and second graders. Geddes found the individual test items on the PPMS to be measuring distinct perceptual-motor tasks. In another study by Neeman [5], four neurological dysfunction patterns were hypothesized in mentally retarded children based on their performance on the PPMS. These dysfunction patterns included problems with posture, shoulder-arm movement, laterality, and ocular-motor control.

Theoretical Constructs and Implications for Intervention

The PPMS is based on the perceptual-motor theory that learning occurs sequentially in stages beginning with generalized movement, which leads to differentiation and refinement of motor responses. More complex perceptual-motor skills develop as a result of interaction of sensory perception with movement patterns. The perceptual skills that develop next are described by the authors as laterality, form perception, directionality, and concept formation. An entire chapter of the manual is dedicated to elaborating on the rationale and development of the survey. In addition, the book *The Slow Learner in the Classroom* by Kephart [3] provides more information of the importance of early motor learning and perceptual concepts on academic learning.

Content and Test Administration

Content

The 22 scorable items on the PPMS are divided into the categories of Balance and Posture, Body Image and Differentiation, Perceptual-Motor Match, Ocular Control, and Form Perception. A checklist of observations is also included for each item. The categories and the items in each category are as follows:

1. Balance and Posture: walking forward, back, and sideways on a walking board, jumping on both feet and one foot, skipping, and hopping

2. Body Image and Differentiation: identification of body parts, imitation of arm postures, maneuvering through an obstacle course, assuming the prone extension posture (Kraus-Weber) in parts (lift chest and lift legs separately), and performing variations of the angels-in-the-snow pattern

3. Perceptual-Motor Match: drawing large circles and lines on a chalkboard (Fig. 6-5) and rhythmic writing patterns including both geometric shapes and letters such as 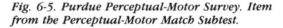 and

4. Ocular Control: ocular pursuits and convergence of the eyes

5. Form Perception: design copying of seven geometric forms and organization of the drawings on the page

Setting and Equipment

No specific setting is described in the manual. Equipment is listed with the procedures for each item. Cards for the form perception items come with the manual. Other required equipment must be obtained by the evaluator, including a walking board, a broom handle, a small pillow and mat, a large chalkboard and two pieces of chalk, a penlight and occluder, and paper and pencils.

Fig. 6-5. Purdue Perceptual-Motor Survey. Item from the Perceptual-Motor Match Subtest.

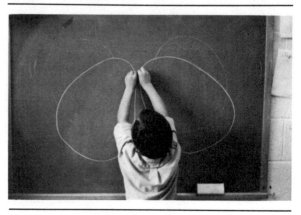

Administration Procedures

In the chapter on administration and scoring, a rationale for including the test items as they relate to perceptual-motor development is presented along with the purpose of each task, specific instructions for administering the items, materials required, and behaviors that should be observed and recorded. There are verbal instructions with each item, and the procedures are very specific.

Scoring

Scoring is fairly elaborate and requires much practice and use to become adept at the scoring criteria for each item. The score sheet lists several observations that can be checked for each item; however, these observations do not easily transfer to the scoring criteria given in the manual. An examiner inexperienced in the use of the PPMS may be quite slow in administering the survey because of the elaborate scoring method. Also, since the scoring criteria are presented within the manual, it becomes somewhat cumbersome to read the directions and find the scoring section while also administering the test and scoring on the score sheet.

Scoring ranges from 1 to 4 points for all items, with the best response a 4. Gradations in performance are considered in all test items, and the scoring criteria take into account the types of difficulties observed in learning-disabled children when performing these types of tasks.

Few guidelines are presented for interpreting test scores. A cutoff score of 65 separated the achievers from the nonachievers, with 15 percent of the nonachievers scoring above this cutoff and 17 percent of the achievers scoring below this score. No further information was given regarding how this cutoff score was derived. The authors caution that this cutoff score should not be used as a criterion for selecting or rejecting children for remedial programs.

Psychometric Properties

Standardization

The PPMS is a criterion-referenced test and was validated on a sample of children. All children in the sample were rated by their classroom teacher in academic performance on a 1 to 5 scale. Nonachievers were given a rating of 1, indicating performance on achievement tests at least 1 year below their current classroom placement. The normal achievers received ratings from 2 (low average) to 5 (superior). The PPMS was administered to a wide range of normal achievers in the early elementary grades to determine if a relationship exists between perceptual-motor skills and academic performance. Two hundred children in Lafayette, Indiana, were used as the normative sample, with 50 students in each grade level, first through fourth. Another sample of 97 nonachievers were matched for grade level and age with the normative group. This sample consisted of 25 children in the first, second, and third grade groups and 22 in the fourth grade group. None of the nonachievers were known to be retarded. No descriptive information or table was given to present the breakdown of the two samples by age, sex, race, and socioeconomic status.

Reliability

Although it is reported in the manual that test-retest stability was examined, two different examiners tested the children rather than the same examiner on two separate occasions; therefore, interobserver reliability was the type of reliability that was really accomplished. Thirty children were randomly selected from the normative sample so that all grades were represented. Retests were completed 1 week after the initial test. A comparison of the two scores yielded a reliability coefficient of .946. Although the manual states that this coefficient represents both a measure of stability of the scoring criteria and the stability between examiners, it is in fact a measure only of the latter. No information is given regarding the training and experience of the examiners. Also, the reliability coefficient was determined only for scores on the entire survey and was not determined for the checklist of observations presented within each of the categories. Jamison [2], in her review of the PPMS, questions the high reliability reported in the manual because the scoring criteria are not specific enough to yield such a high coefficient. She speculates that the examiners may have had extensive training.

Validity

Data from the normative sample were analyzed with respect to grade level, socioeconomic status, and sex. The means and standard deviations for each item are presented in Table 1 in the manual. The overall performance of the normative sample was fairly homogeneous from grades 1 through 4, with the exception of five of the test items which showed a significant difference in scores between age levels. The items showing significant differences included the walking board: backward; chalkboard: circles; chalkboard: lines, lateral; Kraus-Weber; and angels-in-the-snow. Of these five items, the walking board and two chalkboard items had larger mean squares for first graders, which accounted for the significant results. No difference in skill level was present in these three items from grades 2 through 4. It can be said then that only the Kraus-Weber and angels-in-the-snow showed developmental trends across grade levels. In addition to this analysis by items, there were significant differences between the performance of children of office workers versus skilled labor but not between any of the other socioeconomic groups, particularly between low- and high-income groups. There were no differences between the scores of males and females.

Items were validated by assigning a "fail" to scores of 1 and 2 and a "pass" to scores of 3 and 4. Differences between the nonachievers and achievers using this criteria of "pass" and "fail" were significant using chi-square analysis for all items with values at the .05 level of significance, except the developmental drawing: organization item which was nonsignificant. Jamison [2] criticizes these findings because the grade level of the children was ignored in the analysis. Intercorrelations between the subtests were .40 or below, with the exception of the chalkboard and rhythmic writing items which correlated at .48. These results indicate a small but definite relationship between the subtests. To examine concurrent validity, teachers rated each child's performance as ranging from a nonachiever, low average, up through superior performance in the classroom on a 5-point scale. These ratings were correlated with the total test score on the PPMS, which yielded a coefficient of .654. This value represents a substantial relationship and implies that results on the Purdue may reflect classroom performance. No other tests were used to examine whether performance on the PPMS correlated with the other measures of academic performance.

In a review of the PPMS, Landis [4] views the successful discrimination of items between groups of achievers and nonachievers (with exception of one item), and the high total test correlation with teacher ratings as evidence of good validity of the instrument. On the other hand, Jamison [2] describes the abilities tested by the survey as overlapping, unrelated to academic success (e.g., Kraus-Weber item), and poorly assessed. She concludes that the validity of the PPMS is inadequate.

Guidelines for Use in a Clinical Setting

The PPMS should be used primarily with children who exhibit learning problems or are considered to be nonachievers. The PPMS may also be useful with mentally retarded children [5]. No particular adaptations are discussed in the manual for administering the PPMS to children with different types of handicaps.

The clinical observations obtained from administering the PPMS may be very useful to the teacher in observing qualitative responses to different perceptual-motor tasks. The clinician should place weight only on his or her observations of specific behaviors during the entire survey rather than on the checklist of behaviors presented on the score sheet, since these additional observations were not included in the reliability study.

It should be stressed that the PPMS is only a survey and not a measurement tool. No diagnostic decisions should be made based on results from the PPMS; however, use of this test may be helpful in delineating which areas the child is having difficulty with in the perceptual-motor domain and as a form for clinical observations for the experienced therapist. The PPMS may also be of use in designing appropriate activities for a perceptual-motor program. Further studies are necessary before confidence is placed in the usefulness of the PPMS as an instrument to document progress over time.

Review

The PPMS presents a survey of perceptual-motor skills that may be useful to teachers and clinicians in observing qualitative behaviors on a group of perceptual-motor tasks with slow learners or learning-disabled children who range in age from 6 to 10 years. The PPMS should not be used for diagnostic or screening purposes since it does not present a comprehensive validation model of cutoff scores for accurate decision making. It also does not present adequate guidelines for interpretation of results, and no training programs are suggested or available in regard to learning to administer and score the survey. Although the survey may be helpful in designing perceptual-motor tasks for the individual child, the examiner must rely heavily on his or her own clinical judgment in determining specific areas of need.

Further studies are required (1) to determine if the content areas examined in the survey are representative of the domain of perceptual-motor skills, (2) to determine if the observations on the scoresheet are comprehensive and depict the types of behaviors typically seen in this population of children, and (3) to examine if the PPMS correlates with other measures of perceptual and academic performance. Test-retest stability and interobserver reliability studies are also necessary on children who exhibit learning difficulties. The interobserver reliability study focused only on normal children who did not display the many behaviors that would occur in the population of slow learners, for whom the test was designed. The selection of test items focuses on the importance of laterality, form perception, and directionality. However, many of the items rely heavily on motor planning and bilateral motor coordination, factors not discussed in the manual. Further investigation of what the items actually measure is needed. In view of the numerous weaknesses identified in this tool, the clinician or educator may choose other assessments that are better developed and researched.

REFERENCES

1. Geddes, D. Factor analytic study of perceptual-motor attributes as measured by two test batteries. *Percept. Mot. Skills* 34 : 227, 1972.
2. Jamison, C. B. Review of the PPMS. In O. K. Buros (ed.), *Seventh Mental Measurements Yearbook (Vol. 2)*. Highland Park, N.J.: Gryphon Press, 1972. P. 874.
3. Kephart, N. C. *The Slow Learner in the Classroom* (2nd ed). Columbus, Oh.: Merrill, 1971.
4. Landis, D. Review of the PPMS. In O. K. Buros (ed.), *Seventh Mental Measurements Yearbook (Vol. 2)*. Highland Park, N.J.: Gryphon Press, 1972. P. 874.
5. Neeman, R. L. Perceptual-motor attributes of mental retardates: A factor analytic study. *Percept. Mot. Skills* 33 : 927, 1971.
6. Neeman, R. L. Perceptual-motor attributes of normal school children: A factor analytic study. *Percept. Mot. Skills* 34 : 471, 1972.

QUICK NEUROLOGICAL SCREENING TEST

Descriptive Information

The title of this test is *Quick Neurological Screening Test* (QNST), Revised Edition, 1978. Its authors are Margaret Mutti, M.A., Harold M. Sterling, M.D., and Norma V. Spalding, Ed.D. Mutti is an educational psychologist, therapist, and clinical director of the Lafayette Family Counseling Services in Lafayette, California. Sterling is a physician in Physical Medicine and Rehabilitation at the University of California, School of Medicine, and Spalding is an associate professor of special education at San Jose State University. Western Psychological Services (12031 Wilshire Blvd., Los Angeles, California 90025) publishes this test at a cost of $28–$35 for the kit, $8–$12 for a set of 25 scoring sheets, and $3–$5 for 25 geometric form reproduction sheets.

Age and Type of Client

The QNST is a series of 15 observed tasks that can be administered to children as young as 5 years of age who are suspected of having learning disabilities. The instrument has been found to be effective in screening adolescents and adults.

Purpose

The QNST is intended as a screening device for early detection of children with learning disabilities. It taps neurological integration as it relates to learning. Children exhibiting definite problems on the QNST should be referred for further diagnostic testing.

Time Required to Administer and Score Test

The QNST takes approximately 20 minutes to administer and score.

Evaluator

The QNST should be administered by trained psychologists and other school personnel. The tasks in this test are easy to master, and no special training is required. It is stressed, however, that a competent tester must be a careful observer. Adequate practice is needed for effective administration, and it is recommended that an examiner practice 25 tests before administering the QNST alone. Until the examiner is proficient, it is recommended that two persons administer the test together, one administering the items while the other observes and records. A videotape demonstrating the test is available for rental from the Special Education Dept., San Jose State University, San Jose, California 95192.

Historical Perspective of Test Construction

Development and Source of Items

The tasks involved in the QNST are adapted from a pediatric neurological examination and from neuropsychological and developmental scales.

Review of Literature in Terms of Test Use

Since the QNST is a recent test, there is little research data available. Sterling and Sterling [2] compared the results from the QNST with a neurological examination administered by a physician and found 96 percent agreement between the two testing methods. Ingolia and colleagues [1] tested forty-three 6- to 8-year-old boys with learning disabilities and choreoathetoid movements and found that the learning-disabled boys performed lower than normal subjects on six selected items on the QNST thought to be affected by choreoathetoid movements.

Theoretical Constructs and Implications for Intervention

The need for this instrument is based on the prevalence of research relating neurological stability to learning achievement. Each item on the QNST is designed to reflect educational implications. An entire section of the manual is devoted to describing each test item and the relevance of adequate performance in that area for efficient learning and classroom performance. Clinical implications of the various neurological signs are discussed in detail. The QNST provides the examiner with a systematic set of observations that reveal how the child integrates various sensory inputs, how he or she controls muscles, and how he or she organizes motion in time and space.

Content and Administration

Content

The QNST consists of 15 tasks that test the child's motor maturity, fine and gross muscle control, motor planning, spatial organization, visual and auditory perception, and balance. Behavioral observations are also noted regarding anxiety, tactile defensiveness, and attentiveness. The test items include the following:

1. Hand skill: The child writes his or her name on the test form.
2. Figure recognition and production: The child names and copies five geometric forms.
3. Palm form recognition: The child identifies numbers drawn on the palm.
4. Eye tracking of a moving object.
5. Sound patterns: The child reproduces a rhythm tapped out by the examiner.
6. Finger to nose: The child alternates between touching the examiner's finger and his or her own nose with eyes open, then closed (Fig. 6-6).
7. Thumb and finger circle: This is a sequence of touching the thumb to each finger, forming a circle shape with the thumb and finger.
8. Double simultaneous stimulation of hand and cheek: The hand and cheek are touched simultaneously, and the child identifies where he or she was touched.

9. Rapidly reversing repetitive hand movements: This item tests diadokokinesis or rapid alternating movements of the hands in a palm up–palm down sequence.
10. Arm and leg extension: While seated, the child extends the arms and legs, spreading the fingers wide and sticking out the tongue.
11. Tandem walk: This task requires the child to perform heel-to-toe walking on a straight line for 10 feet.
12. Stand on one leg: The child balances on one foot up to 10 seconds with eyes open, then closed up to 5 seconds.
13. Skip: The task is skipping across the room.
14. Left-right discrimination: This item is observed while administering items 6 and 7 when the child is requested to use the right hand. It is also observed in item 12.
15. Behavioral irregularities: Behaviors such as perseveration, excessive talking, fidgeting, tactile defensiveness, anxiety, and distractibility are observed.

Setting and Equipment

The only materials needed are a pencil, ballpoint pen, recording form, and a comfortable writing table. The examining room should be

Fig. 6-6. Quick Neurological Screening Test. Item from the Finger-to-Nose Subtest.

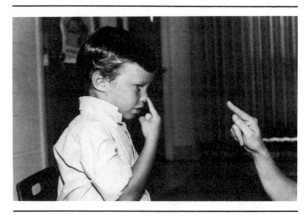

quiet, distraction-free, and large enough to observe the skipping item.

Administration Procedures

Before beginning the test, an introduction is given to the child about what the examiner will be doing with him or her. For each item there are procedures and verbal directions. Scoring considerations are discussed in the manual after each item's procedures. In addition, they are also listed on the recording form. The test items emphasize observations of the child's qualitative performance. The procedures are fairly simple to administer, but the examiner must be familiar with the types of observations that need to be made on each item. The examiner also must have practiced correct administration of the test items. Items such as the double simultaneous stimulation of hand and cheek require precise coordination on the part of the examiner and need to be well practiced.

Scoring

A set of observations is included with each test item, and each observation is scored. A variety of observations reflecting neurological immaturity are included such as observable tremor, moves head while eye tracking, and poor balance. Some of the observations are more quantitative in nature than others; for instance, on the finger-to-nose task, one of the observations is "misses tip of nose by ½ to 1 inch." A description for each of these observations is given under scoring considerations.

The total number of observations is added up for each item; then scores for the 15 items are tabulated. A score exceeding 50 is considered high and is interpreted as indicating that the child is likely to have learning problems in the classroom. A score between 26 and 50 is suspicious, whereas scores of 25 or below are considered normal performance. It is reported in the manual that a child over 7 should have little difficulty performing any of the tasks on the QNST.

Psychometric Properties

Standardization

The QNST was standardized on 1231 subjects defined as undifferentiated and attending "normal" schools and on 1008 learning-disabled children. Subjects ranged in age from under 6 years to over 17 years. The two samples have unequal numbers of children in each age group, with a predominance of children in the under 6 and 6 year age groups in the undifferentiated sample. There were over 100 children in the 8 and 9 year samples, and anywhere from 12 to 77 subjects in the 10 to 17 year age groups (1-year intervals for groups). Unfortunately, the under 6 age group is not defined so it is not possible to know how young the youngest child was in the sample. In the learning-disabled population, there were relatively few subjects in the under 6 to 12 year age groups, with anywhere from 7 to 35 subjects in each age group (1-year intervals). Most of the subjects were in the 13 to 17-plus age groups. All of the subjects were from California.

Reliability

Test-retest reliability using a single examiner was performed on 33 learning-disabled children with a 1-month interval between tests. A reliability coefficient of .81 was obtained. A low but significant correlation of .71 was obtained between two examiners after a 1-month interval. It is unclear if the same 33 subjects were used for both interobserver reliability and test-retest. The most reliable items in the QNST were figure recognition and production, double simultaneous stimulation of hand and cheek, and behavioral irregularities, the total test score, and hand and foot preference.

Validity

In examining both the ability of teachers to administer the QNST in a reliable fashion and also the accuracy with which decisions are made between teachers and persons skilled in administering the QNST, a study was conducted using four teachers who were minimally trained in the test's use and four experts. A sample of 24 children, some with learning disabilities and some without, were tested by both the four experts and four teachers. The scores of the two groups of observers correlated at .69 using the Spearman Rho test. The teachers and experts reached agreement on 93 percent of the children, identifying them as normal neurologically. They agreed on 70 percent of the children who were identified as learning disabled.

Eighty-eight learning-disabled children were matched with 88 normal children for age, sex, socioeconomic status, and intelligence and represented children from 6½ to 18 years of age. Analysis of variance of individual items revealed that the finger-to-nose item is the best single item in discriminating between learning-disabled and normal children. No other single item discriminates between the two groups at all age levels. Another validation study with 14 learning-disabled and 17 normal children found, using a *t* test, that the two groups differed significantly at the .05 level on the various items on the QNST.

Tables 6 and 7 in the manual present data on the number of subjects in the undifferentiated and learning-disabled groups who had performed successfully on the various items. Comparison of performance of the two groups shows marked differences. For instance, on hand skill, 75 percent of the undifferentiated group had attained this skill under 5 years of age, while 75 percent of the learning-disabled group had attained it by 7 years of age. In all items except left-right discrimination and double simultaneous stimulation (where performance was somewhat equivalent), the learning-disabled sample showed a delay of at least 1 year in comparison with the normal subjects in attaining 75 percent in the item. Caution must be expressed in weighting these observations, as the percent successful is not well quantified in the analysis and the number of subjects in the learning-disabled population is very small for the under 6 and 6 year age groups. This information, however, is useful in identifying developmental trends in the various items on the QNST.

Several studies are discussed in the manual regarding the correlation of the QNST with other tests. Using a sample of 30 kindergarten children, E. Landon (no source given) found a low but positive correlation of .51 between the total score on the QNST and the Bender Brain Injury factors on the Bender Visual-Motor Gestalt Test for Children. Correlations of scores between the QNST and the Wide-Range Achievement Test subscores on reading and spelling were found to be .50 and .48 when scores on 21 learning-disabled children were examined. Although the results are not high, they were significant.

To examine if the QNST is valuable as a predictive indicator of reading abilities in first grade, 198 kindergarten children, ages 5½ to 7 years, were tested at 6-month intervals. It was found that the QNST had too many items in which the children had not matured enough for it to be useful in differentiating normal and learning-disabled children at 6 years of age. It was found, however, that children who performed well on the QNST also demonstrated average or better reading scores at the end of first grade; thus, the QNST is useful in identifying normal children with average or better reading skills.

Guidelines for Use in a Clinical Setting

The QNST can be useful in screening school-aged children with learning disabilities. It should, however, be administered in conjunction with a motor and perceptual development screening tool in light of data showing that 30 percent of learning-disabled children may be misdiagnosed. Children who demonstrate definite problems on the QNST should be referred to a neurologist, psychologist, and/or occupational or physical therapist for further testing as needed to provide more in-depth assessment of neurological maturation and its relationship to learning and behavior.

Review

The QNST is a screening tool designed to detect children ranging in age from 6 to 17 years who exhibit soft neurological signs that place them at risk for learning disabilities. It is quick and easy to administer, although the examiner must be skilled in making qualitative observations required in this type of assessment. The test contains a sample of tasks that are often representative of typical behaviors exhibited by learning-disabled children with neurological immaturity. The finger-to-nose test item can also be indicative of cerebellar dysfunction. The instrument is standardized although there were relatively few subjects (i.e., 7–35) in the 6 to 12 year age groups for the learning-disabled population. Test-retest stability was good (r = .81), although interobserver reliability was only fair (r = .71).

A validity study examining the consistency of decision making among four teachers and four experts using the QNST revealed that normal children could be identified with 93 percent accuracy, whereas learning-disabled children were identified with 70 percent accuracy. The test items were found to discriminate between a sample of normal and learning-disabled children, although the sample sizes were very small in the study. Correlations between the Bender-Gestalt, The Wide Range Achievement Test, and the QNST were moderate. A predictive validity study found that the QNST was not necessarily accurate in detecting 6-year-old children with reading problems; however, those who scored high on the test also demonstrated average or better reading scores at the end of first grade. The QNST is useful as a screening instrument for school-aged children; however, some learning-disabled children may not be adequately screened, especially at 6 years of age. Other instruments should be used for 5 and 6 year olds rather than relying solely on results from the QNST for this age group.

REFERENCES

1. Ingolia, P., Cermak, S. A., and Nelson, D. The effect of choreoathetoid movements on the Quick Neuro-logical Screening Test. *Am. J. Occup. Ther.* 36 : 801, 1983.
2. Sterling, P. J., and Sterling, H. M. Neurological status vs. QNST status in 557 students. *Acad. Ther.* 15 : 317, 1980.

SOUTHERN CALIFORNIA POSTROTARY NYSTAGMUS TEST

Descriptive Information

Test Identification

The title of this test is *Southern California Postrotary Nystagmus Test* (SCPNT), 1975. Its author is A. Jean Ayres, Ph.D. Ayres is an occupational therapist with advanced degrees in educational psychology from the University of Southern California and the Brain Research Institute at the University of California at Los Angeles. She has pioneered the development of the theory of sensory integrative dysfunction and has described symptoms of children with vestibular dysfunction. Much of her research has centered around learning-disabled, autistic, and aphasic children. Western Psychological Services (12031 Wilshire Blvd., Los Angeles, California 90025) publishes the test at a cost of $95–$105 per kit, which includes the rotation board, record sheets, angle guide card, and manual.

Age and Type of Client

SCPNT is designed for children ranging in age from 5 to 9 years. It was designed to assess vestibular functioning as measured by postrotary nystagmus.

Purpose

The SCPNT is used to evaluate the normalcy of the child's postrotary nystagmus, a reflex of the eyes that occurs in response to semicircular canal stimulation. Atypical responses on the test may denote inadequate vestibular processing or poor cortical inhibition of vestibular processing.

This test is frequently administered in conjunction with the Southern California Sensory Integration Tests and with various clinical observations of postural mechanisms described by Ayres [1] and Dunn [8].

Time Required to Administer and Score Test

The time required to administer the test is less than 5 minutes. Scoring is accomplished during administration.

Evaluator

Although it is not stated in the manual, professionals who administer this test must have a background in the neurological mechanisms of the vestibular-ocular reflexes and their relationship to vestibular dysfunction. The examiner must also be skilled in administering the test and in interpreting responses. Typically, the SCPNT is administered by occupational and physical therapists experienced in assessment and treatment of sensory integrative dysfunction. Training on the SCPNT is provided as part of the certification course to administer and interpret the Southern California Sensory Integration Tests.

Historical Perspective of Test Construction

Development of Items

Several methods have been used over the years to measure nystagmus of the eyes such as electronystagmography (ENG) on the Bárány test, torsion swing test, and caloric irrigation. These tests are difficult to use clinically as part of developmental or sensorimotor testing. The SCPNT was developed because it can be administered quickly and easily by a skilled examiner within the context of clinical evaluation.

Review of Literature in Terms of Test Use

Considerable research has been conducted on the SCPNT regarding its usefulness with various populations, in expanding the normative data base for the preschool population, and in identifying factors that affect postrotary nystagmus responses as well as the relationship of postrotary nystagmus to postural responses. The various responses of learning-disabled children when tested using postrotary nystagmus have been described by Ayres [3] in a research study measuring vestibular functioning. Approximately 50 percent of learning-disabled children who were studied exhibited depressed postrotary nystagmus when tested using the SCPNT. In another study [16], learning-disabled children with excessive postrotary nystagmus durations had relatively greater sensory integrative dysfunction (as measured by six tests on the Southern California Sensory Integration Tests assumed to measure cortical level functions) than learning-disabled children with normal or depressed SCPNT scores. Results from this study support Ayres' assertion that learning-disabled children with excessive postrotary nystagmus have more cortical level dysfunction as compared with learning-disabled children with normal or depressed nystagmus who demonstrate more evidence of brain stem level dysfunction. Ottenbacher and colleagues [17] tested 26 learning-disabled children with hyporeactive postrotary nystagmus on four measures of vestibular-proprioceptive function. Two types of vestibular abnormalities were described based on their findings: a vestibular-proprioceptive deficit with poor balance and postural mechanisms and a vestibular-oculomotor deficit with poor oculomotor control. Children with depressed postrotary nystagmus and associated vestibular-proprioceptive deficits (i.e., poor standing balance and poor prone extension) were more apt to demonstrate an improvement in nystagmus following sensory integrative therapy. The authors conclude that the SCPNT is useful in delineating different vestibular abnormalities.

Studies have also been conducted on children with mental retardation and on infants with motor delays. Down's syndrome children (ages 5 through 9) have been reported to demonstrate low-average nystagmus when compared with normal subjects [21], although Kantner and colleagues [9] found increased postrotary nystagmus in a sample of Down's syndrome infants. In a study by DeGangi [6], a significant proportion of high-risk infants with abnormal or suspect neurological functions and with delayed motor skills exhibited nystagmus of lesser or greater duration than that seen in the normal infants.

Several other observations have been made regarding the use of the SCPNT. Siegner, Crowe, and Deitz [20] noted more behavioral observations such as poor balance and head control during and after rotation for 4 and 5 year olds with developmental delays as compared with their normal counterparts. The effects of the child's state on duration of nystagmus was investigated by Montgomery and Rodel [13]. Although there were not significant differences, results suggested that arousal or relaxation had an inhibiting influence on nystagmus scores over an alert state.

Several studies have examined the relationship of postrotary nystagmus to other vestibular functions. Ottenbacher [15] found that prone extension, standing balance with eyes closed (SBC), standing balance with eyes open (SBO), and muscle tone were predictors of SCPNT scores in learning-disabled children. Clyse and Short [4] found that walking on the floor with eyes closed, a test of dynamic balance, was the best predictor of postrotary nystagmus duration in learning-disabled children.

Theoretical Constructs and Implications for Intervention

Ayres describes in detail in the test manual the neurological substrates underlying postrotary nystagmus as well as the differences in emotional-physiological responses to testing seen in children with vestibular dysfunction. Learning-disabled children and others with neurological deficits frequently exhibit diminished nystagmus, although some children may demonstrate a prolonged duration. Either response is considered atypical and indicative of vestibular dysfunction. Ayres [3] reported that learning-disabled children with diminished nystagmus were more responsive to sensory integrative therapy in conjunction with special education than learning-disabled children with normal or hyperreactive nystagmus; thus, the use of the SCPNT as a diagnostic tool is valuable in delineating which types of vestibular dysfunction will respond favorably to therapy. Since vestibular stimulation (i.e., spinning, linear acceleration, and movement of the head and body in space) is very effective as a sensory integrative therapy technique, it is important to know how efficiently the child is able to process vestibular input. The SCPNT, along with other measures of vestibular function, provide this information.

Content and Test Administration

Content

The SCPNT measures the duration of nystagmus of the eyes after rotation to the right and left body sides while the child is seated with the head positioned in 30 degrees of flexion (Fig. 6-7). Observations are also made regarding the amount of eye excursion, balance and head control while spinning, and presence of such emotional-psysiological responses as nausea, dizziness, and pleasure or alarm experienced from the rotation.

Setting and Equipment

The equipment accompanying the SCPNT manual are a nystagmus board, on which the child sits and which can be rotated freely to either side, and a cardboard angle guide used to position the head. Besides the nystagmus board and angle guide, the examiner will also need a switchback stopwatch. Facing windows and other sources of light should be avoided because light has a tendency to shorten nystagmus. It is recommended that the child be seated on the board in front of a blank wall so that visual stimuli do

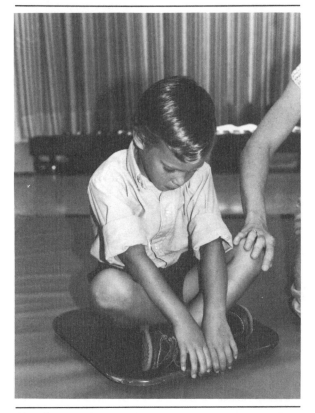

Fig. 6-7. Southern California Postrotary Nystagmus Test. Test administration.

not cause the child to focus the eyes. The light should also be dimmed.

Administration Procedures

Standardized verbal directions are used when administering the SCPNT. These directions instruct the child to sit on the board, to hold the head tilted throughout the test until he or she is stopped, at which time the child should look at the wall, not the examiner. After the child is positioned correctly on the nystagmus board with the head angled in 30 degrees of neck flexion, the examiner, kneeling on the child's left side, pushes the child 10 times in a 20-second period to the left, keeping a steady rhythm. The examiner uses the stopwatch to time the rotations as the child is turned on the board. After 10 rota-

tions, the examiner stops the child suddenly and measures the duration of nystagmus of the eyes using the stopwatch while the child faces the blank wall. The examiner notes balance and head control during and after spinning, excursion of the eyes, and asks the child such questions as (1) "Are you dizzy?" (2) "Is the room moving around and around?"; and (3) "How did you like the ride?" to determine emotional-physiological responses. After completing this procedure for the child's left side, it is repeated for the right unless the child had an adverse reaction to the movement.

The directions are clearly presented and procedures are relatively simple; however, the examiner must have a great deal of experience in rotating the board at a steady rate, and in observing nystagmus and the other observations such as excursion of the eyes. The examiner must also be aware of atypical responses such as orbital nystagmus (i.e., circular movement of eyes) and secondary nystagmus (i.e., after primary nystagmus ends, there is a brief pause and nystagmus begins again, usually with the slow component in the opposite direction) and be able to judge when an adverse response has occurred to the spinning and the test should be discontinued.

Scoring

The duration of nystagmus to the left and right and total number of seconds for both directions are noted on the record sheet and are then interpreted based on standard deviation scores presented in Table 4 of the manual for boys and girls. Although excursion of the eyes and other observations are noted on the record sheet, they are used only for interpretation of response to spinning. No norms are presented on these observations; however, Ayres discusses atypical responses seen in children who are hypo- or hypersensitive to vestibular stimulation. For instance, children who have a depressed duration of nystagmus typically do not express dizziness, alarm, feel nauseated, and may not lose their balance when rotated. They usually enjoy the spinning considerably and wish to continue the rotation after the testing is over.

Psychometric Properties

Standardization

The normative sample for the SCPNT includes 111 males and 115 females, ranging in age from 5 through 9 years, living in the Los Angeles metropolitan area. The number of children in each age group ranges from 15 to 29 for both sexes. No additional information is given regarding socioeconomic or racial background. The means and standard deviations by age level for both sexes were computed for nystagmus. The difference between male and female scores was not statistically significant for a two-tailed t test, but was for a one-tailed t test. In addition to the normative sample including 226 subjects, the duration of nystagmus is presented in a table for 68 learning-disabled children. No information is presented regarding this sample in terms of age, sex, IQ levels, and other identifying characteristics.

Kimball [12] collected normative data on 222 normal children, with approximately 40 children in each age level from 5 to 9 years. No significant differences were obtained by sex or age. Her results indicated significantly different means and standard deviations from the data presented by Ayres, with a higher cutoff point for diagnosis of hyperreactive nystagmus.

Two studies that expand on the norms presented in the SCPNT have been completed. Punwar [18] collected data on 372 subjects aged 3 through 10 years using the SCPNT. There was close agreement between data presented in this study and those presented in the test manual. No significant differences were found for age or sex. A study by Crowe, Deitz, and Siegner [5] provides data on forty-one 4-year-old normal children in the SCPNT. Again, no significant differences were found between these data and those presented in the SCPNT test manual. The mean postrotary nystagmus duration score for males was found to be significantly longer than that for females.

Reliability

Interobserver reliability was obtained on 42 children who were tested 1 week apart by two different examiners. The reliability coefficient was .834 for duration of nystagmus and .485 for excursion for this sample.

Several studies have examined the reliability of the SCPNT and its relationship to other measures of nystagmus. Keating [10] found a significant correlation between scores obtained on postrotary nystagmus testing and electronystagmography (ENG) for duration and excursion of nystagmus in a group of normal and learning-disabled children. Keating states, however, that reliability using postrotary nystagmus may be poor for children who exhibit barely perceptible nystagmus. Royeen [19] found high test-retest reliability on 24 normal grade-school children and found that time of day or sex did not affect test results. Generally acceptable reliability results are substantiated by other studies. Kimball [11] obtained stability of SCPNT scores over 2½ years with retest correlations of .80. Deitz, Siegner, and Crowe [7] also obtained test-retest reliability of .83 for 4 year olds over a period of 5 weeks, but a reliability coefficient of .62 for 3 year olds. Since these studies have centered on the reliability of the SCPNT on normal children, Morrison and Sublett [14] examined its reliability on learning-disabled children. Their findings revealed that learning-disabled children had significantly lower nystagmus durations and more variability over time in their scores compared with normal subjects.

Validity

The only validity study presented in the test manual is the presentation of nystagmus durations for learning-disabled children as they compare with normal subjects. Unfortunately, the sample of learning-disabled children is not defined; therefore, conclusions regarding how this sample differed from the normal subjects cannot be drawn. For example, it is not known if these children had postural vestibular integration deficits, developmental dyspraxia, or other types of sensory integrative disorders. From the table presented in the manual, it can be seen that approximately 52.9 percent of the learning-disabled children had hyporeactive nystagmus ($n = 36$) and 1.5 percent had hyperreactive nystagmus ($n = 1$) in comparison to the normal sample with 9.3 percent who had hyporeactive nystagmus ($n = 21$) and 10.6 percent who had hyperreactive nystagmus ($n = 24$). If conclusions were to be drawn regarding comparisons between these two samples, one could say that approximately 20 percent of normal children would demonstrate hypo- or hyperreactive nystagmus. Because of this high false-positive error rate, other measures of vestibular function are necessary in order to substantiate vestibular dysfunction. In other words, a reading of hypo- or hyperreactive nystagmus may not necessarily denote vestibular dysfunction or poor cortical inhibition of vestibular responses.

Ayres has conducted validity studies of the SCPNT in her research report [2]. In her study of 128 learning-disabled children, it was found that children with average or hyporeactive nystagmus scored better than those with hyperreactive nystagmus on various tests of intelligence, auditory-language processes, and academic performance. The children with prolonged nystagmus had more extensive neurological problems. Also, children with hyporeactive nystagmus made greater gains in sensory integrative therapy than those with normal or hyperreactive nystagmus. Those with hyporeactive nystagmus were less able to benefit from special education in comparison with the other learning-disabled children. Ayres concludes that a disorder in the vestibular system causing the hyporeactive nystagmus interferes with academic learning and that sensory integrative therapy can reduce this disorder.

Guidelines for Use in a Clinical Setting

The SCPNT is most appropriate for 5- through 9-year-old children who exhibit sensory integrative dysfunction. The test can also be administered to 3 to 10 year olds using Punwar's data [18]. The test is not appropriate for children who cannot maintain their heads in a tilted position of 30 degrees of neck flexion throughout the test because of either motor impairments or an inability to follow directions. Young children may need to be instructed to "look at their hands" while being rotated in order to keep their heads tilted correctly. Since 20 percent of normal children obtain scores that are considered hypo- or hyperreactive nystagmus duration, other measures of vestibular functions should be administered such as tests for dynamic balance (with eyes closed) and prone extension. Children with definitive problems with balance, poor prone extension, and other signs of vestibular dysfunction in conjunction with hyporeactive nystagmus can be more assuredly diagnosed as having vestibular dysfunction. These children are most apt to benefit from sensory integrative therapy than those with normal or hyperreactive nystagmus. This is not to say that children with normal or hyperreactive nystagmus will not demonstrate vestibular dysfunction (i.e., gravitational insecurity and poor balance); however, determination of their ability to benefit from sensory integrative therapy may be based on a trial of therapy. Decisions regarding vestibular functioning on the SCPNT should be based primarily on the duration of nystagmus rather than excursion or other observations, such as losing balance while rotating, since the duration of nystagmus is the only measure that demonstrated acceptable reliability.

Review

The SCPNT is a test designed to measure the normalcy of postrotary nystagmus in 5- to 9-year-old children. It can be administered in a short period of time; however, the examiner must be experienced in its administration and be knowledgeable about conditions that may affect test results. The examiner must also have a great deal of experience in the interpretation of test results. The SCPNT can be used with children with learning disabilities, autism, or mental retardation as well as children with vestibular dysfunction who are able to follow the test directions and maintain the test position. Test results of autistic and mentally retarded children should be interpreted with caution since there are no reliability studies on these populations. Good interobserver reliability was obtained on the normative sample on the duration of nystagmus. Other studies have also found good test-retest and interobserver reliability with normal and learning-disabled children on duration measures. Although validity studies were not well-defined or described in the test manual, many studies have been completed that substantiate the use of the SCPNT with different populations and that describe varying responses and changes in nystagmus as a result of intervention. Since 20 percent of the normative sample is likely to demonstrate hypo- or hyperreactive nystagmus, it is important to administer other measures of vestibular function in conjunction with the SCPNT to make a definitive diagnosis of vestibular dysfunction. Overall, the SCPNT provides valuable information regarding the child's vestibular functioning.

REFERENCES

1. Ayres, A. J. *Sensory Integration and Learning Disorders.* Los Angeles: Western Psychological Services, 1972.
2. Ayres, A. J. *The Effect of Sensory Integrative Therapy on Learning Disabled Children.* Pasadena, Calif.: Center for the Study of Sensory Integrative Dysfunctions, 1976.
3. Ayres, A. J. Learning disabilities and the vestibular system. *J. Learn. Disabil.* 11 : 30, 1978.
4. Clyse, S. J., and Short, M. A. The relationship between dynamic balance and postrotary nystagmus in learning disabled children. *Phys. Occup. Ther. Pediatr.* 3 : 25, 1983.
5. Crowe, T. K., Deitz, J. C., and Siegner, C. B. Postrotary nystagmus response of normal four-year-old children. *Phys. Occup. Ther. Pediatr.* 4 : 19, 1984.
6. DeGangi, G. A. The relationship of vestibular responses and developmental functions in high-risk infants. *Phys. Occup. Ther. Pediatr.* 2 : 35, 1982.
7. Dietz, J. C., Siegner, C. B., and Crowe, T. K. The

8. Southern California Postrotary Nystagmus Test: Test-retest reliability for preschool children. *Occup. Ther. J. Res.* 1 : 165, 1981.
8. Dunn, W. *A Guide to Testing Clinical Observations in Kindergartners.* Rockville, Md.: American Occupational Therapy Association, Inc., 1981.
9. Kantner, R. M., et al. Effects of vestibular stimulation on nystagmus response and motor performance in developmentally delayed infants. *Phys. Ther.* 56 : 414, 1976.
10. Keating, N. R. A comparison of duration of nystagmus as measured by the Southern California Postrotary Nystagmus Test and electronystagmography. *Am. J. Occup. Ther.* 33 : 92, 1979.
11. Kimball, J. G. The Southern California Postrotary Nystagmus Test: Stability Over Time. In N. Tyler (ed.), *Integration Topics: Faculty Reviews.* Los Angeles: CSSID Publication, 1980.
12. Kimball, J. Normative comparison of the Southern California Postrotary Nystagmus Test: Los Angeles vs. Syracuse data. *Am. J. Occup. Ther.* 35 : 21, 1981.
13. Montgomery, P. C., and Rodel, D. M. Effect of state on nystagmus duration on the Southern California Postrotary Nystagmus Test. *Am. J. Occup. Ther.* 36 : 177, 1982.
14. Morrison, D., and Sublett, J. Reliability of the Southern California Postrotary Nystagmus Test with learning-disabled children. *Am. J. Occup. Ther.* 37 : 694, 1983.
15. Ottenbacher, K. Identifying vestibular processing dysfunction in learning-disabled children. *Am. J. Occup. Ther.* 32 : 217, 1978.
16. Ottenbacher, K. Excessive postrotary nystagmus duration in learning-disabled children. *Am. J. Occup. Ther.* 34 : 40, 1980.
17. Ottenbacher, K., Short, M. A., and Watson, P. J. The use of selected clinical observations to predict postrotary nystagmus change in learning disabled children. *Phys. Occup. Ther. Pediatr.* 1 : 31, 1980.
18. Punwar, A. Expanded normative data: Southern California Postrotary Nystagmus Test. *Am. J. Occup. Ther.* 36 : 183, 1982.
19. Royeen, C. B. Factors affecting test-retest reliability of the Southern California Postrotary Nystagmus Test. *Am. J. Occup. Ther.* 34 : 37, 1980.
20. Siegner, C. B., Crowe, T. K., and Deitz, J. C. Interrater reliability of the Southern California Postrotary Nystagmus Test. *Phys. Occup. Ther. Pediatr.* 2 : 83, 1982.
21. Zee-Chen, E. L., and Hardman, M. L. Postrotary nystagmus response in children with Down's syndrome. *Am. J. Occup. Ther.* 37 : 260, 1983.

SOUTHERN CALIFORNIA SENSORY INTEGRATION TESTS

Descriptive Information

Test Identification

The title of this test is *Southern California Sensory Integration Tests,* Revised (SCSIT), 1980.*
Its author is A. Jean Ayres, Ph.D. Dr. A. Jean Ayres is an occupational therapist with advanced degrees in educational psychology. She is currently at the University of Southern California and the Brain Research Institute at the University of California at Los Angeles. Ayres has pioneered the development of the theory of sensory integrative dysfunction [5] and has conducted much research involving its application in the diagnosis and treatment of learning-disabled, autistic, and aphasic children. Western Psychological Services (12031 Wilshire Blvd., Los Angeles, California 90025) publishes this test at a cost of $197–$220 per test kit, which includes 10 protocol booklets, 10 design copying and motor accuracy tests, profiles, and test manual; each manual costs $23–$26. The interpretation manual costs $15–$17.

Age and Type of Client

The Southern California Sensory Integration Tests (SCSIT) were designed to be administered to children ranging in age from 4.0 to 8 years, 11 months of age with learning problems, with some tests normed up through 10 years, 11 months of age.

*EDITORS' NOTE: Dr. Ayres has substantially revised the SCSIT into a new test called the *Sensory Integration and Praxis Test* (SIPT), which is currently undergoing a national standardization. Western Psychological Services and Dr. A. Jean Ayres are working together to have the test available by 1987. All therapists currently certified in SCSIT will need to be recertified in the SIPT. The time lag necessary for certified therapists to be recertified and for uncertified therapists to become certified in the SIPT will be considerable. Therefore, it is expected that the 1980 SCSIT will be used for evaluation and diagnosis beyond 1987 and is therefore included in this chapter.

Purpose

The SCSIT is specifically intended to be used in identifying sensory integrative disorders involving form and space perception, praxis, vestibular-bilateral integration, and tactile discrimination functions.

Time Required to Administer and Score Test

The tests can be administered in 1½ hours by an experienced therapist. However, it is recommended in the manual that the test be administered in two 45-minute sessions. Time required to score the tests is not given. However, it generally takes an individual trained and certified in the SCSIT approximately 30 minutes to score the test, and an additional 30 to 45 minutes to interpret the scores.

Evaluator

To effectively administer the SCSIT, a process of certification is required. Persons who seek certification must be familiar with statistics and have a working knowledge of the theory of sensory integrative dysfunction. Occupational therapists and physical therapists are eligible to become certified in the SCSIT. The certification process involves a review of sensory integrative theory, learning of the test mechanics and interpretation of test findings, administration of the test to at least 20 subjects, and an observation of test mechanics by a member of the certification faculty. Written protocols are submitted to certification faculty for review to assure accurate interpretation of test results. Further information regarding certification can be obtained from Sensory Integration International (1402 Cravens Ave., Torrance, California 90501).†

†EDITORS' NOTE: Certification courses for the SCSIT are no longer being offered. SIPT certification is now in process and is similar to the SCSIT process outlined above.

Historical Perspective of Test Construction

Development of Test Items

The SCSIT consists of 17 tests, including the former Ayres Space Test (published in 1962), Southern California Motor Accuracy Test (published in 1964), Southern California Figure-Ground Visual Perception Test (published in 1966), Southern California Kinesthesia and Tactile Perception Tests (published in 1966), and the Southern California Perceptual-Motor Tests (published in 1968). Since the development of these particular tests, Position in Space and Design Copying (both published in 1972) were also added to the 1972 edition of SCSIT. In the 1980 edition, the manual underwent revision, and the Motor Accuracy Test was completely revised with new procedures and normative data.

Review of Literature in Terms of Test Use

Ayres conducted a series of factor analytic studies [1–3, 6, 8] that identified four syndromes based on clustering of scores on the SCSIT. These studies have been criticized because too many tests were administered to too few subjects [16]. The disorders described by Ayres in these studies included deficits involving form and space perception, praxis, postural and bilateral integration, and tactile defensiveness. Since the publication of these studies, further research and theory development have focused on two predominant syndromes, developmental dyspraxia and vestibular-bilateral integration dysfunction, rather than on the earlier syndromes.

Ayres [7] has published an interpretation manual which provides examples of typical cases, test scores on the SCSIT, and interpretations of these results. Ayres recommends supplementing test results on the SCSIT with results on various academic tests (e.g., reading, spelling, and math scores), intelligence tests, and dichotic listening responses when making an interpretation of the child's sensory integrative functioning as it af-

fects learning performance. Since the SCSIT measures only a component of behaviors (i.e., various neurological and perceptual-motor functions) which contribute to learning processes, the diagnostician must employ other evaluative tools in order to delineate the nature of the learning disorder.

The SCSIT was designed to be a diagnostic tool and is not recommended as a measure of progress. A child may make progress that is not apparent from retest scores, since the child must make more than the usual progress between test and retest for an increase in the standard deviation score to occur. Other tests including academic, motor, perceptual-motor, and behavioral observations are better indicators of progress.

Theoretical Constructs and Implications for Intervention

Three levels of functioning are formally assessed by the SCSIT. The first level measures the child's ability to process input from the three basic sensory channels—tactile, proprioceptive (kinesthetic), and vestibular. These functions mature very early in children and are both phylogenetically and ontogenetically the oldest sensory systems. The second level of functioning includes the integration of these basic senses into more complex skills, including lateralization of function, bilateral integration, and motor planning or praxis. The third level of functioning tests the end products of sensory integration, specifically visual-spatial skills and eye-motor coordination. The SCSIT provides information about these three levels of sensory integrative functioning, which are interpreted based on clusters of test scores. For instance, the tactile-kinesthetic tests are interpreted as a group rather than as individual tests. Results from the SCSIT provide the clinician with valuable information regarding the child's responses to sensory input and his or her ability to make adaptive responses, which readily translates into treatment goals and activities described by Ayres [4].

Content and Test Administration

Content

The SCSIT includes tests that measure the child's functioning in the areas of form and space perception, tactile and kinesthetic perception, motor planning and accuracy, and postural and bilateral integration (Figs. 6-8 and 6-9). Table 6-4 presents a list of the tests and what they measure.

Setting and Equipment

A test kit accompanies the test manual and interpretation manual and contains the following equipment: two plastic formboards, four egg- and four diamond-shaped blocks, two pegs, and placement card for blocks for the Space Visualization (SV) test; book of test plates for Figure-Ground (FG) perception; test booklet with eight additional stimulus cards for the Position in Space (PS) test; Kinesthesia (KIN) chart; ten plastic geometric forms, cardboard with 12 printed forms for Manual Form Perception (MFP) and test sheets for Design Copying (DC) and Motor Accuracy-Revised (MAC-R). Protocol booklets for administration and scoring of items for all tests except DC and MAC-R and testing and recording protocol sheets for DC and MAC-R are also included.

In addition to the above, the examiner must

Table 6-4. A description of the tests on the Southern California Sensory Integration Tests

1. **Space Visualization (SV)**: measures visual perception of simple forms rotated in space and the ability to mentally manipulate forms in space
2. **Figure-Ground (FG) Perception**: measures the ability to distinguish a set of superimposed or imbedded visual figures from a distracting background
3. **Position in Space (PS)**: requires the child to recognize simple geometric forms presented in different orientations and sequences; the third section of the test measures visual memory of a sequence of forms presented in various orientations
4. **Design Copying (DC)**: a visual-motor test that requires the child to copy a geometric design on a dot grid; the task measures not only visual perception of the line configurations, but also the ability to accurately duplicate those lines
5. **Motor Accuracy-Revised (MAC-R)**: involves the child's ability to draw accurately on a heavy black line presented as a large butterfly-shaped design; left- and right-hand scores are compared in terms of accuracy and speed; results on this test may provide information regarding hand dominance as well as eye-hand coordination
6. **Kinesthesia (KIN)**: measures kinesthesia primarily of the elbow and shoulder joints in a task where the child must place a finger on a spot previously placed with his or her vision occluded
7. **Manual Form Perception (MFP)**: examines the ability to identify geometric forms by feel and to match the shape felt in the hand to a visual display of forms.
8. **Finger Identification (FI)**: the child must

Fig. 6-8. Southern California Sensory Integration Tests. Space Visualization Test.

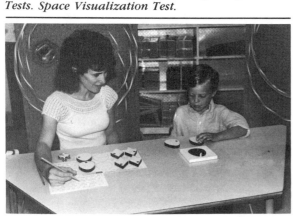

Fig. 6-9. Southern California Sensory Integration Tests. Manual Form Perception Test.

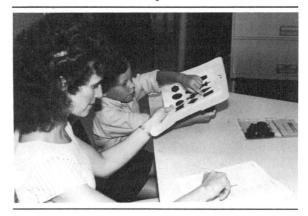

Table 6-4 (continued)

point to whichever finger or fingers were touched while vision is occluded

    9. Graphesthesia (GRA): measures the child's ability to perceive line drawings drawn on the back of one of the child's hands and his or her ability to duplicate the drawing with the other hand on the same place

    10. Localization of Tactile Stimuli (LTS): measures the child's ability to localize touch on the hands and forearms with vision occluded

    11. Double Tactile Stimuli Perception (DTS): the child must identify two tactile stimuli applied simultaneously to the child's cheeks and/or hands

    12. Imitation of Postures (IP): measures the child's ability to imitate hand and body postures demonstrated by the examiner as quickly as possible

    13. Crossing Midline of Body (CMB): the child imitates the examiner in touching the ipsilateral or contralateral eye or ear.

    14. Bilateral Motor Coordination (BMC): the child imitates a series of hand drumming and clapping patterns in a smooth and coordinated manner

    15. Right-Left Discrimination (RLD): examines the ability to discriminate right and left body sides on self and others

    16. Standing Balance: Eyes Open (SBO): the child stands on one foot for as long as possible with eyes open

    17. Standing Balance: Eyes Closed (SBC): reflects cerebellar and vestibular functions of balance; the child stands on one foot with eyes closed as long as possible

provide pencils, a plastic centimeter ruler, cardboard shield to occlude vision for the tactile subtests, a cut cardboard shield for the PS test, two red medium ball-point pens, a felt-tip pen, and a continuous running switch-back stopwatch. A child-sized table and chair large enough to position equipment for testing are needed.

Administration Procedures

Each test item includes specific procedures for presenting the test materials with standardized verbal directions. The test items are sequenced beginning with SV. It is important to administer the tactile-kinesthetic tests as a group since the

examiner observes for an avoidance or discomfort with touch, which is indicative of tactile defensiveness based on the cumulative effect of tactile stimulation. It is important that the tests Imitation of Postures (IP), Crossing Midline of Body (CML), Bilateral Motor Coordination (BMC), Right-Left Discrimination (RLD), Standing Balance: Eyes Open (SBO), and Standing Balance: Eyes Closed (SBC) also be administered as a group since they were standardized in this way. Suggestions as to the order of other tests (FG, PS, DC, and MAC-R) are given in the manual if the examiner finds the child too distractible to proceed with all the testing.

    Test procedures and verbal directions are clearly presented in the revised manual. There is considerable detail, and the examiner must be well practiced to administer the procedures correctly and accurately. Many of the test items require a great deal of perceptual-motor skill from the examiner to administer properly. For instance, on the tactile tests, the examiner must take care to hold the shield without touching the child, administer the tactile stimulus with the exact amount of pressure required, time the response, and record the response quickly to minimize the child's fatigue during testing. The directions include procedures for trial items and additional instructions for varying responses from the child on the tests. For instance, on the MAC-R test, directions are given for what to do when the child stops drawing, goes back over his or her line, or draws too fast or too slow. All of the tests include trial items that teach the child what is expected before the scored items begin.

Scoring

Scores are recorded on the protocol booklet as the child completes each test item. Scoring is complex for some of the tests, necessitating practice (i.e., recording several responses simultaneously as well as knowledge regarding what constitutes a pass or fail). For instance, on the SV test, the examiner must record hand used, number of seconds to respond, and whether the response was correct or not. On the tests measuring motor responses (e.g., IP, BMC) the examiner must know what constitutes a smoothly executed movement pattern or accurate placement of hands and body during imitation (drawing of the test posture for later reference for scoring is recommended in certification courses) since these tests require scoring of the quality of the response. Detailed descriptions are provided in the manual so that the examiner can interpret a variety of responses seen when performing these items. Some of the test items require measuring the distance from the point touched by the examiner or the point where the child's finger was originally placed. Others measure number of seconds, or number of correct responses made. Many of the tests use a graded scoring criteria ranging from 0 to 2 points, allowing for measurement of the skill's development on a continuum. This also makes some of the tests more sensitive to developmental trends.

The scores for each test are added and interpreted based on tables of standard scores. These are presented in terms of standard deviations for each age level. A score of − 1.0 standard deviation or below is suggestive of dysfunction. Most of the test scores are presented for 3- or 6-month increments. There are a total of 57 tables of standard scores for the tests included on the SCSIT. Some of the standard scores were derived by extrapolation. In a review of the SCSIT, Westman [17] stresses that the tester should use caution in interpreting standard scores because the method by which they were calculated is unclear, especially the extrapolations, and adjusted values often differ substantially from the data values.

Psychometric Properties

Standardization

The SCSIT was standardized on normal children ranging in age from 4.0 through 8 years 11 months of age and through 10 years 11 months of age on three visual perception tests, DC, and MAC-R. All children in the sample were from the Los Angeles metropolitan area. The subject pools vary somewhat for different groups of tests since data were collected on four separate occasions. For the MAC-R test, there are 395 right-handed subjects and 60 left-handed subjects with fairly equal size age groups (6-month intervals) ranging from 4 years through 10 years 11 months. There were slightly more males than females in the sample. Distributions of race are provided for right-handed subjects. For the tests of SV, FG, PS, and DC, there were 30 males and females for each age group consisting of 3-month intervals from 4 years through 8 years 11 months, and a total of 60 subjects for each 6-month interval from 9 years through 10 years 11 months, with fairly equal distributions by sex. The total sample size for the visual perception tests was 720 males and 720 females. The normative sample for the remaining tests includes data for children from 4 years through 8 years 11 months with the number of subjects ranging from 71 to 125 for each 6-month interval, again with fairly equal distributions by sex. The sample size for the tactile and kinesthetic tests was 953, and there was a total of 1004 subjects for the perceptual-motor tests. Demographic information is not well-described, and subjects are not identified in terms of academic performance or intelligence test scores. This has been identified as a major weakness by several authors [12, 15, 17].

Mean scores and standard deviations were computed for each age level by test. Tables 62 through 74 in the manual present these data along with right- and left-hand scores where appropriate. Corrections for sampling error were made by computing the curve for the best fit of scores for all tests except KIN and the tactile perception tests. No rationale is offered for why this procedure was not applied to the tactile and kinesthetic tests as well. Statistically significant mean differences were found between males and females for some age levels and some tests. The tests representing significant differences between males and females over more than one age interval (3-month interval) were SV, FG, IP, BMC, and SBO. Although significant differences were found for sex on these subtests, the tables do not list different scores and standard deviations reflecting this difference. Mean scores for 4 and 5 year olds on the RLD test fell below chance level performance; therefore, this test is not recommended for this age group.

Reliability

Although the reliability collected on all tests was reported to be test-retest stability, the type of reliability actually collected was interobserver reliability since the same child was tested on two occasions by two different examiners. The interval of time between the two tests is not reported in the manual. In addition to calculations of reliability coefficients, the standard error of measurement was also computed. Tables 77 through 83 present these data. Reliability studies were completed on 36 right-handed and 3 left-handed children on the MAC-R. For SV, PS, and DC, there were 40 children in each age level and for FG, KIN, MFP, FI, GRA, LTS, and double tactile stimuli (DTS) perception, there were between 36 and 49 children at each age level. For the remaining tests, there were between 36 and 54 children at each age level in the study. Poor to fair reliabilities were obtained on all tests except MAC-R and DC, which had fair to good reliability for most ages. These two tests have more objective scoring procedures and also measure visual-motor skills, which may account for the higher reliabilities obtained in relation to the other subtests. Subtests with fair to good reliability (in the .70s) are reported below. Those not reported had unacceptable reliability coefficients (< .70). The range of reliability for these tests was .01 to .68.

SV: .72–.77 for 6 to 8.11 year olds
PS: .73–.78 for 4 to 5.11 year olds and 10 to 10.11 year olds
DC: .76 to .89 for all age ranges except 7 to 8.11 year olds
FI: .75 for 6 to 6.11 year olds
IP: .71 to .74 for 4 to 5.11 year olds

BMC: .78 for 4 year olds
SBO: .72 for 5 year olds
MAC-R: .73 to .83 (Quotients in the .80s were obtained for 60-second speed and for 120-second accuracy but not the adjusted scores which include the time factor. Test instructions indicate that the 60-second speed should be achieved whenever possible due to the high reliability at this speed.)

Ayres provides a discussion in the manual regarding the low reliability coefficients for many of the tests. She hypothesizes that the test itself measures very unstable neurophysiological processes. However, given low reliability and unstable neurophysiological processes, therapists need to be carefully trained and test results need to be cautiously interpreted. Ayres reminds test users that the SCSIT is designed to determine the nature of the child's sensory integrative dysfunction and is intended for use with children with suspected neurological deficits. Scores should be interpreted based on the standard error of measurement before making a clinical judgment. Ayres also stresses that the SCSIT should be used only in its entirety. The scores are not additive; however, performance on all of the tests should be considered together in making clinical judgments. Test scores are clustered together so that the various sensory integrative functions (e.g., tactile-kinesthetic) can be interpreted for diagnosis.

The poor reliability of the SCSIT is considered to be one of the major weaknesses of the tests [12, 15, 17]. Ayres reports that if the reliability of each test were only .35, the overall reliability of the test would be higher than .90, if one assumes that all the tests are of equal length and computes it as one intact battery. This interpretation assumes that the individual tests in the SCSIT are of equal length and are equivalent in item difficulty, scoring criteria, and demonstrate high item intercorrelations and similar variances. Since none of these assumptions are met, one cannot accept a tentative estimate of overall reliability of the SCSIT as exceeding .90.

Validity

There is no specific information in the manual regarding the test's validity. Ayres has devoted an entire chapter to the description of the tests presented in the SCSIT and documented through a review of the literature the clinical importance of examining the specific content areas included in the SCSIT. No intercorrelations of tests, item discriminations, or studies of learning-disabled children and their performance on the SCSIT are included in the manual. There is no discussion of the developmental sensitivity of the tests (i.e., when one would expect no difference in performance of an 8 and 9 year old based on norms). Some of the tests are too difficult for younger children (e.g., DC for 4 year olds and BMC and SBC for 4 and 5 year olds), while others are too easy for older children (e.g., CML for 8 year olds). There are also no contraindications except that RLD is only administered to ages 5 and up. In inspecting the standard scores, it is apparent that on BMC a four year old can attain a score of 0 and still be considered normal, thus, the tasks involved in this particular test are not developmentally sensitive to the status of 4 year olds. It is interesting that interobserver reliability for BMC for 4 year olds was the only age level for this test that reached a somewhat acceptable level of reliability.

Factor analytic studies are reported in Ayres' research report entitled "The Effect of Sensory Integrative Therapy on Learning Disabled Children" [6]. In this report, 128 subjects were given the SCSIT, the Southern California Postrotary Nystagmus Test, and an intelligence test. Clinical observations were also administered to assess various postural reflexes and neuromuscular mechanisms which affect learning. Of those factors on the SCSIT, it was found that MFP, SV, FG, PS, and DC loaded together as a visual perception factor; KIN, FI, Graphesthesia (GRA), and LTS loaded together as a tactile-proprioception factor; and CML (crossed items only), RLD, and MAC (less accurate hand) shared variance as related factors.

Two studies correlating the SCSIT to other instruments have been conducted. Kimball [13] correlated the SCSIT and the Bender-Gestalt to evaluate children with perceptual-motor deficits. Scores on the Bender were found to be predictive of grouped scores on the Form and Space Perception and Praxis-Tactile tests of the SCSIT. The Bender may be useful then in screening children with sensory integrative dysfunction if problems exist in visual-spatial and tactile perception, and/or motor planning, but it does not tap postural mechanisms. Children with these problems may be overlooked. Ziviani and colleagues [18] correlated scores of 49 learning-disabled children on the Bruininks-Oseretsky Test of Motor Proficiency and the SCSIT. They found that those SCSIT tests which include a motor component (SV, DC, KIN, MFP, IP, BMC, MAC, SBO, and SBC) had a significant correlation with the battery composite scores on the BOTMP. The fine motor composite scores on the BOTMP demonstrated the highest correlation with the SCSIT tests (all tests except FGP, KIN, LTS, and RLD). They concluded that the BOTMP would be useful in screening children who may demonstrate sensory integrative dysfunction.

Guidelines for Use in a Clinical Setting

No specific criteria are offered in the test manual for the type of child who would most benefit from sensory integrative testing. It is a test that is not appropriate for children falling below a low average IQ. Based on the clinical experience of this writer, it appears that the SCSIT should be administered to children whose IQ scores (Wechsler Intelligence Scale for Children-Revised [WISC-R]) show a discrepancy between verbal and performance scores (performance lower than verbal by 13 points or more), which is often indicative of a learning disability, and are manifesting clinical signs of sensory motor dysfunction (i.e., react adversely to touch, clumsy and awkward movements). The SCSIT is designed to be used solely for diagnosis and it is not recommended for reevaluation of progress although it is frequently used for this purpose. The only tests that can be used for evaluation of progress are possibly MAC-Revised, and DC (except for 7 and 8 year olds) due to their higher reliability. Children with motor handicaps, severe auditory processing dysfunction, and severe hyperactivity or distractibility are inappropriate for the tests. Children with severe tactile defensiveness often cannot tolerate completing the tactile subtests. Generally, the SCSIT is not administered to 4 year olds because their behavior does not allow for an accurate assessment of sensory integrative dysfunction, reliability scores are especially low, and many of the tests are not sensitive enough to indicate dysfunction.

Review

The SCSIT is a group of 17 tests designed to be administered to children ranging in age from 4.0 to 10 years 11 months of age with learning disabilities. The tests are useful in delineating sensory integrative dysfunction involving disorders of form and space perception, praxis, vestibular-bilateral integration, and tactile discrimination functions. It should be given by an occupational or physical therapist trained and certified in its administration and interpretation, since procedures, scoring, and interpretation are complex. Since there is strong evidence that some learning-disabled children have sensory integrative dysfunction and that sensory integrative therapy facilitates learning, allowing them to progress educationally, it is important to identify children with sensory integrative dysfunction. The SCSIT provide the clinician with information that allows them to make this judgment.

Limitations of the SCSIT include inadequate standardization procedures (e.g., no information regarding subjects' academic and intellectual level, poor geographic and socioeconomic status representation), poor reliability on the majority of the tests, and inadequate validity studies. Ayres reports that the overall reliability of the entire test would be greater than .90 if the reliability of each test were .35 and if one considers all of the tests to be of equal length. This inter-

pretation cannot be justified in light of many unmet assumptions (e.g., equivalent item difficulty and similar variances). Since the SCSIT is designed to be given to learning-disabled children, it is critical that additional data be collected on a well-defined sample of learning-disabled children so that their performance can be compared with normal age-matched children. Without this comparison, it is impossible to determine how accurate decisions can be made in diagnosing sensory integrative deficits. Despite these major weaknesses in the SCSIT, the tests provide the clinician with valuable information regarding the child's responses to sensory input and his or her ability to make adaptive responses. This information can be used to delineate which children appear to exhibit sensory integrative dysfunction and would most likely benefit from sensory integrative therapy. Test results on the SCSIT may be useful in developing treatment goals.

Findings on the SCSIT should not be used exclusively without support from other tests or behavioral observations from parents and teachers in light of the poor reliability coefficients and inadequate validity studies. The Bruininks-Oseretsky Test of Motor Proficiency [9], the Bender-Gestalt Test for Young Children [14], the clinical observations described by Ayres [4] and quantified by Dunn [11] for kindergartners are recommended to be administered in conjunction with the Southern California Postrotary Nystagmus Test in order to make a comprehensive diagnosis. Psychological testing in conjunction with tests of academic performance should be considered in interpreting the test results. It may also be useful for the child to be evaluated by a neuropsychologist using such tests as the Halstead-Reitan Neuropsychological Battery for Children, the Reitan-Indiana Neuropsychological Test Battery for Children, or the Luria-Nebraska Neuropsychological Battery for Children in order to confirm diagnosis of tactile, visual-spatial, auditory-language, praxis, and laterality deficits.

Restandardization of the SCSIT with revisions in content (i.e., elaboration of praxis tests) is being initiated at the time of this writing. The new test will be called Sensory Integration and Praxis Tests (SIPT). There is a great need for a reliable and valid instrument of sensory integrative function for school-aged children. Until an instrument that meets the criteria for adequacy as an acceptable evaluation tool is available, the SCSIT should be used only in conjunction with findings from other tests in making decisions regarding the child's sensory integrative dysfunction. The test user should take great caution in interpreting test results with poor reliability when a child's performance indicates dysfunction. Because the SCSIT will be replaced by the SIPT during the latter years of the 1980s, therapists must make professional judgments regarding the future use of this test.

REFERENCES

1. Ayres, A. J. Patterns of perceptual-motor dysfunction in children: A factor analytic study. *Percept. Mot. Skills* 20 : 335, 1965.
2. Ayres, A. J. Deficits in sensory integration in educationally handicapped children. *J. Learn. Disabil.* 2 : 160, 1969.
3. Ayres, A. J. Characteristics of types of sensory integrative dysfunction. *Am. J. Occup. Ther.* 25 : 7, 1971.
4. Ayres, A. J. *Sensory Integration and Learning Disorders.* Los Angeles: Western Psychological Services, 1972.
5. Ayres, A. J. *The Development of Sensory Integrative Theory and Practice.* Dubuque, Ia.: Kendall/Hunt, 1974.
6. Ayres, A. J. *The Effect of Sensory Integrative Therapy on Learning Disabled Children.* Pasadena, Calif.: Center for the Study of Sensory Integrative Dysfunctions, 1976a.
7. Ayres, A. J. *Interpreting the Southern California Sensory Integration Tests.* Los Angeles: Western Psychological Services, 1976b.
8. Ayres, A. J. Cluster analyses of measures of sensory integration. *Am. J. Occup. Ther.* 31 : 362, 1977.
9. Bruininks, R. H. *Bruininks-Oseretsky Test of Motor Proficiency.* Circle Pines, Minn.: American Guidance Service, 1978.
10. Clark, F., Mailloux, Z., and Parham, D. Sensory Integration and Children with Learning Disabilities. In P. N. Clark and A. S. Allen (eds.), *Occupa-tional Therapy for Children.* St. Louis: Mosby, 1985.
11. Dunn, W. *A Guide to Testing Clinical Observations in Kindergartners.* Rockville, Md.: American Occupational Therapy Association, 1981.
12. Evans, P. R., and Peham, M. A. S. *Testing and Measurement in Occupational Therapy: A Review of Current Practice with Special Emphasis on the Southern California Sensory Integration Tests.* Monograph No. 15. University of Minnesota, 1981.
13. Kimball, J. G. The Southern California Sensory Integration Tests (Ayres) and the Bender-Gestalt: A correlative study. *Am. J. Occup. Ther.* 31 : 294, 1977.
14. Koppitz, E. M. *The Bender-Gestalt Test for Young Children.* New York: Grune & Stratton, 1964.
15. Ottenbacher, K. Review of testing and measurement in occupational therapy: A review of current practice with special emphasis on the Southern California Sensory Integration Tests. *Occup. Ther. J. Res.* 2 : 248, 1982.
16. Reed, H. B. Review of the SCSIT. In O. K. Buros (ed.), *The Eighth Mental Measurements Yearbook* (Vol. 2). Highland Park, N.J.: Gryphon Press, 1978. P. 875.
17. Westman, A. S. Review of the SCSIT. In O. K. Buros (ed.), *The Eighth Mental Measurements Yearbook* (Vol. 2). Highland Park, N.J.: Gryphon Press, 1978. P. 875.
18. Ziviani, J., Poulsen, A., and O'Brien, A. Correlation of the Bruininks-Oseretsky Test of Motor Proficiency with the Southern California Sensory Integration Tests. *Am. J. Occup. Ther.* 36 : 519, 1982.

TEST OF VISUAL-PERCEPTUAL SKILLS (NON-MOTOR)

Descriptive Information

Test Identification

The title of this test is *Test of Visual-Perceptual Skills (Non-Motor), 1982.* Its author is Morrison F. Gardner. Special Child Publications (P.O. Box 33548, Seattle, Washington 98133) publishes the test manual at a cost of $10–$12; TVPS test plates, $38–$42; and TVPS Record Forms, $8–$10 for 25.

Ages and Type of Client

The Test of Visual-Perceptual Skills (TVPS) was designed for children ranging in age from 4 years through 12 years, 11 months. It can be used with learning-disabled children to determine their level of functioning in visual-perceptual skills.

Purpose

The TVPS was designed as a diagnostic tool to measure the child's strengths and weaknesses in visual perception in terms of seven component areas including visual discrimination, visual memory, visual-spatial relationships, visual form constancy, visual sequential memory, visual figure-ground, and visual closure.

Time Required to Administer and Score Test

The test manual indicates that the time needed to administer the TVPS may vary depending on the age of the child. However, that range might be from 7 minutes for the younger child to 15 minutes for the older child. Scoring time is not addressed in the manual but is judged to be minimal.

Evaluator

The manual did not indicate that any special training was needed to administer the TVPS. Specialists who might use the evaluation results to develop a remediation program are occupational therapists, learning specialists, teachers of special education, psychologists, and optometrists.

Historical Perspective of Test Construction

Development and Source of Test Items

Two versions of the test were developed before the final standardized version. The visual-perceptual forms not biased according to race, culture, sex, language, education, or occupa-tions, social, or economic levels of the parents were selected. The directions were intended to be understandable and culture-free. Initially 659 forms were generated and administered to 10 children. A total of 267 items were administered to 50 children for the second revision. An item analysis narrowed the items to 112, with 16 items selected for each of the 7 subtests. The items within each subtest were arranged in order of difficulty.

Review of Literature in Terms of Test Use

Since the TVPS is a new instrument, no studies have been conducted on its use other than those described in the test manual.

Theoretical Constructs and Implications for Intervention

The theoretical background relating the importance of visual perception to learning is not provided in the manual. No rationale is presented for inclusion of the seven components of visual perception comprising the different subtests and their relative importance to the domain of visual perception. In addition, the author does not necessarily support claims that dysfunction in visual perception is specifically related to reading or spelling disorders; and, as a result, determination of the usefulness of a test of visual perception is left up to the reader. The author does, however, state that visual-perceptual disorders may or may not be related to visual-motor dysfunction. The need for a nonmotor test of visual-perception is not well supported, and there is no discussion regarding how the TVPS should be used in conjunction with other instruments such as the Developmental Test of Visual Perception (VMI) in making a differential diagnosis. Gardner states that remediation should be directed toward subtests in which the child shows a significant deficit. No particular remediation methods are advocated; they are left up to the examiner's experience and training.

Content and Test Administration

Content

The TVPS contains seven subtests of visual perception, each containing 16 items of progressive difficulty. The different subtests include the following:

1. Visual Discrimination: ability to match a form or configuration of forms with one of several similar forms
2. Visual Memory: ability to recall a form and find it among an array of similar forms
3. Visual-Spatial Relationships: ability to distinguish a form or part of a form with a different spatial orientation from five forms of identical configuration
4. Visual Form Constancy: ability to distinguish a form that may be presented in a different size, rotation, reversed, and/or hidden display
5. Visual Sequential Memory: ability to recall a series of forms from among four separate series of forms
6. Visual Figure-Ground: ability to find a form hidden in a distracting background
7. Visual Closure: ability to match a completed form with one of four incomplete forms

In examining the content of the TVPS, it appears that there may be some overlap in the Visual Form Constancy and Visual Figure-Ground Subtests as both contain hidden figures or distracting backgrounds. Likewise, the Visual Sequential Memory Subtest requires that the child use visual-spatial abilities along with visual memory.

Setting and Equipment

The TVPS should be administered in a well-illuminated distraction-free environment. The only materials needed are the record form, the test plates, and a pencil to record the child's responses.

Administration Procedures

The TVPS is easy to administer. The child is shown the test plates and is then asked to point to the correct response. Each of the subtests includes directions for administering the items. The verbal directions are simple and easy to understand. The instructions stress that the child should understand the directions before proceeding with the items. Although the test items are not timed, some of the directions suggest that the examiner may prod the child if a choice has not been made in a certain time period. All items are presented in sequential order until the child makes a determined number of consecutive errors for that particular subtest (i.e., three failures out of four consecutive items for subtests with four choices).

Scoring

Care is taken in the scoring so that the child is not aware of failures. The examiner records in the space provided the number of the child's response. The correct answer is in parentheses to the right of this space to allow for quick scoring. The testing is discontinued once the child has attained the ceiling level for each subtest. The number correct for each subtest is then determined and recorded on the front page of the record form in the spaces provided. An example of a completed protocol is presented in Appendix A of the manual. After the raw scores have been calculated for each of the subtests, a perceptual age, scaled scores, and percentiles based on the raw scores are determined for each of the subtests using Tables 17 through 19. The perceptual quotient, percentile rank, and median perceptual age are determined based on the sum of the scaled scores for the total subtest scores. Table 20 is used in these calculations. Although the test was standardized on children up through 12 years 11 months, a section of Table 17 provides scaled scores for individuals 13 years and older. Since performance levels on the TVPS leveled off by 12 years, it was projected that no further changes occur in visual perception after that time.

The interpretation of derived scores is described in the manual. A scaled score of 10 and a perceptual quotient of 100 are suggestive of average performance. The standard error of measurements are described for the scaled scores and perceptual quotients. In addition, the standard error of measurement difference is discussed. A scaled score difference of 3 or more between any pair of the subtests is considered to be a significant difference in performance ability. The interpretation part of the manual also includes a brief discussion of how the scores obtained on the TVPS might be compared with other standardized test scores.

Psychometric Properties

Standardization

The TVPS was standardized on 962 children between the ages of 4 years and 12 years 11 months. The children were all from the San Francisco Bay area and attended private or parochial schools. The sample sizes are fairly equally distributed across age and sex. Table 4 in the manual presents the breakdown for age, sex, and race (white and nonwhite only). A weighted sample was selected using the Picture Completion Test of the Wechsler Preschool and Primary Scale of Intelligence (WPPSI) or Wechsler Intelligence Scale for Children—Revised (WISC-R), which was used to establish a normative group. All subjects in the sample were normal functioning, and children with learning or sensory disorders were excluded from the sample. The sample does not include any criterion group to compare the performance of normals. The sample is broken down into 1-year intervals; however, the norm tables present interpolations for 4-month intervals for 4 years through 6 years 11 months, and 6-month intervals for 7 years through 9 years 11 months. It is not clear why the standardization sample was not grouped accordingly, rather

than using interpolations. An analysis using sex as a factor did not reveal any significant sex differences for any of the subtests; therefore, the norms were not broken down by sex.

Reliability

Reliability was determined by using measures of internal consistency (Cronbach's alpha-coefficients) for the subtests and the test as a whole. These reliability coefficients range from low to fair for most of the subtests, with generally poorer reliabilities for the 10 to 12 year olds. The use of the TVPS with older children is therefore questionable. The ranges for reliability are as follows:

1. Visual Discrimination: .46 to .76
2. Visual Memory: .49 to .72
3. Visual-Spatial Relationships: .24 to .83
4. Visual Form Constancy: .48 to .79
5. Visual Sequential Memory: .48 to .85
6. Visual Figure-Ground: .56 to .82
7. Visual Closure: .72 to .85

Overall, the latter three subtests demonstrated fair (> .70) to good (> .80) reliability for most of the age groups, and visual form constancy had fair reliability for most of the age groups while the other subtests were less reliable overall. The total test reliability was good, however, with ranges from .83 to .92. No test-retest reliability measures were obtained to examine stability of measures over time.

Validity

Five types of validity were examined in the development of the TVPS, including content, item, diagnostic, criterion-related, and predictive. The content validity was determined by designing items for the seven factors included on the TVPS. No factor analyses were done to assess if the seven factors do indeed measure seven distinct subdomains of visual perception. In addition, no theoretical basis was provided to justify inclusion of the seven factors within the test. Evidence of content validity is therefore considered to be weak. Item validity was established by calculating item correlations with subtest and total test scores. Item difficulty was also considered in the development of test items.

In order to assess diagnostic validity, subtest intercorrelations based on scaled scores were computed to determine if the different subtests measure unique characteristics of visual perception. Moderate intercorrelations were obtained, ranging from .54 to .65, which lends support for inclusion of the different subtests in the total test. A group of 45 learning-disabled children ranging in age from 5 to 12 years were also selected to determine if the TVPS can discriminate children with deficits in visual perception. The characteristics of this sample were not described (i.e., type of learning disability) other than age, sex, and race. The results of their tests were compared with a matched sample of children from the standardization sample. Analysis of variance revealed highly significant differences in performance on the total test; however, the data were not examined in terms of criterion-group performance. Since it appears that one of the major intents of the instrument is to identify children with visual perceptual deficits, cutoff scores and classification accuracies should have been calculated.

Criterion-related validity was examined by comparing the performance on the TVPS with other tests of visual perception, including the Picture Completion subtest of the WPPSI and WISC-R, the Bender Visual-Motor Gestalt Test (BVMGT), and the Developmental Test of Visual-Motor Integration (VMI). All children in the standardization sample received the Picture Completion subtest. A sample of one-hundred eight 5 to 8 year olds was tested on the BVMGT, and fifty-one 4 to 6 year olds were tested on the VMI. Results of these analyses revealed moderate correlations between these tests and the TVPS. One must consider, however, that validation between the TVPS and the BVMGT and VMI was con-

ducted only on younger children, and generalizations cannot be extended for 9 to 12 year olds. Strong correlations were also obtained between TVPS performance and chronological age. The items on the TVPS were purposely selected to correlate with chronological age; therefore, the high correlations obtained between the TVPS and age do not constitute criterion validity.

Predictive validity was also determined by comparing scores on the TVPS to the reading and spelling subtests of the Wide Range Achievement Test (WRAT) on 184 seven to nine year olds. Low correlations were obtained between the TVPS and WRAT subtests. An overall correlation of .36 was obtained for the reading subtest and .41 for the spelling subtest. Gardner concluded that the TVPS may be useful in predicting levels of achievement when used together with other tests, although the evidence presented is not strong to support this claim.

The validity of the TVPS has been criticized by both Busch-Rossnagel [1]* and Denison [2] in their reviews of the TVPS. Busch-Rossnagel points out that there are no criteria for predicting which subtests will differentiate the performance of learning-disabled and normal children. In addition, she states that there is a lack of discussion regarding why visual perception should predict achievement scores. Along these lines, Denison also points out that there is no research supporting the rationale for the construct of visual perception or the components selected for the subtests. Busch-Rossnagel concludes that validity studies should focus on diagnostic and predictive validity since the presumed intent of the TVPS is to diagnose learning problems in visual perception.

Guidelines for Use in a Clinical Setting

The TVPS is a test of visual perception that may prove useful in the assessment of motor-impaired children and children with learning disabilities;

*Electronic data base is available on-line through BRS Information Technologies.

however, since no validity studies were conducted on children with motor impairments, the usefulness of the TVPS with this population has not been determined. Since the TVPS is a nonmotor test of visual perception, it would be expected that the TVPS would be useful with children with cerebral palsy and motor incoordination. When using the TVPS with children with motor impairments or learning disabilities, the test user must exercise caution in interpreting test results until studies have been completed on these populations. The TVPS may be used in conjunction with the Motor-Free Visual Perception Test (MVPT), Developmental Test of Visual-Motor Integration (VMI), and/or BVMGT to arrive at a differential diagnosis. It is important to determine if the child has a visual perception and/or visual-motor integration deficit, as this will affect remediation strategies.

Review

The TVPS is designed to measure nonmotor visual perception. Although it is not clearly stated, the intent of the test is to diagnose children with visual perception deficits. A major problem underlying the use of the TVPS is that the rationale for development of the instrument is not presented, which leaves justification for use of the tool up to the test user. Similarly, the rationale for inclusion of the seven factors of visual perception is not presented nor are there factor analytic studies to support their inclusion as separate subtests. The TVPS is quick and easy to administer and score. Interpretation of scores is based on standard scores, perceptual ages, and percentiles. In determining if a child has a visual perceptual problem, guidelines are presented in the manual based on scaled score differences. The test user must bear in mind that no comparisons were made between the normative sample and a criterion group of children with visual perceptual deficits; therefore, decisions made regarding the classification of a child as delayed in visual perception should be made with caution.

The test is well standardized but has a limited geographic representation. Because performance was found to level off between the ages of 10 and 12 years, the author presents a table of scaled scores for use with individuals 13 years and older. Since internal reliability coefficients were the poorest for 10 to 12 year olds, the test is not recommended for use with children 10 years and older by this reviewer. Likewise, extending the scaled scores for older children is not based on sufficient empirical support.

The major problem with the TVPS lies in its weak validity, especially in the areas of diagnostic and predictive validity. The predictive validity of the test for achievement scores in reading and spelling is not strong, and the rationale for this prediction is not discussed. In addition, the predictive validity of visual perception should be examined in relation to relevant domains (i.e., motor planning and reading). Further studies are also needed in diagnostic validity to determine the performance of children with visual perceptual deficits on the TVPS in comparison to the normative sample.

There are problems with the reliability of the TVPS as well. Reliability included only measures of internal consistency, and these were poor to fair for four of the seven subtests, with poorer reliabilities for the 10 to 12 year olds. The total test reliability coefficients were good, and reliabilities were fair to good for the Visual Sequential Memory, Visual Figure-Ground, and Visual Closure Subtests. The test is best interpreted as a total test; however, scores on these three particular subtests may also be examined in diagnosis. Test-retest reliability studies are also needed.

REFERENCES

1. Busch-Rossnagel, N. A. Review of the TVPS. In O. K. Buros (ed.), *The Ninth Mental Measurements Yearbook.* Highland Park, N.J.: Gryphon Press, 1985.
2. Denison, J. W. Review of the TVPS. In O. K. Buros (ed.), *The Ninth Mental Measurements Yearbook.* Highland Park, N.J.: Gryphon Press, 1985.

CHAPTER REVIEW

Before summarizing the tests critiqued in this chapter, several questions are posed in evaluating the effectiveness of the instruments reviewed in assessing the domain of sensorimotor functions: (1) Are the available sensorimotor instruments appropriate in testing the various age and disability groups most typically seen by therapists, educators, and psychologists? (2) Do the available tests tap behaviors characteristic of the domain of sensorimotor functions? and (3) Can accurate and reliable decisions be made based on findings derived from the available instruments? To evaluate the adequacy of the tests reviewed in this chapter, several tables were constructed to summarize information related to these three questions.

The majority of instruments available for assessment of sensorimotor functions reviewed in this chapter were developed for children with learning disabilities and perceptual and motor delays. Very few of the instruments can actually be used with mentally retarded and cerebral-palsied children. None of the instruments were validated on autistic or emotionally disturbed children. All of the tests included samples of normal children, but only 8 of the 14 tests reviewed actually considered the performance of a criterion group in comparison with normals or completed validity studies on a sample or samples of delayed children. Since the primary reason that a child may be tested in sensorimotor functions is usually to determine the type and extent of delay, it is critical that the test be validated on a sample of children with delays in that area. If the test has been validated or standardized only on normal children, it is difficult to determine if the test actually discriminates between the performance of delayed and normal children. Tests that have not been validated on samples of delayed children may also not be sensitive to the distinct problems presented by that particular disability.

All the tests reviewed were designed to be administered to preschool or school-aged children. Table 6-5 presents the list of instruments

reviewed and the age group and disability for which the test was intended.

In testing any content area, it is always helpful to have tests that can be used for screening as well as diagnosis. About half of the instruments reviewed were intended to be used as screening tools. Another nine instruments were designed to be used for diagnosis. Four of the tests listed were recommended by the authors to be used as both a screening and diagnostic tool. With the Bruininks-Oseretsky Test of Motor Proficiency (BOTMP), a short form is available for screening and a long version of the test is used for diagnosis. With the other three instruments, an experienced professional skilled in that particular content area is needed to make definitive diagnostic decisions using the tool, whereas a paraprofessional or teacher who has not necessarily been trained in sensorimotor functions may administer the test for screening purposes. When making diagnostic decisions using such a tool, the expert clinician will examine quality of performance on test items, clustering of subtest scores, and performance in relation to other areas of development to determine the impact of the delay. Two of the instruments reviewed, Dunn's Guide to Testing Clinical Observations in Kindergartners and the Purdue Perceptual-Motor Survey (PPMS), were intended to be used for clinical observation only. A set of clinical observations such as these should always be administered in conjunction with other instruments. Three other assessments also allow the test examiner to make clinical observations in addition to test items administered. Oftentimes these clinical observations can only be interpreted based on the examiner's experience and training. It is critical then to consider the credentials of the examiner when a tool is used for diagnosis and when clinical judgments are made based on observations derived from the tool, especially with the Southern California Tests of Sensory Integration (SCSIT). In addition, seven of the instruments lend themselves to either therapeutic intervention or educational programming. Activity programs are available as

Table 6-5. Age and disability groups for which test is intended

Name of test	Age groups			Disability				Validation or sampling (includes criterion group)
	Infants	Preschool	School age	LD	MR	Motor handicap	Perceptual or motor delay	
1. Beery (VMI)		✓	✓	✓				
2. BOTMP		✓	✓	✓	✓	✓	✓	✓
3. DeGangi-Berk (TSI)		✓		✓	✓		✓	✓
4. DTVP (Frostig)		✓	✓	✓			✓	
5. Dunn's Guide		✓	✓	✓			✓	
6. Imitation of Gestures		✓	✓	✓				
7. Jordan		✓	✓	✓				✓
8. MVPT		✓	✓	✓	✓	✓	✓	
9. Peabody (PDMS)	✓	✓	✓			✓	✓	✓
10. Purdue (PPMS)			✓	✓			✓	✓
11. QNST		✓	✓	✓				✓
12. SCPNT		✓	✓	✓				✓
13. SCSIT		✓	✓	✓				✓
14. TVPS		✓	✓	✓				✓

Key: VMI, Beery-Buktenica Developmental Test of Visual-Motor Integration; BOTMP, Bruininks-Oseretsky Test of Motor Proficiency; DTVP, The Marianne Frostig Developmental Test of Visual Perception; MVPT, Motor-Free Visual Perception Test; PDMS, Peabody Developmental Motor Scales (Revised); PPMS, Purdue Perceptual Motor Survey; QNST, Quick Neurological Screening Test (Revised); SCPNT, Southern California Postrotary Nystagmus Test; SCSIT, Southern California Sensory Integration Tests; TVPS, Test of Visual-Perceptual Skills (Non-Motor).

part of the Frostig Developmental Test of Visual Perception and the Peabody Developmental Motor Scales (PDMS). Table 6-6 summarizes the recommended uses of the tests reviewed.

Although the tests reviewed in this chapter fall under the domain of sensorimotor functions, the test content may vary considerably from one test to the next. The area of postural mechanisms, reflexes, and balance was included in the majority of the instruments. The other areas most typically covered were bilateral integration, fine motor control, eye-hand coordination, praxis, visual perception, and visual-motor integration. The content areas least tapped by the instruments were tactile, vestibular, gross motor skills, and cross-modal integration (i.e., stereognosis). Gross motor skills can frequently be tested using motor development tests; therefore, the reader is referred to those tests. Table 6-7 presents the content areas examined by the different tests reviewed.

Last, but certainly not least, are evidence of the reliability and validity of the instruments reviewed. Only six of the fourteen instruments reviewed demonstrated good interobserver reliability. Although the DTVP test manual reports good interobserver reliability, one study reported poor to fair interobserver reliability on the DTVP. Two other tests, the Beery-Buktenica Developmental Test of Visual-Motor Integration (VMI) and Peabody (PDMS) demonstrated good interrater agreement (two examiners scoring the same set of responses). The other six instruments reviewed either demonstrated poor to fair interobserver reliability or studies were not completed. Test-retest reliability studies are more promising. Nine of the tests reviewed demonstrated good stability over time. The SCSIT had good test-retest reliability for only two subtests; thus, it is not included among the nine tests mentioned. The remaining four tests did not have any test-retest reliability studies

Table 6-6. Recommended use of test*

Name of test	Screening	Diagnosis	Clinical observations	Programming or intervention
1. Beery (VMI)	✔			
2. BOTMP	✔	✔		
3. DeGangi-Berk (TSI)	✔	✔		✔
4. DTVP (Frostig)	✔	✔		✔
5. Dunn's Guide			✔	✔
6. Imitation of Gestures		✔		
7. Jordan	✔			
8. MVPT	✔	✔		
9. Peabody (PDMS)	✔	✔		✔
10. Purdue (PPMS)			✔	✔
11. QNST	✔		✔	
12. SCPNT		✔	✔	✔
13. SCSIT		✔	✔	✔
14. TVPS		✔		

*Based on recommendations in manual.
Key: VMI, Beery-Buktenica Developmental Test of Visual-Motor Integration; BOTMP, Bruininks-Oseretsky Test of Motor Proficiency; DTVP, The Marianne Frostig Developmental Test of Visual Perception; MVPT, Motor-Free Visual Perception Test; PDMS, Peabody Developmental Motor Scales (Revised); PPMS, Purdue Perceptual Motor Survey; QNST, Quick Neurological Screening Test (Revised); SCPNT, Southern California Postrotary Nystagmus Test; SCSIT, Southern California Sensory Integration Tests; TVPS, Test of Visual-Perceptual Skills (Non-Motor).

performed. Of the tests reviewed, only one completed decision-making reliability, the DeGangi-Berk Test of Sensory Integration (TSI). This type of reliability is critical as it assures the diagnostician that decisions regarding the child's performance would be accurate on retesting performance. Based on reliability studies completed, only three of the tests reviewed can be used for interpreting scores by subtest as well as total test score: the DeGangi Berk (except for the Reflex Integration Subtest), the TVPS (on only three of the seven subtests), and the Peabody (PDMS). Only three of the tests reviewed completed reliability studies on samples of delayed children as well as normal subjects: the VMI, DeGangi-Berk, and Quick Neurological Screening Test (QNST). Since sensorimotor tests are most likely to be administered to children with delays in this area, it is important that reliability studies be completed on children with sensorimotor deficits as well as on normal children. Table 6-8 presents reliability studies completed on the tests reviewed.

Several aspects of validity were considered in evaluating the assessments reviewed in this chapter. Only six of the instruments provide evidence that accurate decisions can be made based on obtained test scores. For the Motor-Free Test of Visual Perception (MVPT) and QNST, decisions are accurate only for normal children. Test results on the VMI have been shown to be deflated in comparison with results on other visual-motor tests; therefore, the examiner should keep this in mind when using this test. Either the other instruments demonstrated poor or questionable accuracy in making decisions or studies were not completed. Ten of the fourteen tests had test items that were sensitive to the age groups for which the test was designed. On six of the tests reviewed, the test items were found to measure what they were intended to measure. For the remaining tests, domain or content validity was poor or questionable, or no studies were completed to support this type of validity. In addition, the ability of the test items to discriminate between normal individuals and a criterion group of delayed subjects was found to be good with only seven

Table 6-7. Sensorimotor functions assessed by test

Name of test	Tactile	Vestibular	Bilateral integration	Postural mechanisms, reflexes, and balance	Praxis	Fine motor and eye-hand coordination	Visual perception	Visual-motor integration	Cross-modal sensory integration	Gross motor
1. Beery (VMI)								✔		
2. BOTMP			✔	✔		✔				✔
3. DeGangi-Berk (TSI)		✔	✔	✔						
4. DTVP (Frostig)						✔	✔	✔		
5. Dunn's Guide		✔		✔						
6. Imitation of Gestures					✔					
7. Jordan							✔			
8. MVPT							✔			
9. Peabody (PDMS)				✔		✔				✔
10. Purdue (PPMS)			✔	✔		✔		✔		
11. QNST	✔		✔	✔	✔			✔	✔	
12. SCPNT		✔								
13. SCSIT	✔		✔	✔	✔	✔	✔	✔	✔	
14. TVPS							✔			

Key: VMI, Beery-Buktenica Developmental Test of Visual-Motor Integration; BOTMP, Bruininks-Oseretsky Test of Motor Proficiency; DTVP, The Marianne Frostig Developmental Test of Visual Perception; MVPT, Motor-Free Visual Perception Test; PDMS, Peabody Developmental Motor Scales (Revised); PPMS, Purdue Perceptual Motor Survey; QNST, Quick Neurological Screening Test (Revised); SCPNT, Southern California Postrotary Nystagmus Test; SCSIT, Southern California Sensory Integration Tests; TVPS, Test of Visual-Perceptual Skills (Non-Motor).

of the tests reviewed. With the remaining tests, these studies were not completed, with the exception of the TVPS which found significant differences between the performance of learning-disabled and normal children on the total test. Table 6-9 presents the information on validity.

After analyzing the various psychometric components of the tests reviewed in this chapter, it is apparent that some of the tests have not provided adequate support for their use through reliability and validity studies. Of the tests reviewed, six tests demonstrate good psychometric evidence supporting their use, although additional studies may be needed in areas such as determining predictive validity and decision-making reliability. Further data collection to strengthen the sample base is also needed with several of these instruments, including the VMI,

BOTMP, DeGangi-Berk, Peabody (PDMS), QNST, and SCPNT. Although adequate evidence of reliability and validity is provided by the Jordan, MVPT, and Purdue (PPMS), further reliability and validity studies are needed on these three instruments. The studies most needed on these three instruments are reliability and validity studies on disability groups for which the test is intended and interobserver reliability studies. Diagnostic and predictive validity studies and test-retest reliability studies are also needed for the TVPS. It is recommended that the DTVP not be used for screening or diagnosis because of poor validity. The Dunn, Imitation of Gestures, and SCSIT should be used only for clinical assessment and not for diagnostic decision making because of lack of reliability and validity studies. It is not to say that these three instru-

*Table 6-8. Reliability studies conducted on tests**

Name of test	Good interobserver reliability (> .80)	Good test-retest reliability (> .80)	Reliability good on both subtest and total test	Reliability studies completed on both criterion group and normals
1. Beery (VMI)	✓	✓		✓
2. BOTMP	✓	✓ (grades 2 and 6 only)		
3. DeGangi-Berk (TSI)	✓ (except reflex integration subtest)	✓	✓ (except reflex integration subtest)	✓
4. DTVP (Frostig)		✓		
5. Dunn's Guide				
6. Imitation of Gestures				
7. Jordan		✓		
8. MVPT		✓		
9. Peabody (PDMS)	✓	✓	✓	
10. Purdue (PPMS)	✓			
11. QNST		✓		✓
12. SCPNT	✓	✓		
13. SCSIT		✓ (on only 2 subtests)		
14. TVPS			✓ (on only 3 of 7 subtests)	

*Based on reliability studies reported in manual and in literature.
Key: VMI, Beery-Buktenica Developmental Test of Visual-Motor Integration; BOTMP, Bruininks-Oseretsky Test of Motor Proficiency; DTVP, The Marianne Frostig Developmental Test of Visual Perception; MVPT, Motor-Free Visual Perception Test; PDMS, Peabody Developmental Motor Scales (Revised); PPMS, Purdue Perceptual Motor Survey; QNST, Quick Neurological Screening Test (Revised); SCPNT, Southern California Postrotary Nystagmus Test; SCSIT, Southern California Sensory Integration Tests; TVPS, Test of Visual-Perceptual Skills (Non-Motor).

ments should not be used, because they do provide occupational and physical therapists with valuable information in determining whether a child may benefit from therapy. It is apparent after reviewing these tests that more systematic and rigorous attention needs to be directed toward the psychometric aspects of test design in constructing sensorimotor tests.

In addition to the psychometric components of test development, several gaps are evident in the availability of sensorimotor tests for particular age and disability groups. Tests of tactile functions are strongly needed, especially for preschool children. A reliable and valid instrument that can assess cross-modal integration of sensory inputs, praxis, laterality, and visual-spatial skills for preschool and school-aged children is also needed. The SCSIT is being revised

and restandardized, which will hopefully fulfill some of these needs. Several neuropsychological batteries are also available, such as the Halstead-Reitan Neuropsychological Battery for Children, which may prove useful in diagnosing skills in some of these areas for school-aged children.

In addition to the need to develop tests for specific content areas, there is a critical need to validate instruments on mentally retarded, cerebral palsied, and autistic children. Since each of these disabilities causes the child to respond differently on a variety of tasks, instruments need to be developed that take into account the child's limitations as a result of the specific disability (i.e., cognitive level) while allowing the accurate detection of sensorimotor dysfunction. Cross-validation studies are urgently needed on many

*Table 6-9. Validity studies conducted on tests**

Name of test	Accurate decision making in detecting criterion group	Items sensitive to age group for which test is intended	Items measure what they are intended to measure	Items discriminate between normals and criterion group
1. Beery (VMI)	✓ (may be deflated)	✓	✓	
2. BOTMP	✓	✓	✓	✓
3. DeGangi-Berk (TSI)	✓	✓	✓	✓
4. DTVP (Frostig)				
5. Dunn's Guide		✓		
6. Imitation of Gestures		✓		
7. Jordan		✓		✓
8. MVPT	✓ (for normals only)			✓
9. Peabody (PDMS)	✓	✓	✓	✓
10. Purdue (PPMS)		✓	✓	✓
11. QNST	✓ (for normals only)	✓		✓
12. SCPNT			✓	
13. SCSIT				
14. TVPS		✓		

*Based on validity studies reported in manual and in literature.
Key: VMI, Beery-Buktenica Developmental Test of Visual-Motor Integration; BOTMP, Bruininks-Oseretsky Test of Motor Proficiency; DTVP, The Marianne Frostig Developmental Test of Visual Perception; MVPT, Motor-Free Visual Perception Test; PDMS, Peabody Developmental Motor Scales (Revised); PPMS, Purdue Perceptual Motor Survey; QNST, Quick Neurological Screening Test (Revised); SCPNT, Southern California Postrotary Nystagmus Test; SCSIT, Southern California Sensory Integration Tests; TVPS, Test of Visual-Perceptual Skills (Non-Motor).

of the instruments reviewed in this chapter in order to make them applicable to disabilities other than learning disorders.

It is apparent from these conclusions and recommendations that extensive research in the development of sensorimotor instruments lies ahead. Several of the instruments show definite promise, and the reliability and validity studies conducted on these are encouraging while other instruments reviewed lack many of the components necessary for their use in making sound screening and diagnostic decisions. Given the difficulty of sampling large numbers of delayed children, the task that lies ahead in validating these instruments is indeed overwhelming. There is an urgent need for developing and refining available sensorimotor instruments so that children with different types of sensorimotor dysfunctions can be identified as early as possible in their development and provided with appropriate therapeutic and educational programs.

REFERENCES

1. Maurer, R. G., and Damasio, A. R. Vestibular dysfunction in autistic children. *Dev. Med. Child. Psychol.* 21 : 656, 1979.
2. McCracken, A. Tactile function of educable mentally retarded children. *Am. J. Occup. Ther.* 29 : 397, 1975.
3. Montgomery, P., and Richter, E. Effect of sensory integrative therapy on the neuromotor development of retarded children. *Phys. Ther.* 57 : 799, 1977.
4. Ornitz, E. Vestibular dysfunction in schizophrenia and childhood autism. *Compr. Psychiatry* 11 : 159, 1970.
5. Piggott, L., et al. Vestibular dysfunction in emotionally disturbed children. *Biol. Psychiatry* 11 : 719, 1976.
6. Stilwell, J. M., Crowe, T. K., and McCallum, L. W. Postrotary nystagmus duration as a function of communication disorders. *Am. J. Occup. Ther.* 32 : 222, 1978.
7. Torok, N., and Perlstein, M. A. Vestibular findings in cerebral palsy. *Ann. Otol. Rhinol. Laryngol.* 71 : 51, 1962.

Language Tests

7

Patricia B. Porter

Language is the system that provides the symbols and the structure for human communication. While the basic definitions of what characterizes a language disorder are often debatable, we know that something is wrong with the system when the message is not getting either from the speaker or to the listener in its proper form. Knowledge of the content and form of normal language development provides the standard against which the language capability of any one child can be measured. Nearly all language assessment procedures distinguish between language comprehension and production, and the four major components of language are measured across these dimensions. The four major components considered in language assessment are

1. Semantics: the understanding and use of vocabulary and concepts
2. Syntax: the understanding and use of grammatical structures
3. Morphology: the smallest meaningful units contained within a language
4. Pragmatics: the situational and interpersonal uses of language

The emphasis placed on any one of these components in the language assessment process depends on the linguistic and learning theories to which one espouses. Certainly the most valuable aspect of the assessment procedure is the knowledgeable diagnostician who keeps up with developments in all areas of language.

A useful language assessment measures a rep-resentative sample of the language understood and used by a child. This sample is then compared with other aspects of the child's developmental profile (e.g., motor development, cognitive status). Ideally, the resultant information should give the diagnostician (1) information about how language comprehension and use corresponds with the child's other developmental aspects and (2) information on which to base a treatment program. Tests presented in this chapter do one or both of these.

No tests can sample all aspects of language and communication. The tests selected for presentation in this chapter are those currently in common use. These tests measure language comprehension and use in children 3 to 15 years of age. While tests of phonology (sound characteristics of a given language), speech articulation, and hearing acuity are often included in the evaluation of communication disorders, they are separate areas of concern and have not been included in this chapter. Consideration, rather, is directed toward tests that measure the four component areas listed above.

The following tests are discussed in this chapter:

Assessment of Children's Language Comprehension
Bankson Language Screening Test
Boehm Test of Basic Concepts
Carrow Elicited Language Inventory
Clinical Evaluation of Language Functions
Environmental Language Inventory
Illinois Test of Psycholinguistic Abilities

Peabody Picture Vocabulary Test

Porch Index of Communicative Ability in Children

Preschool Language Scale

Sequenced Inventory of Communication Development

Test for Auditory Comprehension of Language

Test of Language Development-Primary

Test of Language Development-Intermediate

The Token Test for Children

Utah Test of Language Development

Language Sampling Techniques

ASSESSMENT OF CHILDREN'S LANGUAGE COMPREHENSION

Descriptive Information

Test Identification

The title of this test is *Assessment of Children's Language Comprehension* (ACLC), 1972. Its authors are Rochana Foster, Jane J. Giddan, and Joel Stark. All three authors are speech and language pathologists. Consulting Psychologist Press (577 College Ave., Palo Alto, California 94306) publishes this test at a cost of $14–$18.

Age and Type of Client

The ACLC can be used to assess normally developing or handicapped children, ages 3 years to 6 years. No speech is required.

Time Required to Administer and Score Test

This test can usually be administered and scored in approximately 20 minutes.

Evaluator

No specific professional credentials are listed as necessary for the administration of this test. The ACLC can be administered by persons other than speech and language pathologists.

Historical Perspective of the Test Construction

Development and Source of Test Items

The authors describe language development and language impairment in the test manual. They list the primary categories of language impairment in children as reduced auditory sensitivity, reduced language comprehension, reduced language production, perceptual impairment, intellectual limitation, and nonrelating behavior. Linguistic maturity, in the view of the authors of the ACLC, involves the child's ability to process an increasing number of syntactic units. They refer to these increments as critical elements. Each time the child understands or produces an utterance that includes an additional morpheme or word, he or she is adding another critical element. While many deficits are part of the profile of language-impaired children, the authors suggest that as a group they have very poor auditory memory. The ACLC is designed to evaluate this element. The test assesses poor vocabulary development, comprehension of an increasing number of items, and consistency of the pattern of words missed within a sequence.

Content and Test Administration

Content

The ACLC consists of a series of plates that present visual stimuli to the child. It is divided into parts, with Part A presenting one critical element for the child's response. These elements include common nouns, the present progressive form of verbs, and some prepositions and modifiers. There are 50 items in this section. In Part B, the child is required to remember two critical elements and respond to one of four items on each of the 10 plates. In Part C, a third critical element is added. The child chooses one picture from an array of four on 10 picture plates. Part D provides the child with four critical elements, and each plate contains five pictures. The choices include the correct answer and pictures, with the first, second, third, and fourth element varying.

Setting and Equipment

The child is seated at a low table where he or she can comfortably see the test plates and is asked to point to the pictures. Only the stimulus items in Part A can be repeated. The only materials necessary are the series of plates and the recording sheet.

Administration Procedures

The examiner is directed to (1) present each picture plate, (2) make sure the child looks at the plate, and (3) say "Show me _____," followed by the stimulus item. The administration procedure is the same for all four steps.

Scoring

To score, the examiner adds the number of correct responses. Part A requires identification of common nouns, present progressive verbs, and some prepositions and modifiers. If the majority of items are missed in Part A, the authors suggest that it is futile to continue with the rest of the test. The remaining parts contain the same vocabulary and longer constructions. The authors do not, however, list the specific cutoff number as pass/fail for Part A. The number of correct responses, divided by 10 then multiplied by 100, equals the score for Parts B, C, and D.

Psychometric Properties

Standardization

The normative group consisted of 311 nursery and elementary school children, 85 percent from Tallahassee, Florida, and the remainder from a rural Vermont Head Start Program. The parents' socioeconomic and educational backgrounds were mixed, and 38 percent of the children were black. The authors point out that the normative data should be considered tentative because they are drawn from such a limited geographical area.

Reliability

Odd-even reliability coefficients were computed for single-element (Part A) items and for Parts B, C, and D combined. The computed correlation coefficients were .86 and .80 for odd and even, respectively. No test of examiner reliability was reported.

Validity

No validity data were reported.

Guidelines for Use in a Clinical Setting

Criteria for Selection

The authors include a section on "Guidelines for Language Training" in the test manual. Also included is a section on "Clinical Applications of the ACLC." This section provides, for the clinician, therapeutic suggestions drawn directly from the test and based specifically on the child's performance on each part. The programming approach, based entirely on the building of critical elements, is systematic and clear. The procedures, however, are not directly functional. That is, they are unrelated to the use of language for communicative purposes. Examiners desiring to assess language comprehension using this instrument would either have to accept the "critical elements" philosophy or spend considerable effort interpreting the results to make them directly applicable for therapy.

Review

The ACLC provides an excellent method for determining a child's understanding of the critical elements that make up language. The normative data are limited, and no validity measures are reported. The test seems inappropriately used as a diagnostic instrument. Given the clinicians' understanding of the critical elements concept put forth by the authors, the instrument can be used to identify points of weakness.

BANKSON LANGUAGE SCREENING TEST

Descriptive Information

Test Identification

The title of this test is *Bankson Language Screening Test* (BLST), 1977. Its author is Nicholas W. Bankson, Ph.D. Bankson is the Chairman of the Department of Speech Pathology and Audiology at Boston University. University Park Press (300 N. Charles St., Baltimore, Maryland 21201) publishes the test at a cost of $15–$20.

Age and Type of Client

The BLST is designed to be used with normally developing and handicapped children between the ages of 4 years 1 month and 8 years 0 months.

Purpose

The BLST was designed to be an efficient, broad-based screening device to identify children who may need language remediation and to determine appropriate areas for further language testing.

Time Required to Administer and Score Test

Approximately 25 minutes is needed to administer and score the BLST.

Evaluator

No specific professional credentials are listed as requisite for administration of this screening test. The author does request, however, that the evaluator practice giving the test approximately 5 times before administering it for screening purposes.

Historical Perspective of Test Construction

Development and Source of Test Items

The development of the BLST was based on a "review of those areas that language interven-

tionists frequently test and remediate in younger children" [1]. The selection of the subtests was predicated on this review.

Content and Test Administration

Content

The BLST is divided into the following five sections and consists of 18 subtests:

Semantic Knowledge
Body parts
Nouns
Verbs
Categories
Functions
Colors
Quantity
Opposites

Morphological Rules
Pronouns
Verb tenses
Plurals
Comparatives-Superlatives

Syntactic Rules
Subject-Verb Agreement/Negation
Sentence Repetition-Judgment

Visual Discrimination
Matching-Discrimination
Association-Sequencing

Auditory Perception
Memory
Sequencing-Discrimination

Setting and Equipment

A comfortable, quiet setting is recommended. Required equipment includes the test booklet, a plain piece of paper, a book, and the score sheet.

Administration Procedures

The child is presented visual or auditory stimuli and is asked to verbally respond to the examiner's questions. Specific instructions for the administration and scoring of each subtest are included opposite each test plate. The author suggests that if the child does not hear or understand a specific instruction, the examiner can repeat or paraphrase the instruction.

Scoring

The items are scored either correct or incorrect. The examiner then tallies the correct responses for each subtest and compares the total with the normed scores at the child's age level on the mean and standard deviation tables included in the test manual. Next, the examiner tallies all correct responses and finds the percentile equivalent of the child's raw score on the percentile table in the test manual. Both of the tables are aged-normed into eight 6-month intervals ranging from 4 years 1 month to 8 years 0 months. Only expressive responses are scored.

Psychometric Properties

Standardization

The BLST was standardized on 637 children ranging in age from 4 years 1 month to 8 years. There were eight age groupings progressing at 6-month intervals, with between 45 and 92 children in each group. The children all lived in a semirural county near Washington, D.C. The total sample ranged from lower middle to upper middle class, with 75 percent of the total sample from the middle middle class. Eighty percent were white, eighteen percent were black, two percent were from other ethnic groups.

Reliability

The author determined the reliability of the BLST in two ways. Test-retest reliability was assessed by administering the test to a group of 70 children two times, with second testing occurring 1 week after the original testing. Pass-fail reliability for all items was established at the .94 level. In addition to test-retest reliability, the Kuder-Richardson 20 (KR-20) test, indicated a .96 overall reliability index. The *KR-20* measures the degree to which the items in a test all measure the same thing. It is a special form of alpha-coefficient used with dichotomous (right or wrong) items.

Validity

Concurrent validity of the BLST was determined by comparing the scores of 70 children on the BLST with their performances on three other widely used language tests. Pearson product-moment correlations, which are correlation coefficients computed for a set of scores in connection with a linear regression, between the BLST and the other tests were as follows:

BLST and the Peabody Picture Vocabulary Test: $r = .54$

BLST and the Boehm Concept Test: $r = .62$

BLST and the Test of Auditory Comprehension of Language: $r = .64$

The author notes that the three comparison instruments differed from the BLST in the following two ways: (1) They assessed receptive as compared with expressive language, and (2) they are more circumscribed in the aspects of language on which they focus. The author suggests that content validity of the BLST is based on the fact that the items included in the instrument were selected as representative of the kinds of tasks that language clinicians assess and remediate. The author reports that additional correlations were obtained between selected subtests of the BLST and tests designed to measure similar language behaviors. He compared the eight Semantic Knowledge subtests with the Boehm Concept Test, with a resulting r value of .82. A comparison was also made between a total score from the five Morphological Rules and Syntactic Rules subtests and the child's score on a 100-utterance spontaneous language sample scored according to the developmental sentence scoring criteria outlined by Lee [2]. A correlation of .76 was obtained.

Guidelines for Use in a Clinical Setting

Criteria for Selection

This instrument is a useful tool to screen for children who may need language remediation and, to a lesser degree, to determine appropriate areas for further language testing.

Value of Clinical Observations

The instrument is designed such that scores obtained on various subtests can be graphed for ease of interpretation of a language profile sheet at the end of the score sheet. The author states that children who score at the thirtieth percentile and below are candidates for further language assessment. Those at the fifteenth percentile and below are those who are most certain to be enrolled for clinical language instruction, while those from the sixteenth through the thirtieth percentile are those for whom a classroom enrichment approach, directed toward specific linguistic weaknesses, may be appropriate. The author correctly notes that the test may not be appropriate for use with urban black populations, on whom the test was not standardized.

Review

The BLST is easy to administer with interesting visual stimuli. With 153 items, however, its administration is a fairly tedious procedure. The author has indicated that, if necessary, the test presentation can be limited to 38 items from the BLST that, according to an item analysis, are most discriminating. The division of items into the five subtest areas allows for easy scoring and readily available visual inspection of expressive language strengths and weaknesses. The selec-

tion of tests used for comparison in the evaluation of concurrent validity seems inadequate, given that each of these tests examines receptive rather than expressive abilities.

REFERENCES

1. Bankson, N. *Bankson Language Screening Test.* Baltimore: University Park Press, 1977. Pp. 1–3.
2. Lee, L. *Developmental Sentence Analyses.* Evanston, Ill.: Northwestern University Press, 1974.

BOEHM TEST OF BASIC CONCEPTS

Descriptive Information

Test Identification

The title of this test is *Boehm Test of Basic Concepts* (BTBC), 1971. Its author is Ann E. Boehm, Ph.D. Dr. Boehm's doctoral dissertation in education [1] provided the initial impetus for development of this instrument. The Psychological Corporation (757 Third Ave., New York, New York 10017) publishes the test at a cost of $16–$20.

Age and Type of Client

The BTBC is designed to assess normally developing or handicapped children between the ages of 4 and 7 years. Physically handicapped children can point to the correct response.

Purpose

The purpose of the BTBC is to assess the mastery of 50 language concepts commonly found in preschool and primary grade instructional materials and essential to understanding and communication.

Time Required to Administer and Score Test

Approximately 25 minutes per booklet is needed to administer and score this test.

Evaluator

This instrument was designed to be administered by teachers.

Historical Perspective of Test Construction

Development and Source of Test Items

The development of the BTBC proceeded from the mistaken assumption held by many educators that children have mastered the basic concepts necessary for understanding and following directions by the time of school entry. The test is composed of two forms. Form A was developed by selecting directions and other terms that occurred with considerable frequency, that were rarely defined, and that represented relatively abstract basic concepts or ideas. These concepts were gathered from a comprehensive selection of preschool and primary grade curriculum materials in the areas of reading, arithmetic, and science. The concepts, selected in this manner, were translated into pictorial, multiple choice items and were presented to appropriate groups on a trial basis. The details of these trials are presented in the section on Standardization. The author selected to omit the items in these trials that children found difficult for reasons *other* than lack of concept knowledge. Also omitted were items that were answered correctly by nearly all of the kindergarten and first grade pupils tested. Items for Form B were written to parallel those included on Form A, with like numbered items on the two forms measuring knowledge of the same basic concept.

Content and Test Administration

Content

Both forms of the BTBC consist of 50 pictorial items arranged in approximate order of increasing difficulty and divided evenly between two booklets, each containing three sample questions followed by 25 test questions. The child is

to respond to the question by marking the appropriate picture. Booklet 2 is more difficult than booklet 1. Each item consists of a set of pictures, about which statements are read aloud to the children by the examiner. The statements briefly describe the pictures and instruct the children to mark the one that illustrates the concept being tested.

Setting and Equipment

The test can be administered to an individual child or to a class of children, in a comfortable, quiet setting. The testing materials are all that is needed for the teacher, and two test booklets plus a crayon or pencil are needed for each child.

Administration Procedures

Booklet 1 is distributed to each of the children taking the test. Directions are given to the children about how and where to mark the correct answer on the booklet. The teacher then begins by administering three sample questions and then checking to see if everyone correctly followed directions. If so, the teacher then begins to administer each item. The following is a sample item: "Look at the table and the boxes. Mark the box that is away from the table . . . Mark the box that is *away* from the table." Booklet 2 is administered in the same fashion. If the children are very young or lack the attention span required to respond to all 50 items of the test at a single sitting, one can administer the test in two sittings. Administer the test booklet 1 in one session and booklet 2 in the second session. Detailed directions are provided for each booklet on both Form A and B. The items in boldface are to be read aloud to the children in the administration process. Italicized items are to be read to the children twice.

Scoring

The total number of items answered correctly is added for each child. The teacher can divide the total of correct answers by the total number of children tested and record the results as a group average. The teacher can also determine the percent of children in the class who answered each item correctly. In addition to this, the percentile correct can be determined for each child, and these percentages can be compared with norms listed in the manual. Dr. Boehm includes a special section on scoring and recording accuracy, noting points at which errors have frequently occurred.

Psychometric Properties

Standardization

The author selected a group of concepts that occur frequently in curriculum materials. The concepts selected were thought to be important for understanding and following instructions, although little or no attention is given to these concepts in their direct instruction. The author then conducted an experimental trial of items to identify those that would be most useful to the teacher. The first trial sample consisted of 267 kindergarten, 306 first grade, 264 second grade, and 297 third grade pupils attending four schools in a city of about 75,000 people located in southeastern New York state. The author notes that one of the participating schools drew its pupils from population areas of relatively high socioeconomic status, one drew from areas of relatively low socioeconomic status, and two drew from mixed areas. Eight 25-item test booklets containing, in all, 200 trial items were administered to the children at each grade level. Each class of pupils was given only four of the eight booklets, with the selection and sequence of booklets rotated to help assure random trial samples for each item. The best 50 items were selected on the basis of the following: (1) each measured a different concept; (2) each item had point-biserial correlation with the subjects' total scores on the booklet in which the item appeared, exceeding .30, (3) each showed fairly even rises in percent, passing values across those

levels, and (4) together they yielded a roughly normal distribution of percent, passing values centered around .50 for kindergarten pupils. After minor revision, a second trial was undertaken. This sample consisted of 651 kindergarten, 823 first grade, and 710 second grade pupils from six schools in a city of about 2 million population located in an eastern state. Based on the results of this trial, several additional revisions were made. The resulting revision of the BTBC was used to secure normative data.

Because the BTBC was designed as a screening and teaching instrument rather than for predictive or administrative purposes, the author considered it unnecessary to select standardization samples representative of children in kindergarten and the first and second grades in the nation as a whole. The normative information presented is intended more as an informal guide than as the essential procedure for interpreting test results. More than 10,000 children were used in the standardization of the BTBC.

Reliability

Both split-half reliability coefficients and standard errors of measurement were computed for Form A and Form B. The split-half reliability coefficients for the total score on Form A ranged from .68 to .90, while the corresponding coefficients for the total score on Form B ranged from .12 to .94. The author notes that the coefficient of .12 was obtained for the second grade, high socioeconomic level sample, a group that had a mean total score of 48.5 and a standard deviation of 0.9. She notes further that such a group forms the extreme upper end of the ability groups for which the BTBC had been presumed applicable. Therefore, at this level, the value of the BTBC would seem to lie only in the identification of children who are far below the group's average ability. Alternate form reliability coefficients were determined for total scores on Forms A and B. These values ranged from .55 to .92, with a median of .76.

Validity

The author suggests that for the BTBC, validity is primarily a matter of the relevance of the test content. The author deems the BTBC valid because the test items were selected from relevant curriculum materials and represent concepts basic to understanding directions and other oral communications from teachers at the preschool and primary grade level.

Guidelines for Use in a Clinical Setting

Criteria for Selection

The BTBC is useful both in determining individual weaknesses in students' understanding of basic concepts as they enter school and in revealing the specific needs of a class in relation to their understanding of basic concepts applicable for use in basic kindergarten and first grade curricula.

Review

Some of the test questions seem a bit dated (e.g., "Look at the clothes hanging on the line . . . "); however, the concepts being tested are basic and timeless. It would appear that the BTBC would be of greatest value when administered in a class setting.

REFERENCE

1. Boehm, A. E. "The Development of Comparative Concepts in Primary School Children," doctoral dissertation, Columbia University, 1967.

CARROW ELICITED LANGUAGE INVENTORY

Descriptive Information

Test Identification

The title of this test is *Carrow Elicited Language Inventory* (CELI), 1974. Its author is Elizabeth Carrow-Woolfolk, Ph.D., a speech and language pathologist currently on the faculty of the University of Texas at Austin. Teaching Resources Corporation (50 Pond Park Rd., Hingham, Massachusetts 02043) publishes the test at a cost of $35–$40.

Age and Type of Client

This test is designed for children ages 3 years 0 months to 7 years 11 months who have the capability to speak.

Purpose

The CELI was developed to provide a means for measuring "productive control of grammar." The child is required to imitate a sequence of sentences representing basic sentence construction types and specific grammatical morphemes. Carrow-Woolfolk suggests that CELI provides a means of identifying children with language problems as well as specific linguistic structures that may be contributing to the child's inadequate linguistic performance.

Time Required to Administer and Score Test

The test is administered individually. It requires about 5 minutes to administer and 20 to 30 minutes to score.

Evaluator

The CELI was developed primarily for use by speech pathologists.

Historical Perspective of Test Construction

Development and Source of Test Items

The CELI was developed to improve on the body of language information elicited in language sampling of a child's spontaneous speech. Dr. Carrow-Woolfolk cites the work of McNeill [10], Menyuk [6, 7], and others to support the drawbacks inherent in language sampling and the relative value of sentence imitation as a source of information about the development of language comprehension and expression in children. Although imitation is well supported as a means to study language-disordered children, Dr. Carrow-Woolfolk found no procedure that systematically assembled widely representative sentence constructions and grammatical morphemes available to be used as stimuli for assessment purposes. The CELI was developed as an attempt to eliminate some of the problems of sampling by including stimulus items representing a wide range of grammatical complexity. Further, the test allows analysis of forms over which the child has productive control but which may not occur in a particular language sample. Finally, the test is designed to measure the deviation of the child's performance against normal adult speech.

Content and Test Administration

Content

The CELI consists of 52 stimuli: 51 sentences and 1 phrase. The stimuli range in length from 2 to 10 words, with an average length of 6 words. Of the 51 sentences, 47 are in the active tense and 4 in the passive tense; 37 are affirmative and 14 are negative; 37 are declarative, 12 are interrogative, and 2 are imperative. The grammatical categories and features covered by the test include articles, adjectives, nouns, noun-plurals, pronouns, verbs, negatives, contractions, adverbs, prepositions, demonstratives, and conjunctions. Within each of these categories, the items range from simple to complex forms.

Setting and Equipment

The author suggests that the child should be tested individually in a quiet room. The stimulus sentences are presented in a live voice; the stimuli and the child's responses are recorded on high-fidelity audio tape equipment. No additional material is required other than that included in the test kit.

Administrative Procedures

After the instructions have been read to the child, the examiner is directed to read the stimulus sentences from the scoring and analysis form and record the child's response. If the child does not imitate a sentence the first time it is given, the clinician is directed to test the next three sentences and then return to the nonimitated sentence to see if the child will repeat it on the second trial. Only two trials for each stimulus sentence can be given. If the child self-corrects a response, the second version is the one used for analysis. Directions are straightforward and easy to follow. Young children can be difficult to test because they are sometimes distracted by the microphone. The author suggests that, in this case, the microphone can be hidden in a hand puppet. The written record of the child's responses made by the examiner, supplemented with the tape-recorded responses, should yield a complete body of elicited responses.

Scoring

Forms provided in the test kit list all the sentences in the order of their occurrence and provide spaces beside each sentence for writing the child's response. The form gives the grammatical classification of all words used in the stimulus sentences. The author suggests that the clinician use phonemic notation for transcribing the child's responses. Columns to the right of the grammar categories on the scoring form can be used to record the types of errors found in the child's response. The author lists five categories of error types: substitutions, omissions, additions, transpositions, and reversals. In scoring, there should be a one-to-one relationship between words and errors. No substitution or other form of error should be counted as two or more errors except as indicated in the rules. Each error should be marked according to type in the appropriate column on the right side of the scoring form. After the sentence has been marked, the total number of errors of each type should be recorded in the grid on the right side of the score sheet. After the entire test has been scored, the examiner should tally the number of errors made in each grammatical category and of each type. The sum of the grammar subcategory totals should match the sum of the types of category totals, and this grand total should be added to the bottom of the last page of the scoring form. The author lists seven pages of rules for scoring, with examples given for each type of error. The raw scores obtained by the child are converted to a derived score, which indicates the child's relative standing as compared with the normative sample of the test. Mean scores for the total error of scores and types of category scores are presented in the test manual for each age group. A child's total score and types of category scores can be located on these curves and evaluated relative to the mean for his or her age group. Percentile ranks corresponding to specific total raw scores and subcategory scores for each age are listed as well. Standard scores are provided by transformation of total raw scores to stanine scores for each age level. The stanine score provides a single-digit system of scores with a mean of 5 and a standard deviation of approximately 2. Children with a stanine of 1 or 2 are more than 1 standard deviation below the mean.

Dr. Carrow-Woolfolk lists cautions in test interpretation. She suggests that a child's performance on the CELI may not be reflective of the status of his or her grammatical system. She points out that the child's motivation and effort may influence test responses. Inconsistency in response should make the examiner question the validity of the test results.

Psychometric Properties

Standardization

The CELI was administered to 475 white children between the ages of 3 years 0 months to 7 years 11 months who came from middle socioeconomic level homes where Standard American English was the sole language spoken. The au-

thor reports that all children in this normative sample were selected from day-care centers and church schools in middle-class neighborhoods of Houston, Texas. All children with apparent speech or language disorders were eliminated from the sample group. All the children were tested by the same examiner using the same directions.

Reliability

In an effort to determine test-retest reliability, the author selected 25 children (five each at the age levels of 3, 4, 5, 6, and 7 years), tested them, and then retested them after a period of 2 weeks. These children were selected at random. The same examiner administered, transcribed, and scored the two test results. The product-moment correlation coefficient obtained was 0.98.

Interexaminer reliability was obtained by correlating the transcriptions and scoring by two examiners with 10 randomly selected tapes. The correlation coefficient was 0.98. A second measure of interexaminer reliability was obtained by the administration, transcription, and scoring of the CELI by two examiners on 20 children. Ten of these children were diagnosed language-disordered children; the correlation coefficient reported by the author was 0.99.

Carrow-Woolfolk reports that an attempt was made to establish an age–raw score equivalency table. She notes, however, that there was considerable instability of the scores across the ages when grouped on a small interval scale. The author fit two linear models to the data in an attempt to smooth out the score difference across ages. An F test of the difference in models yielded an F of 121.193, with a probability of $<.0000$ that the two models fit the data equally well. The author concluded, then, that the relationship between age-in-months and the test scores was curvilinear. The scores show a gradual increase in errors beginning at age 6 to 7 years to the upper limit. The author notes that the test ceiling is at about 79 months (6 years 7 months) and that the increase in errors past that age is due to chance.

Validity

The author reports that three methods were used to determine the validity of the CELI. Two of these methods involve concurrent validity, or the agreement between the test score and temporarily identical but independent indicators of the same phenomena; and one method involves congruent validity, or the agreement between the test score and the values obtained on similar but separate indicators administered at the same time. Since language has been shown to be a developmental phenomena, as children mature chronologically one would expect that their skills in all aspects of language would improve as well. The author indicates that an analysis of variance of tests in the age differences in total scores and in subscores on the CELI were significant. This finding indicated that the test scores did improve with age and that they followed a developmental pattern. The product-moment correlation coefficient between age and total score was .62. The author suggests one can conclude that the CELI has concurrent validity. In an effort to investigate the manner in which this instrument could correctly classify individuals who differ with respect to the language variables being measured, the author cites a 1974 study that used the CELI to separate language-disordered children from children with normal language. She found that the instrument reflected a significant difference in total language score between the two groups, with significant differences found between the groups in grammar subcategory scores ranging from $p < .00$ to $p < .0047$. In this same study, the CELI was compared with the *Developmental Sentence Scoring* (DSS) procedure developed by Lee and Canter [5]. The correlation between the CELI and the DSS, an instrument widely used in the assessment of language, was – .79. The author proposes, then, that the CELI has congruent validity.

McDade, Simpson, and Lamb [9] have suggested, however, that Dr. Carrow-Woolfolk's data relate to the test's norm-referenced capabilities rather than its validity. That is, "they support the test's ability to identify children with language impairment but say nothing about its capacity to go beyond summary scores to describe those specific components of grammar that need remediation" [9]. They suggest that a criterion-referenced rather than norm-referenced test of validity would be the most appropriate measure. The comments were made in a reply to Dr. Carrow-Woolfolk's response [3] to their initial article [8].

Guidelines for Use in a Clinical Setting

Criteria for Selection

This instrument provides a well-structured mechanism for the elicitation of maximum information on a child's basic sentence construction types and specific grammatical morphemes. The test is diagnostic. It is useful not only in identifying children with language problems but also in determining the specific linguistic structures that may be contributing to the child's language difficulty. The latter is of great value in determination of specific language therapy goals. Use of this instrument implies that the examiner believes that assessment through imitation of an utterance is a reasonable way to elicit language from a child.

Value of Clinical Observations

The author provides considerable support for assessment through imitation in the test manual. Other studies of language-impaired children, however, have reported that children's imitations are semantically and grammatically more advanced than their spontaneous speech [2, 12]. Further, Bartel [1] concluded, following a study of 40 preschool, language-impaired children, that the CELI provided inaccurate representations of the children's linguistic capabilities. She suggests that the CELI, by itself, does not provide the clinician with information on which to plan a therapeutic intervention program.

Review

The CELI provides the opportunity to elicit an elaborate, comprehensive body of language from a child. The strength of the instrument, however, depends totally on the willingness of the child to imitate fairly complex sentences such as "Couldn't Daddy have been coming?" Many young children may have great difficulty remaining interested in the task through the imitation of 52 sentences. The lack of any visual stimuli may be a liability in terms of engaging the child in the task at hand. Finally, McDade et al. [9] and others [4] question the use of imitative performance as a basis for any clinical decisions.

REFERENCES

1. Bartel, K. "Elicited Imitation: Caution When Assessing Preschoolers with Auditory Processing Deficiencies." Presentation to the American Speech-Language-Hearing Association Annual Conference, San Francisco, November 1984.
2. Bloom, L., Hood, L., and Lightbrown, P. Imitation in language development: If, when and why. *Cognitive Psychol.* 6 : 380, 1974.
3. Carrow-Woolfolk, E. CELI validity reviewed: A response to McDade, Simpson and Lamb. *J. Speech Hear. Disord.* 48 : 328, 1983.
4. Connell, P., and Myles-Zitzer, C. An analysis of elicited imitation as a language evaluation procedure. *J. Speech Hear. Disord.* 47 : 390, 1982.
5. Lee, L., and Canter, S. Developmental sentence scoring: A clinical procedure for estimating syntactic development in children's spontaneous speech. *J. Speech Hear. Disord.* 36 : 315, 1971.
6. Menyuk, P. Alternation of rules in children's grammar. *J. Verbal Learn. Verbal Behav.* 3 : 480, 1964.
7. Menyuk, P. *The Acquisition and Development of Language.* Englewood Cliffs, N.J.: Prentice-Hall, 1971.
8. McDade, H. L., Simpson, M. A., and Lamb, D. E. The use of elicited imitation as a measure of expressive grammar: A question of validity. *J. Speech Hear. Disord.* 47 : 19, 1982.
9. McDade, H. L., Simpson, M. A., and Lamb, D. E. Reply to Carrow-Woolfolk. *J. Speech Hear. Disord.* 48 : 334, 1983.
10. McNeill, D. *The Acquisition of Language: The Study of Developmental Psycholinguistics.* New York: Harper and Row, 1970.
11. Prutting, C., and Connelly, J. Imitation: A closer look. *J. Speech Hear. Disord.* 41 : 412, 1976.
12. Ramar, A. Syntactic styles in emerging language. *J. Child. Lang.* 3 : 49, 1976.

CLINICAL EVALUATION OF LANGUAGE FUNCTION

Descriptive Information

Test Identification

The title of this test is *Clinical Evaluation of Language Function* (CELF)—Diagnostic Battery, 1980. Its authors are Eleanor Messing Semel, Ph.D., and Elisabeth H. Wiig, Ph.D. Dr. Semel is a speech and language pathologist. Dr. Wiig is also a speech and language pathologist and is Professor of Communication Disorders at Boston University. Charles E. Merrill Publishing Company (1300 Alum Creek Dr., Columbus, Ohio 43216) publishes the test at a cost of approximately $75–$100 for the diagnostic battery.

Age and Type of Client

The test is designed for individuals between the ages of 4 and 18 years.

Purpose

The CELF-Diagnostic Battery is designed to provide differentiated measures of selective language functions in the areas of phonology, syntax, semantics, memory, and word finding and retrieval. The subtests assist in the identification of children in grades kindergarten through 12 with language disabilities (1) to provide a differential diagnosis of the areas involved through selected language probes and (2) to identify areas for follow-up language intervention. The authors note that the CELF is not designed to provide in-depth assessment at the levels of phonology or pragmatics.

Time Required to Administer and Score Test

Approximately 76 minutes is needed for administration and scoring of this test.

Evaluator

The CELF can be administered without formal training if the examiner is experienced in administering, scoring, and interpreting psychological, clinical, or individual educational tests. The test authors suggest that the examiner be trained by using the CELF training videotape available from the publisher. The results of the administration of the CELF should not be considered valid until the examiner has administered at least 10 tests under supervision.

Historical Perspective of Test Construction

Development and Source of Test Items

The CELF was developed as an outgrowth of a large study on the prevalence and nature of learning and language disabilities in children and adolescents developed by Wiig and Semel [3, 4]. The authors have noted prevalence of language disorders in children and adolescents who have been identified as learning disabled. This language disorder syndrome is characterized by disorders of comprehension at the word and sentence levels; deficits in the immediate recall of spoken digits, words, sentences, and oral directions; and word-finding problems and dysnomia. The CELF was designed to probe aspects of the language disorder syndrome observed among children and adolescents with learning disabilities and learning handicaps.

Content and Test Administration

Content

The CELF features 11 subtests that probe selected aspects of language functioning in the areas of word meaning, sentence structure, recall, and retrieval; two supplementary subtests are designed to probe aspects of processing and production at the level of speech sounds. The subtests are as follows:

    Processing Subtests
        Processing Word and Sentence Structure
        Processing Word Classes
        Processing Linguistic Concepts
        Processing Relationships and Ambiguities
        Processing Oral Directions
        Processing Spoken Paragraph
    Production Subtests
        Producing Word Series
        Producing Names on Confrontation
        Producing Word Association
        Producing Model Sentences
        Producing Formulated Sentences
    Supplementary
        Processing Speech Sounds
        Producing Speech Sounds

These subtests have been grouped by response mode. Six of the subtests in one supplementary subtest require recognition, interpretation, and/or recall and asks for pointing, yes/no responses, or Wh-questions/answers (i.e., who, what, when, where or why questions). These are the Processing Subtests. The five remaining subtests in one supplementary subtest require active naming, word or sentence recall, or sentence formulation and production. These subtests have been grouped to form the Production Subtests. The statement of purpose and design for each of the subtests is elaborately discussed in the test manual.

Setting and Equipment

The CELF subtest should be administered in a quiet room with adequate illumination and ventilation. If the examiner is right-handed, he or she should be seated next to the child on the child's right side. If the examiner is left-handed, he or she should be on the child's left. These seating arrangements allow the examiner maximum control of the presentation of visual stimuli and ease in recording the child's response. They also assure that the child cannot see what the examiner records on the score form.

Materials needed for administration of the CELF include the examiner's manual, stimulus/ score form, picture stimuli for several of the subtests, stopwatch, and cassette recorder if possible.

Administration Procedures

Guidelines for administration of each of the subtests are listed in the test manual. Ten of the subtests are untimed and are scored for the accuracy of responses. Three of the subtests—Producing Word Series, Producing Names on Confrontation, and Producing Word Association—are timed and assess the speech or quantity of response as well as their accuracy. The test items themselves are presented on the score form for ease of administration. Each of the subtests begins with presentation of trial items. These trial items act as a manner of screening for the test items themselves. The examiner is directed to discontinue with a particular subtest if the child fails to respond correctly to the trial item. Following successful completion of the trial items, the examiner is assessed using the test items for that particular subtest.

Scoring

Procedures are listed for scoring each of the subtests in the test manual. In most instances the examiner is directed to check whether the child's response was incorrect in the appropriate columns on the score form. The score forms also include error analysis grids for the majority of the subtests, to permit a more detailed evaluation of the error response patterns. The error analysis grids follow a general design in which the items are grouped on the basis of semantic category or relationship, syntactic structure, or the like. Item numbers are presented for each grouping. The error analysis grids also allow for the derivation of the error percentage on the basis of the specific number of items failed. Criterion raw scores for pass (above criterion raw score) or fail (at or below criterion raw score) are presented for each subtest by grade level in the test manual.

Psychometric Properties

Standardization

The authors note that the CELF Diagnostic Battery was standardized concurrently with the CELF Screening Test. The screening tests are not described in detail in this review. The screening tests, developed for both elementary and advanced levels, were designed to provide a measure for screening the language processing and production abilities of school-aged children over a wide range of grade levels. The authors note that it is appropriate to evaluate children who performed poorly on the screening test via the CELF-Diagnostic Battery. The standardization sample for the CELF Screening Test was stratified to reflect the 1970 U.S. census data as closely as possible according to grade level, sex, racio-ethnic background, and geographic region. The residence of the children and the parents' occupations were also taken into consideration. The target sample size for each grade level was a minimum of 100 children. The authors note that this number was approximated at all grade levels except fifth grade, where a total of 132 children were given the screening, 56 with the elementary-level test and 76 with the advanced-level test. The total size of the standardization sample was 1405 children. Children selected for inclusion in the screening standardization were selected to show patterns of normal development in academic achievement. Grade level, rather than age level, was used to stratify the normative sample along the age continuum. The authors note that the primary goal of the standardization of the Diagnostic Battery of the CELF was to establish criteria for determining which children given the Diagnostic Battery should be recommended for extension testing. The purpose of extension testing, according to the authors, is to explore the variables that seemed to be primary in contributing to the child's incorrect responses. It is important to identify a baseline at which the child can respond correctly in order to make judgments about the degree of difference between the conditions at that basal level and the conditions under which the child might normally be expected to perform. The degree of these differences will indicate the seriousness of the child's deficit. Following the scoring directions for each of the subtests in the test battery, the authors list procedures for extension testing. Many of these procedures include reference to other diagnostic tests.

In standardization of the Diagnostic Battery, performances of 159 children, ranging in grade level from kindergarten through twelfth grade, were analyzed to establish criteria for determining which children, given the Diagnostic Battery, should be recommended for extension testing. The number of children at any grade level ranged from 6 to 37. Approximately 30 percent of this sample was drawn from among low scoring children in the Screening Test norming sample. An additional 20 percent were children identified or at least referred as having potential language or learning problems. These children came from eight different states and were not included in the norm sample for the screening test. An additional 20 percent of this sample had not been diagnosed as learning or language disabled but were attending a university-sponsored summer school for help with reading and math difficulties. These children were not part of the screening sample either. Thirty percent of the children were regarded as normal to above average in school abilities and performance, and one-fourth of these children were included in the screening sample.

Reliability

Interrelationships among the various subtests of the Diagnostic Battery were evaluated. The correlation coefficients for subtest relationships were assessed; several of the correlations among subtests were significant at the .05 or .01 level, but most were not. The authors noted that significant positive correlations existed among the subtests that probe the processing, recall, and formulation of sentence structure. Measures of accuracy and time of the naming and serial recall subtests correlated negatively.

The authors evaluated test-retest reliability by administering the Diagnostic Battery twice to a group of 30 randomly selected academically achieving children with normal language development, with a 6-week time interval between tests. The same team of three trained examiners evaluated the children on the two occasions, but no child was evaluated twice by the same examiner. All test-retest reliability coefficients proved significant at the .01 level. The range of measures reflecting the magnitude of the correlation coefficients was from .56 to .98. The authors note that relatively low test-retest reliability correlations for individual subtests could be expected with samples of children who are all about the same age. They suggest that this is a problem of restricted range. They noted that when the subtests of the CELF were combined, the test-retest reliability coefficient increased ($r = .96$). The authors cautioned that administration of only selected individual subtests may result in less reliable diagnoses with the CELF. They recommend that to be most reliable, subtests should be administered as a total battery, or at least in sections containing the processing and/or production subtest.

Validity

The authors evaluated concurrent validity by comparing the performances on the Diagnostic Battery with performances on existing criterion measures of speech and language ability based on the test protocols of 30 children with learning disabilities. These children all attended the fifth and sixth grades and ranged in age from 12 years 2 months to 12 years 7 months. They exhibited academic deficits of two or more grade levels in two or more academic areas. The authors compared various subtests of the CELF to the verbal subtest of the Illinois Test of Psycholinguistic Abilities (ITPA), selective verbal subtest of the Detroit Test of Learning Aptitude (DTLA), the Wepman Test of Auditory Discrimination, The Fisher-Logemann Test of Articulation, the Northwestern Syntax Screening Test (NSST), The Token Test, and the Spache Reading Passage. The authors listed only concurrent validity coefficients of magnitudes at or greater than .40.

All subtests of the CELF correlated at .87 with the verbal subtests of the ITPA and at .52 with the DTLA subtests. The Processing Speech Sounds Subtest correlated at .76 with the Wepman, and the Producing Speech Sounds Subtest correlated at .59 with the Fisher-Logemann. Processing Linguistic Concepts correlated at .62 with Part V of the Token Test, and Processing Word and Sentence Structure correlated at .53 with the NSST Receptive Section. The various subtests of the CELF were correlated individually with similar subtests of the DTLA and ITPA. Correlations ranged from .42 to .94. More specific correlation information can be found in the CELF test manual [2].

Additional Standardization Information

The test authors requested feedback from examiners in the test manual. They received feedback and have modified parts of the test accordingly. One of the frequent comments was that grade level criteria seemed too low; some children who passed the Diagnostic Battery nevertheless appeared to exhibit language disabilities. Norms for the various subtests of the Diagnostic Battery were requested. Semel-Mintz and Wiig published a report in a *CELF Update* in 1982 [1] that was distributed to all persons who had purchased the original test. The authors reported a norming study implemented to develop age and grade level norms for the Diagnostic Battery. The Diagnostic Battery was administered to 1378 students during the fall of 1981. The children were in kindergarten through twelfth grade and ages 6 to 18 years. All were considered normal. From this sample, the authors developed norms for the Diagnostic Battery available in three forms: (1) language age scores for total processing and for total production, (2) percentile ranks by grade level for total processing and for total production, and (3) individual subtests pass/fail criterion scores for each grade level. Some changes in scoring of various subtests in the Diagnostic Battery were necessitated by these new forms. The authors list these scoring changes in the 1982 *Update*. The authors note that all three scores are easily converted from raw scores, and while language age scores are available, examiners are urged to consider all three measures in evaluating a student's performance on the Diagnostic Battery.

Guidelines for Use in a Clinical Setting

Value of Clinical Observations

Use of the Extension Testing concept is very useful for the clinician. The examiner is not left with just a diagnosis, but rather with an understanding of the child's performance in language understanding and use under various conditions. With this understanding as to what the child both can and cannot do, the clinician can plan specific intervention strategies. The CELF is well supported by the authors' comprehensive handbook, *Language Assessment and Intervention for the Learning Disabled* [4].

Review

The picture stimuli used in administration of the CELF are clear and colorful. Their content, however, is not particularly engaging for kindergarten and first grade children. Questions remain regarding what many examiners consider to be the inflated norms of the CELF. The authors and Charles E. Merrill Publishing Company should be congratulated for their continuing attempt to address these concerns via the periodic publication of the *CELF Update* series [1]. These booklets contain items such as raw score–percentile rank tables for the Diagnostic Battery subtests and answers to some of the more frequent questions submitted to the test authors by examiners in the field.

REFERENCES

1. Hutchinson, T. (ed.). *CELF Updates 1, 2 and 3.* Columbus, Oh.: Merrill, 1981, 1982, and 1983.
2. Semel, E. M., and Wiig, E. H. *Clinical Evaluation of Language Function—Diagnostic Battery Examiner's Manual.* Columbus, Oh.: Merrill, 1980.
3. Wiig, E. H., and Semel, E. M. *Language Disabilities in Children and Adolescents.* Columbus, Oh.: Merrill, 1976.
4. Wiig, E. H., and Semel, E. M. *Language Assessment and Intervention for the Learning Disabled.* Columbus, Oh.: Merrill, 1980.

ENVIRONMENTAL LANGUAGE INVENTORY

Descriptive Information

Test Identification

The title of this test is *Environmental Language Inventory* (ELI), 1978. Its author is James D. MacDonald, Ph.D. Dr. MacDonald is the Director of the Language Program at the Nisonger Center, Ohio State University, and Associate Professor of Speech and Hearing Science at Ohio State University, Columbus. Charles E. Merrill Publishing Company, Test Division (1300 Alum Creek Dr., Box 508, Columbus, Ohio 43216) publishes the test at a cost of $11–$15 for the ELI Manual and $11–$15 for ELI Score Forms.

Age and Type of Client

The test is designed for young children or developmentally delayed individuals.

Purpose

The ELI was developed as a model of training and service for severely language delayed clients. The Inventory can be used for experimental or diagnostic purposes. The ELI assesses expressive language from the first word combinations through four-word sentences. In addition, the ELI assesses the rules in the production modes of imitation, conversation, and play.

Time Required to Administer and Score Test

The author suggests that there are two major uses of the ELI: experimental (comparing child's total score against others of his or her own baseline) and diagnostic (analyzing subtest data to determine a child's strengths or weaknesses). The diagnostic form should take approximately 30 minutes to complete, whereas the experimental form may require 45 minutes. For diagnostic use, the test may be administered in parts on separate days. For experimental use, administration should be accomplished in a single day. Time needed for scoring the test is variable.

Evaluator

The ELI was developed primarily for use by speech and language pathologists. Heavy emphasis, however, is placed on recruiting parents, teachers, and paraprofessionals to assist in information gathering and subsequent language training.

Historical Perspective of Test Construction

Development and Source of Test Items

The development of the ELI follows the movement, in the study of child language, away from the focus on the structure of adult grammar toward an emphasis on the rules governing the structure of early utterances and the concepts specifying the semantic function of those structures in child language. The foundation of the

ELI was determined in the identification of language classes to be sampled and trained with the clinical objective of expansion of the child's utterances, semantic intent of the language classes identified, and strategies designed to provide the information and procedures necessary for training immediate generalization of the language classes to spontaneous use. The author draws heavily on the work of Schlesinger [5] and Brown [1] in his definitions of the semantic relations in emerging language and the range of structural meanings in children's first two-word utterances.

Content and Test Administration

Content

The ELI consists of procedures to assess expressive language in three modes: conversation, imitation, and play. Conversation and imitation are evaluated in a single procedure, while a separate procedure is provided for assessment in free play. The test consists of 24 stimulus sets, three of which assess each of the eight semantic-grammatical rules. Each stimulus set includes one nonlinguistic cue and two linguistic cues. The nonlinguistic cue provides the environmental event that specifies the meaning expressed by the rule; the same nonlinguistic cue is used to access both the conversational and imitative production of a rule. Separate linguistic cues are used, one to elicit the rule in conversation, the other in imitation. For the conversation-imitation-conversation procedure the author presents the following sample procedure for one item. This task illustrates the elicitation of the three-word production of the rule "action plus object."

Example: Action plus object
    Nonlinguistic cue: Kick large ball in air.
    Conversation cue: "What am I doing?"
    Imitation cue: "Say, kick big ball."
    Conversation cue: "What am I doing?"

In the free play sample, parents, teachers, or work associates are asked to describe situations in which the client verbalizes most readily. The clinician is directed to record 50 utterances as a free production language sample. In cases where it is impossible to obtain a 50-utterance free production sample, the author directs that the examiner should obtain as many utterances as possible within a reasonable amount of time. Dr. MacDonald lists specific directions in the manual as to how to record the free play sample.

Setting and Equipment

MacDonald suggests that for the conversation-imitation-conversation procedure, all test materials should be within the examiner's reach but out of sight of the child. Pretest items are to be administered first to acclimate the examiner and the child to each other. For the free play sample, the setting should be structured to stimulate conditions within which the client has been found to verbalize most readily. Materials necessary for administration include the following:

1. One administration and recording form for the conversation-imitation-conversation procedure
2. A separate recording form for free play
3. Tokens and food bits if tangible reinforcement is to be applied (Dr. MacDonald encourages the reinforcement of all responses, not just correct responses)
4. The test manual
5. The following objects:

Paper	Bag	Bed for doll
Large ball	Baby doll bottle	Small book
Dry cereal	Pin	Cup
bits	Small ball	Regular-sized
Small car	Large car	chair
Dog	Doll	Raisins
Blocks		

In the manual, the author notes that these objects are only suggested stimuli and that the examiner may substitute items to meet the needs of each client. However, he notes further, that the items should be kept constant if the test is being administered for experimental use.

Administration Procedures

The procedure for administration of the Conversation-Imitation-Conversation Test includes presentation of all 24 stimulus sets. If a client makes no response to four consecutive conversation tasks, Dr. MacDonald suggests that the examiner continue with the imitation tasks alone in order not to frustrate the client with extensive failure experience. The examiner is then directed to return to the conversation task if the client responds to all of the imitated tasks. As is noted throughout the test manual, the author suggests that the ELI can be adapted in creative response to the particular client in order to obtain an optimal language performance if it is being administered for diagnostic use.

During the free play sample portion of the test, the examiner is encouraged to record the child's utterances while attempting to keep conversation to a minimum. If the child is silent, however, the author suggests that modeling an imitation may be useful. He suggests further, however, that each of the child's comments that follows modeling or imitation should be marked as such. When utterances are recorded, the examiner is directed to also record the accompanying contextual cues. Such cues, the author notes, are often valuable pieces of information in understanding the meaning of the client's utterance.

Scoring

The ELI can yield several scores for three language modes: conversation, imitation, and play. All possible scores will not usually be needed for a given study or client. The range of scores available are as follows:

Semantic-grammatical rules
  Frequencies of rules in imitation-
    conversation-play

Rank order of rules in imitation-conversation-play
Proportions of rules in imitation-conversation-play
Utterance length
  Mean length utterance as total words in imitation-conversation-play
  Mean length of utterance (MLU) for intelligible words only in imitation-conversation-play
Intelligibility
  Proportion of intelligible words in imitation-conversation-play
  Frequency of unintelligible multiple-word utterances in imitation-conversation-play

The author gives elaborate scoring procedures for each of the scoring categories.

Psychometric Properties

Standardization

MacDonald states in the test manual that "Experimental support of the psychological validity and reliability of the Environmental Language Inventory is a complex issue" [3]. He then supports this contention with 33 detailed pages covering validity and reliability. The author lists multiple field studies of the test instrument with both normally developing and developmentally delayed children. The author notes that, while the ELI has not been submitted to traditional normative testing, data on test performance (imitation and conversation) are available for 25 normally developing children, and data on free speech distributions are available for 40 normal children, 10 normal first graders, and 10 normal adults. He notes further that two studies were conducted with mentally retarded children in order to assess both the instrument's test-retest reliability and its comparison to rule usage in Mean Length of Utterance in the three modes: imitation, conversation, and play. These studies conducted by Rich [4] and Conrad [2] are discussed at length in the test manual. Briefly, 10 mentally retarded subjects, 5 between 5 and 7 years old, and 5 between 6 and 9 years old, were evaluated by Rich and Conrad. In Rich's study, ELI demonstrated reliable quantitative language assessment (MLU) on two administrations one week apart. Conrad showed that the ELI is a reliable instrument for assessing a child's MLU and semantic-gramatic rule patterns.

Reliability

In a study of temporal reliability of mean length of utterance, group means for ELI imitation, conversation, and play showed that the ELI yielded a relatively consistent mean length of utterance over a 1-week interval for two groups of delayed children. Intratest reliability was studied by examining mean length of utterance comparisons. The mean length of utterance in ELI conversation and that used in free play were not significantly different. The mean length of utterance used in imitation, however, was significantly greater than that in ELI conversation.

Validity

Validity was examined by reviewing the correspondence between the rules tested by the ELI and those used spontaneously by normal and delayed children. The author reports that the ELI yielded patterns of rules that reflected the patterns occurring in the children's free speech, for both normal and delayed subjects.

Guidelines for Use in Clinical Settings

Criteria for Selection and Value of Clinical Observations

The author includes a section in the manual entitled "Application to Clinical Treatment of Delayed Language." He notes within this section that the ELI was designed as both a testing and teaching model. The author cites that since the initial program development in 1973–1974, over 100 environmental language programs have been conducted at the Nisonger Center. There is broad experience in application of the ELI to clinical treatment. There is no question that regardless of the nature of a client's language delay, the essential feature of the ELI (i.e., environmental context and generalization focus) allows the test substantial use in development of environmental language treatment.

Review

The strength of this inventory is direct applicability for use in language training. The testing is done in a natural setting using both structured stimuli and spontaneous language sampling. This method allows the clinician to assess a broad spectrum of the client's communicative ability. The test is designed such that the results can be easily interpreted and readily used to develop a training program. A significant strength of the inventory is the removal of the sterile test setting. Examiners often hear parents say "He talks much more at home, and would do better if he could say what he means in his own words." The ELI provides the examiner with flexibility to respond to this frequent criticism in language testing.

REFERENCES

1. Brown, R. *Development of First Language: The Early Stages*. Cambridge, Mass.: Harvard University Press, 1973.
2. Conrad, T. T. "Reliability and Validity of Language Measures in School-aged Retarded Children," unpublished master's thesis, Ohio State University, Columbus, 1975.
3. MacDonald, J. D. *Environmental Language Inventory Manual*. Columbus, Oh.: Merrill, 1978.
4. Rich, J. "Semantic Performance of Retarded Children in Imitation, Conversation and Play," unpublished master's thesis, Ohio State University, Columbus, 1976.
5. Schlesinger, I. N. Production of Utterances and Language Acquisition. In E. I. Slobin (ed.), *The Ontogenesis of Grammar*. New York: Academic Press, 1971.

ILLINOIS TEST OF PSYCHOLINGUISTIC ABILITIES

Descriptive Information

Test Identification

The title of this test is *Illinois Test of Psycholinguistic Abilities* (ITPA), Revised Edition, 1968. Its authors are Samuel A. Kirk, Ph.D., James J. McCarthy, Ph.D., and Winifred D. Kirk, Ph.D. The authors are special educators. Dr. S. Kirk is the former Director of the Institute for Research on Exceptional Children, University of Illinois. Dr. McCarthy is a Professor in the Department of Studies in Behavioral Disabilities; Dr. W. D. Kirk is former Adjunct Professor in the Department of Speech and Hearing, University of Arizona. University of Illinois Press (Urbana, Illinois 61801) publishes the test at a cost of $65–$75.

Age and Type of Client

The test is designed to assess children 2 to 10 years of age. More specific information about the type of child who could appropriately be tested with the ITPA is unavailable.

Purpose

The ITPA has as its purpose assessment of six representational levels and six automatic levels of receptive and expressive language abilities. The representational levels are auditory reception, visual reception, auditory association, visual association, verbal expression, and manual expression. The automatic levels include grammatic closure, visual closure, auditory sequential memory, visual sequential memory, auditory closure, and sound blending.

Time Required to Administer and Score Test

Approximately 60 to 90 minutes is needed for administration and scoring of this test.

Evaluator

The authors direct that examiners appreciate the significance of the scientific method in test administration before using the ITPA. The examiner must be acquainted with the general directions for administration of standardized tests such as those listed for the Stanford-Binet Intelligence Scale [18]. The ITPA authors suggest that a new examiner should have adequate background and should administer a minimum of 10 practice tests before being considered a valid examiner. Further, they direct that it is preferable to be observed by an experienced examiner and to reread the manual frequently during this period so as to avoid unwittingly practicing the same errors.

Development and Source of Test Items

The first edition of the ITPA was an experimental edition published in 1961. The revised version is an attempt to improve the subtest and to add tests for abilities not tapped by the original battery. The ITPA was conceived as an instrument to delineate specific abilities and disabilities in children in order that remediation might be undertaken when needed. The seed for the development of the original ITPA is found in the work of Dr. Samuel Kirk. In his early work with young disadvantaged mentally retarded children, he noticed that they displayed wide discrepancies among their abilities. He felt there was a need for a systematic, diagnostic device which would tap and differentiate various facets of cognitive ability.

Theoretical Constructs

Dr. S. Kirk used as the theoretical basis for these measures Osgood's principles concerning the communication process [15]. The outgrowth of this model postulates three dimensions of cognitive abilities: channels of communication, psycholinguistic processes, and levels of organization. Psycholinguistics are the psychological functions of the individual that operate in communication activities. The subtests of the ITPA are designed to tap each of these functions [16].

Content and Test Administration

Content

The ITPA consists of 12 subtests: Auditory Reception, Visual Reception, Visual Sequential Memory, Auditory Association, Auditory Sequential Memory, Visual Association, Visual Closure, Verbal Expression, Grammatic Closure, Manual Expression, Auditory Closure, and Sound Blending. Each of these subtests has directions for materials, procedure, and recording. A trial item is also provided for each of the subtests.

Setting and Equipment

The examiner is directed to ensure good environmental conditions for the child, such as adequate lighting free from glare reflection from the page, avoidance of distracting noises or interruptions, and freedom from fatigue. Where verbal responses are required, the child's hands, toys, and so forth should be kept away from the mouth; on visual items the child should be seated high enough and close enough to the materials to have a clear and undistorted view. Standardized procedures must be followed rigidly.

Separate materials are listed for each of the subtests and include the test manual, recording forms for each of the subtests, picture book one, visual sequential memory booklet, 17 plastic chips, visual sequential memory tray, stopwatch, picture book two, five visual closure picture strips, red felt-tip pen, and five objects (nail, ball, block, envelope, and button).

Administration Procedures

The administration procedure differs for each of the subtests. The procedure is clearly listed under the heading of each subtest in the test manual. The authors suggest that the 12 subtests of the ITPA should be given in the order presented on the record form (i.e., the order presented under Content, above). The authors have also specified starting points for children of differing ability levels for each of the 12 subtests. For the majority of children, this level is chronological age.

Scoring

Each of the subtests has its own established basal and ceiling levels, as well as its own recording and scoring procedure. Many of the directions for establishment of basal and ceiling levels are divided on the subtests for subjects below age 6 and above age 6. Demonstrations provided for each of the subtests vary according to the age level of the child as well. A detailed section in the manual provides scoring instructions for verbal expression. The scoring standards provide specific examples of creditable and noncreditable responses in each of 10 categories (e.g., label and classification, color, function or action). The summary record form allows the recording of raw score, age score, and scaled score for each of the 12 subtests. In addition, there is a section for the sum of raw scores, mean scaled score, and median scaled score. Tables in the Appendix of the manual provide norms for securing the psycholinguistic age for each subject as well as scaled scores and composite psycholinguistic age. There is an additional table, which allows the examiner to secure a Stanford-Binet mental age estimate.

Psychometric Properties

Standardization

The ITPA was originally standardized on 932 middle-class children residing in the vicinity of suburban Chicago. Few children from the central city were represented in the sample. Norms were computed for children 2 years 5 months of age to 10 years of age. Kirk and Kirk [8] maintained, however, that "the norms at both [age] extremes were obtained to increase the ceiling for 8 year olds, or to show a deficit for 3 to 4 year olds."

Reliability

The authors measured internal consistency for each subtest and for the composite score according to age, with and without intelligence range corrected. Composite reliability for all age groups was above .87. Interscore reliability for verbal expression was found to be between .98 and .99; the resultant value appeared to depend on whether the coefficients were calculated on simultaneous ratings of experienced or naive examiners and also on the age of the subjects. Measures of test-retest reliability were not particularly impressive; standard error of measurement and stability of coefficients were used to examine this measurement. Stability coefficients for 4-, 6-, and 8-year-old children over 5 months were computed for subtests, supplementary tests, composite score, and psycholinguistic quotient. Subtest coefficients ranged from .42 to .87. The authors corrected for restriction in the range of intelligence score in the sample. The psycholinguistic quotient ranged from .87 to .91. Clark [3] in a review of the ITPA suggested that it appears to be "one of the more stable measures within a category of tests generally lacking in this kind of precision. While some of the subtests of the ITPA are of questionable stability for some age groups, the composite test score is adequate."

Validity

The authors have made no effort to present information on the test validity. They do report, however, that they have attempted to maintain a high degree of face validity in selecting items. Many other studies have been made of the validity of the ITPA. Hammill and Larsen [5] and Hare, Hammill, and Bartel [6] conducted an analytic

study using 126 third grade children. They factor-analyzed the ITPA data along with other reference tests and reported that seven factors emerged and accounted for 66 percent of the variance. They concluded, in this study, that the ITPA does have construct validity.

Another study undertaken by Newcomer et al. [14] factor-analyzed the ITPA using 20 other tests that matched subtests of the ITPA on respective constructs measured. Results of this analysis showed, once again, that the ITPA does have construct validity. It should be noted, however, that numerous other studies have not supported the findings of these studies. Clark [3] points out that the Osgood [15] model, on which the ITPA was based, is considered somewhat outmoded. It has, in fact, been severely criticized as a model of human language. Clark notes that "The lack of acceptance of Osgood's theory within the discipline of psycholinguistics in cognitive psychology militate against the validity of the ITPA." Predictive validity of the ITPA was measured in a study by Hirshoren [7]. In this study, 41 white children were tested in kindergarten with the Stanford-Binet and the experimental edition of the ITPA. These children were then followed up 2 years later in the second grade with the California Achievement Test. Hirshoren [7] reported that the ITPA was at least as valid as the Stanford-Binet in predicting school achievement of kindergarten children. Ten Brink [17] maintains, however, that neither instrument predicts school achievement of kindergarten children with much precision.

Hammill and Larsen [5] included the ITPA in a review of 33 studies to determine whether auditory perceptual skills were related to reading ability. In this review, it was found that the median coefficient between reading and combined auditory skills was not statistically significant. Larsen, Rogers, and Sowell [10] administered the Auditory and Visual Sequential Memory and Sound Blending subtests of the ITPA, the Wepman Auditory Discrimination Test, and the Bender Visual-Motor Gestalt Test to a sample of

59 learning-disabled and 30 normal children. Results showed that none of the tests differentiated between the groups.

Guidelines for Use in a Clinical Setting

Criteria for Selection

The ITPA is a useful diagnostic instrument if the evaluator seeks to investigate a child's information processing abilities. It is a lengthy test, and fatigue is often a factor in its administration.

Value of Clinical Observations

The ITPA has been widely used as the basis on which educational programs have been implemented. Hammill and Larsen [4] reviewed 38 studies of such educational programs. Their findings indicated that the effectiveness of psycholinguistic programs for the retarded had not been demonstrated. They suggested, however, that approximately 50 percent of the studies using psycholinguistic training with disadvantaged children reported significant gains in the associational and representative areas. The authors concluded that there had not been any conclusive demonstration of the efficacy of training psycholinguistic functions. It should be noted that exception has been taken to the authors' conclusions in the Hammill and Larsen study [11, 12]. Critical review, however, has shown that the study was able to withstand all counterpositions published [3]. Ayres [1] has incorporated the ITPA in her sensory integrative theory to help clarify which neural systems were apt to be most associated with auditory language problems. Clark [3] points out that the syndromes or neural systems so constructed were helpful in differentiating children who would from those who would not make gains as a consequence of sensory integrative procedures. In most of the recent effectiveness studies, however, Ayres [2] found that changes on the ITPA in a group receiving sensory integrative therapy were not significant, although these same children made academic gains. In attempting to measure therapeutic gains, teachers, occupational therapists, and speech and language pathologists may wish to use a more sensitive measure than the ITPA.

Review

The ITPA is widely used and reported. It is one of the most comprehensive tests available using, as its base, an informational processing model. Properly used, with children whose ages are within the normative range for the test, an abundance of information can be determined. This information yields a profile of the child's strengths and weaknesses in areas of verbal communication, reception of visual symbolic material, motor expression by gestures and writing, auditory and visual memory, auditory and visual closure as well as some information about responses requiring the child to see relationships and integrate concepts.

REFERENCES

1. Ayres, A. J. *Interpretation Manual of the Southern California Sensory Integrative Tests.* Los Angeles: Western Psychological Services, 1976.
2. Ayres, A. J. Cluster analyses of measures of sensory integration. *Am. J. Occup. Ther.* 31 : 362, 1977.
3. Clark, F. A. The Illinois Test of Psycholinguistic Abilities: Considerations of its use in occupational and physical therapy practice. *Phys. Occup. Ther. Pediatr.* 2 : 29, 1982.
4. Hammill, D. D., and Larsen, S. C. The effectiveness of psycholinguistic training. *Except. Child.* 41 : 5, 1974.
5. Hammill, D. D., and Larsen, S. C. The relationship of selected auditory perceptional skills and reading ability. *J. Learn. Disabil.* 7 : 429, 1974.
6. Hare, B., Hammill, D., and Bartel, N. Construct validity of selected subtests of the Illinois Test of Psycholinguistic Abilities. *Except. Child.* 40 : 13, 1973.
7. Hirshoren, A. A comparison of the predictive validity of the Revised Stanford-Binet Intelligence Scale and the Illinois Test of Psycholinguistic Abilities. *Except. Child.* 35 : 517, 1969.

8. Kirk, S. A., and Kirk, W. D. Uses and abuses of the ITPA. *J. Speech Hear. Dis.* 43 : 58, 1978.
9. Kirk, S. A., McCarthy, J. J., and Kirk, W. D. *The Illinois Test of Psycholinguistic Abilities—Revised Edition.* Urbana, Ill.: University of Illinois Press, 1968.
10. Larsen, S. C., Rogers, D., and Sowell, V. The use of selected perceptual tests in differentiating between normal and learning disabled children. *J. Learn. Disabil.* 2 : 85, 1976.
11. Lund, K. A., Foster, D. E., and McCall-Perex, D. The effectiveness of psycholinguistic training: A reevaluation. *Except. Child.* 44 : 310, 1978.
12. Minscoff, E. Research on psycholinguistic training. *Except. Child.* 42 : 144, 1975.
13. Newcomer, P. L., and Hammill, D. D. ITPA and academic achievement: A survey. *Read. Teach.* 28 : 731, 1975.
14. Newcomer, P. L., et al. Construct validity of the Illinois Test of Psycholinguistic Abilities. *J. Learn. Disabil.* 8 : 220, 1978.
15. Osgood, C. E. Motivational Dynamics of Language Behavior. In M. R. Jones (ed.), *Nebraska Symposium on Motivation.* Lincoln, Nebr.: University of Nebraska Press, 1957.
16. Paraskevopoulos, J. N., and Kirk, S. A. *The Development and Psychometric Characteristics of the Revised Illinois Test of Psycholinguistic Abilities.* Chicago: University of Illinois Press, 1969.
17. Ten Brink, T. A critique of Hirshoren's ITPA validity study. *Except. Child.* 36 : 351, 1970.
18. Terman, L. M., and Merrill, M. E. *Stanford-Binet Intelligence Scale: Manual for the Third Revision.* Boston: Houghton Mifflin, 1960.

PEABODY PICTURE VOCABULARY TEST

Descriptive Information

Test Identification

The title of this test is *Peabody Picture Vocabulary Test,* Revised Edition (PPVT-R), Forms L and M, 1981. Its authors are Lloyd M. Dunn, Ph.D., and Leota M. Dunn. Dr. Dunn is an Affiliate Professor of Special Education at the Manoa campus of the University of Hawaii. For 20 years, he was on the faculty of the Peabody College, which is now part of Vanderbilt University. He served there as Chairman of the Special Education Department and later as the first research director of the institute on mental retardation and intellectual development. Dr. Dunn holds a doctorate in special education and psychology. Leota Dunn has a bachelor's degree in elementary education. She taught for 12 years in the primary grades of Canadian schools. She collaborated with her husband, Lloyd, in developing the original PPVT but was not then recognized as a coauthor. She is currently a free-lance author and psychometrician in Honolulu, Hawaii. American Guidance Service (Circle Pines, Minnesota 55014) publishes the test at a cost of $30–$40 for Form A or Form B and $50–$60 for both forms.

Age and Type of Client

The PPVT-R is recommended for individuals between 2½ and 40 years of age. It is appropriate for nonspeaking persons as well as nonreaders. A pointing response is all that is required.

Purpose

The PPVT-R is designed primarily to measure receptive vocabulary for Standard American English. It is not a comprehensive test of general intelligence; instead, it measures only one facet of general intelligence, namely, vocabulary.

Time Required to Administer and Score Test

Approximately 10 to 20 minutes is needed to administer and score this test.

Evaluator

No formal course work is necessary to administer the PPVT-R. The author suggests that the examiner become thoroughly familiar with the test material and practice administering and scoring the test, preferably under the supervision of an experienced examiner, before administering it to a client.

Historical Perspective of Test Construction

Development

The Dunns suggest, as they did in the original version of the PPVT, that although far from perfect, vocabulary is the best single index of school success [1, 2]. They note, however, that performance on a receptive vocabulary test cannot be equated with innate or fixed ability. Therefore, the PPVT should not be considered a comprehensive test of general intelligence. Dr. and Mrs. Dunn suggest that the revised version of the PPVT can be appropriately used as an initial screening device in scanning for bright, low-ability, and language-impaired children who may need special attention.

Content and Test Administration

Content

The PPVT-R contains two parallel forms, now designated *Form L* and *Form M*. Each form contains five training items, followed by 175 test items arranged in order of increasing difficulty. Each item has four simple black-and-white illustrations arranged in a multiple choice format. The subject's task is to select the picture considered to illustrate the best meaning of the stimulus word presented orally by the examiner.

Setting and Equipment

The authors suggest that the test should be given in a quiet room away from other people. Two chairs, one a comfortable size for the subject, and a table or flat-topped desk of appropriate height are needed. The authors discuss recommended seating arrangements in the test manual.

Test equipment necessary for administration include the following: the appropriate series of plates for Form L or Form M, an individual test record appropriate for the form used, the test manual, and an optional technical supplement to the manual which elaborates on standardization and development of the norms for the revised version of the PPVT [5].

Administration Procedures

The test examiner is directed to the starting point coded to the left of the item numbers on the score sheet. The starting points correlate to the chronological age of the subject and are derived so that the middle 50 percent of any age group will obtain a basal without having to either work backward or respond to too many easy items. From the starting point the examiner works forward until the subject makes the first error. If eight or more consecutive correct responses have been made, a basal has been established. (If a basal is not established, the examiner will need to work backward until achieved.) The examiner continues to test forward until the subject makes six errors in eight consecutive items. The last item is the ceiling item.

The authors give two separate sets of instructions, one for young children under the age of 8 years and the other for older children, adolescents, and adults. Essentially, the subject is directed to look at the pictures and to "put your finger on," "point to," or "tell me the number" of the word said by the examiner.

Scoring

The total raw score is the number of correct responses over the critical range. That is, all items below the basal are counted as correct, and all items above the ceiling are counted as incorrect. The raw score is obtained by subtracting the number of errors over the critical range from the number of the ceiling item. The raw score is then converted to a derived score. The PPVT-R was standardized on both age and grade reference groups; thus, an individual score can be compared with a large group of persons of the same chronological age or in the same grade. Three deviation-type age norms are reported:

standard score equivalence, percentile ranks, and stanines. Also reported are developmental-type age norms or age equivalence. The Dunns point out that interpretation of derived scores is difficult. They include in their manual a section on finding errors of measurement. In the original edition of the PPVT and also in the 1965 edition, raw scores could be converted to mental ages and intelligence quotients [3, 4]. No such conversion directions are given in the newest revision.

Psychometric Properties

Standardization

The PPVT-R was standardized on two populations. The first, ages 2½ through 18 years, included 4200 children and youth. The authors considered chronological age, sex balance, geographic representation, occupation of the major wage earner in the family, ethnic representation, and community size. The sampling plan was based on population data from the 1970 U.S. census. Such rigorous controls were not used to ensure the representative national sample of the second population, which was comprised of individuals between 19 and 40 years of age. The authors state that it was difficult to obtain a sample of adults willing to take the PPVT-R. Summary information for 828 persons, however, were obtained and attention was given to age and sex balance, geographic representation, and occupational representation. The Dunns discuss, in great detail, the development of the items for the original edition of the PPVT and the development of the new item pool. In addition, attention is given to the item field testing and calibration for the revised version of the PPVT.

Reliability

Split-half correlations based on all subjects in the standardization sample were obtained. The authors selected to use the Rach-Wright Latent Trait methodology for split-half analyses. The standard procedure for calculating split-half reliability was rejected because each set of items (odd and even) would include items below the basal, which are counted as correct, and items above the ceiling, which are counted as incorrect. Using the new methodology, for each subject, the number of items answered correctly between the basal and ceiling items was obtained separately for the odd and even items. For children ages 2½ through 18, the coefficients ranged from .67 to .88 on Form L, and from .61 to .86 on Form M. The median split-half reliability for the adult standardization sample was .82. The authors also calculated immediate retest alternate-forms reliability coefficients. For the various age groups, the reliability for raw scores ranged from .73 to .91, with a median of .82. Delayed retest alternate-forms reliability coefficients were determined, with a minimum of 9 days and a maximum of 31 days elapsing between the first and second testings. For the various age groups, the reliability coefficients for raw scores ranged from .52 to .90, with a median value of .78. The authors describe the reliability of the PPVT-R as "satisfactory."

Approximately 100 published studies have reported reliability data on the original PPVT. The authors summarized some of these studies in the test manual. No reliability studies, other than those performed by the authors and listed above, are currently reported for the revised version of the PPVT.

Validity

The authors report that content validity was built into both editions of the PPVT when the test was originally designed. A complete search was made of *Webster's New Collegiate Dictionary* [8] for all words whose meanings could be depicted by a picture. This dictionary was assumed by the authors to represent the content universe for receptive vocabulary. They assume then that both versions meet adequate standards for picture vocabulary test measurements.

Construct validity is supported, by the authors, by citing information from the Stanford-

Binet Test of Intelligence [10]. Their rationale is that studies investigating the measurement of intelligence have shown that vocabulary is the best single type of test for predicting school success [9]. The authors note, however, that the process of measuring receptive vocabulary by picture selection, as in the case of the PPVT, is not equivalent to defining words orally, as in the case of the Stanford-Binet Test of Intelligence.

In a review of the literature over the period 1959 to 1979, the Dunns found over 300 validity studies of the original PPVT [6]. They summarized several of these studies in the test manual and abstracted 286 of these reports in the technical supplement to the manual. The studies show that the original PPVT correlates quite strongly with other vocabulary tests, and with vocabulary subtests of individual intelligence and psycholinguistic tests. These correlations range from a median value of .30 with the Wechsler Preschool and Primary Scale of Intelligence [11] to a median value of .86 for the Full Range Picture Vocabulary Test. In correlation with achievement tests, concurrent validity correlation ranged from a median of .38 for the Reading Subtest of the Wide Range Achievement Test [7] to .68 for the median of the total test score for the Peabody Individual Achievement Test [5]. Predictive validity studies with the PPVT were sparse in number. The correlations ranged from a median of .24 for the Reading Subtest of the Wide Range Achievement Test to .62 for the total test median for the California Achievement Test.

Guidelines for Use

The PPVT-R is a measure of receptive vocabulary. The test is easily administered, easily scored, and adaptable for use with many handicapped populations.

The authors suggest that because the test does not require subjects to read or write, it is especially fair for nonreaders or other persons with written language problems. Since responses can be gestural, the authors suggest that it is appropriate for the seriously impaired, especially

"expressive aphasics and stutterers." In addition, it can be used successfully with certain autistic, withdrawn, and even psychotic persons because extensive verbal interaction between the examiner and subject is not required. The subject must have hearing adequate to receive the stimulus word. Neither pointing nor oral responses are essential; therefore, the authors suggest that even severely cerebral-palsied individuals are less handicapped in the testing situation. Only a yes/no signal to the examiner's pointing is actually required to respond to the test items.

Review

Results obtained in administration of the PPVT-R should not be overgeneralized. In the past, the test has been interpreted as rendering an intelligence quotient or a mental age score. The authors have noted the limitations of the instrument and have cautioned against expanding on the test results. Rather, they stress that the PPVT-R is best used as part of a test battery in a comprehensive evaluation of an individual. The strength of the test is its flexibility. It can be used as a measure of receptive vocabulary with severely impaired populations. Many of the vocabulary items pictured, however, are not particularly relevant to severely handicapped populations.

REFERENCES

1. Childers, P. R. Concurrent validity of a group administered the Peabody Picture Vocabulary Test. *J. Educ. Res.* 60 : 92, 1966.
2. Dale, E., and Reichert, D. *Bibliography of Vocabulary Studies.* Columbus, Oh.: Ohio State University, Bureau of Educational Research, 1957.
3. Dunn, L. M. *Peabody Picture Vocabulary Test* (original edition). Circle Pines, Minn.: American Guidance Service, 1959.
4. Dunn, L. M. *Peabody Picture Vocabulary Test, Expanded Manual.* Circle Pines, Minn.: American Guidance Service, 1965.
5. Dunn, L. M., and Markwardt, S. C. *Peabody Individual Achievement Test Manual.* Circle Pines, Minn.: American Guidance Service, 1970.
6. Hufano, L. "Validity Studies on the Peabody Pic-

ture Vocabulary Test, Published Between 1965 and 1974," unpublished manuscript, University of Hawaii, 1977.

7. Jastak, J. S., and Jastak, S. D. *Wide Range Achievement Test Manual* (1976, Revised Edition). Wilmington, Del.: Guidance Associates of Delaware, 1976.

8. Merriam, G., and Merriam, C. *Webster's New Collegiate Dictionary.* Springfield, Mass.: Merriam, 1953.

9. Terman, L. M., and Merrill, M. A. *Measuring Intelligence.* Boston: Houghton Mifflin, 1937.

10. Terman, L. N., and Merrill, N. A. *Stanford-Binet Intelligence Scale: Form L-M* (3rd ed.). Boston: Houghton Mifflin, 1960.

11. Wechsler, D. *Wechsler Preschool and Primary Scale of Intelligence Manual.* New York: The Psychological Corporation, 1967.

PORCH INDEX OF COMMUNICATIVE ABILITY IN CHILDREN

Descriptive Information

Test Identification

The title of this test is *Porch Index of Communicative Ability in Children* (PICAC), 1974. Its author is Bruce E. Porch, Ph.D. Dr. Porch is a speech and language pathologist at the Veterans Administration Hospital, Albuquerque, New Mexico. Consulting Psychologists Press (577 College Ave., P.O. Box 11636, Palo Alto, California 94306) publishes the test at a cost of $52–$65.

Age and Type of Client

The test is designed to be used with 4- to 12-year-old children. Children functioning at kindergarten level or below should be given the Basic Battery; children at the first grade level and above should be administered the Advanced Battery.

Purpose

The PICAC is designed to assess and quantify certain verbal, gestural, and graphic abilities. Through its use, the clinician may obtain general and specific levels of output ability and make inferences about input and integrative ability.

Time Required to Administer and Score Test

About 60 to 120 minutes is needed to administer and score this test.

Evaluator

No professional qualifications are listed as essential for administration of the PICAC. The author notes that prior to his completion of the test manual, about 40 hours of instruction and practice were required to train testers to the point where they were scoring with good agreement. He notes that the effectiveness of the test manual in replacing or supplementing direct instruction has not been fully established, but it appears that the PICAC can be learned adequately enough for general clinical use without direct instruction if the clinician will use the 40 hours to accomplish the following:

1. Become thoroughly familiar with the scoring method in the manual.
2. Practice administration of the battery and scoring responses until the scoring categories and test format are fully memorized.
3. Test at least 10 subjects of varying degrees of communicative involvement.

The author directs that, whenever possible, these steps should be carried out under the supervision of someone trained or presently being trained in use of the PICAC. The trainee should always have at least one other person trained or training in the method with whom to compare results. In cases where clinicians are planning to use the PICAC for research purposes, Dr. Porch recommends that at least one member of the research group have direct training with someone thoroughly familiar with the battery, so that there will be some assurance that the results can be compared with those of other centers.

Historical Perspective of Test Construction

Development and Source of Test Items

Dr. Porch developed the Porch Index of Communicative Abilities in 1964. The purpose of the development of this test was the study of the adult aphasic patient. The test became widely known for its binary choice scoring system, concept of task and response continua, profile analysis, and especially for the continuous efforts to maintain high intrascore and test-retest reliability through comprehensive training of all examiners. Dr. Porch later developed PICAC with these same principles and methods in mind.

Theoretical Constructs and Implications for Intervention

The PICAC is sensitive to changes in behavior and the processes by which a child produces a communicative product as well as the product itself. The test is maximally designed to allow for intermodality and intersubtest comparisons. It does not emphasize measurements of psycholinguistic and linguistic abilities.

Content and Test Administration

Content

The PICAC consists of two batteries. The basic battery is to be used for the child functioning at the preeducation level and is best used for children who have not completed kindergarten. The advanced battery is for children who are at the 6-year-old or first grade level or above. There are 15 subtests in the Basic Battery and an additional five (III, IV, VII, A, and B) in the Advanced Battery. All subtests, except one, revolve around 10 common objects. The subject responds by talking, gesturing, and/or writing as directed in that particular subtest. The following is a list of all subtests:

The Basic PICAC Battery
  Basic Test I (verbal: function)
  Basic Test II (gestural: function)
  Basic Test V (auditory: function)
  Basic Test VI (verbal: naming)
  Basic Test VIII (verbal: completion)
  Basic Test IX (reading: names)
  Basic Test X (auditory: commands)
  Basic Test XI (visual: pictures)
  Basic Test XII (auditory: names)
  Basic Test XIII (verbal: imitation)
  Basic Test XIV (visual: matching)
  Basic Test C (graphic: dictation)
  Basic Test D (graphic: spelling)
  Basic Test E (graphic: copying)
  Basic Test F (graphic: geometric form)
The Advanced PICAC Battery
  Advanced Test I (verbal: function)
  Advanced Test II (gestural: function)
  Advanced Test III (reading: function)
  Advanced Test IV (verbal: description)
  Advanced Test V (auditory: function)
  Advanced Test VI (verbal: naming)
  Advanced Test VII (reading: backward)
  Advanced Test VIII (verbal: completion)
  Advanced Test IX (reading: names)
  Advanced Test X (auditory: command)
  Advanced Test XI (visual: pictures)
  Advanced Test XII (auditory: names)
  Advanced Test XIII (verbal: imitation)
  Advanced Test A (graphic: function)
  Advanced Test B (graphic: names)
  Advanced Test C (graphic: dictation)
  Advanced Test D (graphic: spelling)
  Advanced Test E (graphic: copying)
  Advanced Test G (graphic: drawing)
  Advanced Test H (drawing: copying)

Setting and Equipment

Testing should be carried out in a room free of distracting noise or movement; the subject should be seated at a large table, preferably with the table facing a blank wall; and the examiner is directed to sit at the subject's right. The purpose of this arrangement is easy access to the materials for both the examiner and the child. The examiner remains largely out of the field of vision where he or she can relaxedly observe the performance without danger of cueing or distracting the child. The test materials necessary for administration of the complete PICAC are

1. The test format, which describes the materials and procedures required for each subtest.
2. Ten pairs of test objects, one set of which should be on the table in front of the child during all subtests. The second set is used for Subtest 14 for matching with the objects on the table and for testing tactile perception. The objects are provided with the test.
3. Stimulus cards in standard list order for subtests requiring reading names, visual pictures, graphic copying, reading function, reading backward, and reading names and prepositions.
4. One score sheet.
5. Graphic test sheets on which the subject writes and draws during the graphic subtest.
6. One black pen for the subject to use during the graphic subtest.
7. A watch or clock.

Administration Procedures

The test objects described above are placed on a blotter directly in front of the subject or slightly toward the child's best field of vision. Dr. Porch directs the examiner to move these objects appropriately during the various subtests of the test. The PICAC is an item competency test rather than a speed test; therefore, the subject is given as much time as he or she feels is necessary to complete each task. The complete test should be given in one session whenever possible. Directions for test administration are clear, and administration is not difficult. Specific and elaborate directions for administration of each of these subtests is included in the test manual.

Scoring

All information and scores pertaining to a given administration of the PICAC are recorded on one score sheet. Scoring procedures are very precise. Each type of response is scored according to one or more of five basic dimensions—accuracy, responsiveness, completeness, promptness, and efficiency. Each response is also evaluated in terms of categories. Representative categories include items such as "complex," "repeated," and "unintelligible." There are 16 category scores. In addition to this score, the examiner is asked to record whether the answer was, in fact, correct or incorrect. Once the items have been scored, several kinds of scores are computed. Mean scores are computed for subtests; for gestural, verbal, and graphic modalities; for overall response level; for general communication level; and for visual and auditory levels. In addition, the examiner notes the total number of minutes required by the subject for completion of each subtest. Because the PICAC is not a speed test, the child is given as much time as he or she needs to complete the test. The child's responses are converted to numbers using this multidimensional binary choice scoring system. The answers are judged correct or incorrect across each of the parameters listed above. These numbers are recorded on a score sheet and are used to compute means and percentiles, which are graphed on summary forms to be analyzed.

Psychometric Properties

Standardization

The construction of the PICAC batteries and the elaborate scoring methods described above were carefully developed over a 3-year period. Dr. Porch notes that during that time numerous revisions and modifications in the content and scoring procedures were made. At the point at which the batteries could be administered with consistency, 615 children were tested in an initial standardization study. These children were drawn from private and parochial schools in California, New Mexico, and Ohio. The children in this sample had to be functioning adequately at a grade level commensurate with their age, with no history of educational problems that necessitated special education, psychiatric treatment, or indication of significant learning or emotional disorders. The sample used for the Basic Battery was composed of 94 girls and 95 boys, for a total of 189 subjects. The sample for the Advanced Battery was composed of 244 girls and 182 boys (n = 426). The author reports that scores in the sample had a fairly equal distribution by sex, although sampling by race was considerably skewed toward the Caucasian group. With this limited sample, however, there was no significant correlation of test scores to race. The author notes that there is considerable speculation as to the effect of various cultural backgrounds on test results, and he recommends further study testing larger samples of various groups to determine whether the PICAC is appropriate for use with various subpopulations. Dr. Porch reports that the adult version of the test, the PICA, has been found to be reasonably tolerant of normal individual variations and group differences and the results amazingly interpretable. It is his hope that the same will prove true of the children's test. The author gives specific directions in the manual to aid the examiner in decisions regarding assessment of children representing subpopulations with this test battery.

Reliability

The author investigated score agreement by having three examiners, all of whom were extensively trained in the PICAC procedures (one of these examiners was Dr. Porch), assess a total of 40 children using the Basic Battery. Ten children at each of the age levels of 3, 4, and 5 years were examined. These children attended nursery school or preschool and were heterogeneous in their abilities and presented a wide range of be-

haviors on the test. They were considered the average sample. A second group of 10 children was added to the sample in order to maximize the range of behavior that the scores would be required to quantify. This group was described by the authors as attendees at a school for severely mentally retarded children. Their IQs were under 30, and they were significantly impaired in communicative abilities. After the testing of the subjects was completed and recorded on videotape, each of the three examiners viewed the tapes independently, scored the behavior, and tabulated their scores. The differences between the means were reported to be very small. The author noted that the potential range of variation was .15 on Subtest 9 to .04 on Subtest 14. The examination of the modality scores from each score revealed the same findings. Results of interscore reliability using the Advanced Battery were essentially the same.

Split-half reliability was examined using the data from two halves of each of the subtests given to the subjects and scored by the three examiners in the interscore reliability examination. An odd-even split was used. Application of the Spearman-Brown formula allowed estimation of reliability for each subtest. Correlations of halves ranged from .86 to .98. Test-retest reliability was carried out with the same subjects as were used in the interscore reliability study. Each child used for that study was tested again within a week. The tester involved in the retest did not refer to the score sheet of the previous test before reviewing the tape, and the author scored the second set of tests for a comparison with the first set. The results of this study for the Basic Battery of the PICAC showed that all the subtests but Subtest 2 have a stability coefficient that exceeds the .90 level. Subtest 2, a gestural task in which the child demonstrates the function of objects, had a stability coefficient of .86. For the Advanced Battery the data show that there was considerable variation among the subjects and relatively little change from test to retest. All coefficients were .94 or higher.

Validity

Because the PICAC batteries were designed to sample a variety of communicative skills at different levels of complexity, it was assumed that the distribution curves for the modality and subtest scores would not be distributed throughout the scoring range. Dr. Porch projected, rather, that the distributions would yield scores centered near the lower part of the scale for the most difficult tasks and toward the top of the scale for the easier tasks. Obviously, the main interest in the distributions was to determine how they changed with the child's age. There is a strong relationship between the PICAC modality scores and the child's age. The major changes noted over time were found to be that as age increases, the means increase and the variation between subjects decreases. The same holds for the relation between the grade and test scores. Distributions are presented in the PICAC test manual. Dr. Porch discusses analyses on the Basic Battery and the Advanced Battery separately in the test manual. In most instances, results for both batteries were similar. Modality scores on the PICAC were found to be highly correlated with the age and grade level of the child in the examination by the author. Interrelationships between the modality scores were found to be significantly correlated at the .001 level. The author noted that this was not surprising since any communicative task reflects the total efficiency of brain circuitry, particularly in the small child. In the Basic Battery the subtest means were found to be highly correlated with the exception of Subtest 14, which is matching objects with objects. This subtest was not significantly correlative with Subtest 9, which is a reading task, and Subtest E, copying the names of 10 objects. Dr. Porch hypothesizes that the relationship is probably related to the fact that the variance on Subtest 14 is very small, and therefore all of the correlations would be lowered to the simplicity of the task.

The author noted the relation of PICAC subtest and modality means to the age, education, and sex of his sample. Subtest means and modality means increased progressively with age and with educational level.

Guidelines for Use in a Clinical Setting

The PICAC provides the examiner with a wealth of information regarding the child's communicative function. Modality comparison is a particularly useful element. The test results provide perhaps the best foundation available on which a therapeutic program can be based.

Review

The common items used as stimuli for the PICAC are regular, household items (e.g., key, pencil, fork). They are interesting and engaging. The small black-and-white cards of pictures representing the common objects and words and letters are much less interesting. The test is reasonably easy to administer but very complex to score. It does, however, yield an abundance of information useful in planning therapeutic intervention. The more the examiner administers the PICAC, the more reliable the results. It is only with this kind of experience, however, that the test can be used to accurately measure small changes in a child's communicative behavior over time. Test validity has not been firmly established. The test will be strengthened considerably when additional reliability data are gathered from examiners who have had varying degrees of training and experience in administration of the PICAC.

REFERENCE

1. Porch, B. E. *Porch Index of Communicative Ability in Children.* Vol. 1: *Theory and Development.* Palo Alto, Calif.: Consulting Psychologists Press, 1979.

PRESCHOOL LANGUAGE SCALE

Description Information

Test Identification

The title of this test is *Preschool Language Scale* (PLS), Revised Edition, 1979. Its authors are Irla Lee Zimmerman, Ph.D., Violette G. Steiner, and Roberta Evatt Pond. Dr. Zimmerman is a clinical psychologist with additional credentials as a school psychologist. She is presently in private practice and is a research psychologist at the UCLA Neuropsychiatric Institute. Steiner is a child development specialist, and Pond is a teacher of psychology, including human development and women's study at the Anchorage Community College in Anchorage, Alaska. She has worked as a speech and language specialist. Charles E. Merrill Publishing Company, Test Division (130 Alum Creek Dr., Box 508, Columbus, Ohio 43216) publishes the test at a cost of $33–$40.

Ages and Type of Client

The test is designed to assess language in 1- to 7-year-old children or persons who are assumed to be functioning at the preschool or primary language level.

Purpose

The PLS is designed as a diagnostic and screening instrument capable of measuring receptive and expressive language strengths and deficiencies. The auditory comprehension and verbal language tasks are classified according to age levels at which most children can complete the task successfully.

Time Required to Administer and Score Test

Thirty minutes is usually needed to administer and score this test.

Evaluator

The PLS is designed for use by classroom teachers, speech clinicians, psychologists, and child development specialists. No specific training requirements are listed.

Historical Perspective of Test Construction

Development and Source of Test Items

Items from the Auditory Comprehension and Verbal Language Scales are drawn from existing developmental literature. The authors cite the work of Doll [2], Kinsler [6], and others to support the use of normative development data to produce a language scale. The authors emphasize that this scale uses a natural dichotomy between auditory comprehension and verbal ability as the basis for its construction. The PLS consists of a series of auditory and verbal language tasks, each based on evidence of the average age of attainment by preschool and early primary children. The authors note that age levels obtained for this test are "not directly comparable to mental ages established on such measures of intelligence as the Wechsler Scales [15], Peabody Picture Vocabulary [3], or Stanford-Binet [13, 14]." This revised edition differs from the original by having clearer instructions, simplified scoring, and repositioning or reconfirming item placement to reflect increased knowledge of children's developmental progression [16].

Content and Test Administration

Content

The two scales of the PLS measure auditory comprehension and verbal language. The Auditory Comprehension Scale provides a measuring instrument to register recognition and comprehension of noun and nonnoun words, the stages of concrete and abstract thought, concept acquisition, and the ability to understand grammatical features of language, according to the test authors. Vision is used as one of the methods for evaluating language development by requiring the child to identify, manipulate, or conceptualize pictures and objects. The authors note that there is minimal use of motor skills, making items suitable for administration to the physically handicapped. The Auditory Comprehension Scale has four test items at 6-month intervals up to 5 years, then yearly up to 7 years. Each test item lists the concept to be tested, the materials needed, procedure, score, rationale, and reference. The following is an example of one of the test items from the PLS Auditory Comprehension Scale [19]:

Two years six months to three years
13. Recognize Action (activity discrimination)
Material: Picture Book plate 8, page 16.
Procedure: Say, "Where is . . ."
a. "washing?"
b. "playing?"
c. "blowing?"
Score: Credit 1 point if the child identifies two actions as named.
Rationale: This item calls for comprehension of a more advanced type of verb form. The distinguishing characteristic of the questions involves knowledge of action words in the sentences, matched with discrimination of the picture.
Reference: Haeussermann (1958) required children at this age level to distinguish portrayed action. Dunn [3] inserted an increasing number of action words in the Peabody Picture Vocabulary Test for this age.

The Verbal Ability Scale provides for measuring such aspects as vocabulary, verbalized memory span, stages of concrete and abstract thought, concept acquisition, articulation, and ability to use grammatical features of the language. As in the Auditory Comprehension Scale, all items are arranged according to the same sequential language progression identified by the authors [12]. The Verbal Ability Scale is divided according to the same age levels as the Auditory Comprehension Scale, and includes four test items under each age level. The following is an example of one test item [19]:

Two years six months
13. Repeats Three Digits (attentive verbal imitation)
Procedure: "Listen. Say 4-2. Now say . . ."
a. "1-4-9"
b. "9-6-1"
c. "2-5-3"
The examiner must pronounce the numbers distinctly and uniformly at the rate of one per second.
Score: Credit 1 point if the child repeats one series of three digits correctly.
Rationale: The child's increasing ability to listen actively and his or her lengthening short-term memory span allow for repetition of a longer series of numbers at this stage of development.
Reference: Digit-span items were used in the earlier Binets and remain at this level on the 1973 version. McCarthy [8] further confirmed the placement of three digits at this age level.

Setting and Equipment

Testing should take place in a comfortable setting, preferably without observers. Presence of the child's mother is accepted if she is needed to ensure cooperation on the part of the younger child. The authors noted, however, that the mother must be warned to stay in the background and to say nothing that might suggest an answer to the child.

To administer the scale, the examiner will need a PLS Booklet for each child to be evaluated and the following materials: one PLS manual, one PLS picture book, twelve 1-inch color blocks, one small piece of coarse sandpaper, one set of coins (half-dollar, quarter, dime, nickel, and penny), and one watch or clock with a second hand. These objects are not included in the test kit.

Administration Procedures

The authors suggest that before attempting to administer the scale, the examiner should become thoroughly familiar with the material described in the manual and should practice giving the items. They also suggest that the child be given positive reinforcement for all efforts, whether or not he or she succeeds. Each scale is begun by administering the four items at an age level slightly below the child's estimated ability. If the child misses an item, it is necessary to go back into the scale until the child succeeds in passing all four items at one age level. This will become the child's basal age. Testing continues forward at this point. If the child passes any item at one age level, the following age level must be administered in full. Each scale is discontinued at the point where the child fails all items at one age level.

Scoring

The basal age for each section is entered on the score sheets, followed by the number of items passed at each succeeding level. Those items passed between 1 year 6 months and 5 years are multiplied by a credit of 1½ months; those at 6 and 7 years are multiplied by a credit of 3 months. The resulting sum is added to the basal age for each section. These age totals represent the equivalent language ages for both the Auditory Comprehension and Verbal Ability Scales. The author suggests that the Auditory Comprehension age and Verbal Ability age can be compared by converting each to a language quotient. To convert, divide each by the chronological age and multiply by 100. An overall language age consists of the average of both Auditory Comprehension and Verbal Ability age. This value can be converted to a language quotient by the same formula.

Psychometric Properties

Standardization

The authors note that the Revised PLS is "ready for rigorous normative studies that would develop means and standard deviations for each level covered" [19]. They encourage examiners to develop their own local norms, thereby making the PLS a more criterion-referenced measure.

Reliability

The authors determined split-half reliability by examining children enrolled in two consecutive year-long Head Start programs. Each child's test results were scored twice, once for odd items only and once for even items only. Using the Spearman-Brown formula, reliability coefficients range from a low of .75 to a high of .92, with a median of .88 [18]. No other reliability testing was reported in the manual.

Validity

Several measures were discussed in the test manual. Content validity is felt, by the authors, to be evidenced from the detailed description and rationale provided for each of the test items. Item analysis of passes and failures shows discriminating value of items at ascending language age levels. The authors note several studies which have shown that item difficulty advances sequentially with age [7, 11, 16]. The authors cite numerous studies of concurrent validity. Correlation coefficients of several tests were reported in the manual and are summarized in Table 7-1.

To measure predictive validity, the authors cite studies comparing results on the PLS and later school success [1, 17]. These studies found that less than 10 percent of the children who scored average or better on the PLS later scored below average on the Lee Clark Reading Readiness test. de Montfort [1] compared the results achieved by 40 above-average 4 year olds on the PLS Auditory Comprehension Scale with results obtained 2 years later on the Burt Reading Test. The correlation was a low $r = .24$.

Guidelines for Use in a Clinical Setting

The PLS is *not* a diagnostic instrument. Too few language components are actually measured, and there are too few items at each age level. Results on the PLS can, however, be used to assist in determining the direction of diagnostic assessment.

Table 7-1. Concurrent validity

Test	Population	Correlation coefficient
Preschool Language Scale (PLS) and Illinois Test of Psycholinguistic Abilities[a]	Children with cerebral palsy, ages 4–10 yr	$r = .97$
PLS and Utah Test of Language Development[b]	32 middle-class 3 and 4 year olds	$r = .70$
PLS and Peabody Picture Vocabulary Test[c]	Children with possible language problems, ages 3–6 yr	$r = .59$
PLS and 1960 Stanford-Binet[d]	60 black Head Start children, ages 3–5 yr	$r = .66$

[a]Data from N. L. Higbee, "A Comparative Study of the Preschool Language Scale and the Illinois Test of Psycholinguistic Abilities When Administered to a Population of Cerebral-Palsied Children," master's thesis, University of Southern California, 1974.
[b]Data from G. H. Scott, "A Comparison of the Utah Test of Language Development and the Preschool Language Scale," master's thesis, Illinois State University, 1973.
[c]Data from A. Roston, "Peabody Picture Vocabulary Test and Preschool Language Scale: Results for Preschool and Kindergarten Children," unpublished paper, 1977.
[d]Data from N. Kassoff, "A Comparison of Various Preschool Scales," master's thesis, University of Southern California, 1972.

Review

The PLS is easy to administer and easy to score. The materials used are appealing to children. There are, however, few test items at each age level, and very few items test understanding or use of language structure. It is of interest to note that in measurements of concurrent validity, the best correlation was found with the ITPA in assessment of young children with cerebral palsy. Neither of these tests is an appropriate instrument to be used in assessment of the language of physically handicapped children. The items on the PLS most closely resemble items from the verbal scale of intelligence tests; consequently, the correlations between the PLS and the Utah Test of Language Development and the PLS and the Stanford-Binet are virtually the same.

REFERENCES

1. de Montfort, M. "The Relationship Between Language Ability and the Acquisition of Reading in a Selected Population Aged Between 4 and 6 Years," master's thesis, Dublin College of Speech Therapy, Dublin, Ireland, 1976.
2. Doll, E. A. *Preschool Attainment Record.* Minneapolis, Minn.: American Guidance Service, 1966.
3. Dunn, L. M. *Manual to the Peabody Picture Vocabulary Test.* Minneapolis, Minn.: American Guidance Service, 1965.
4. Higbee, N. L. "A Comparative Study of the Preschool Language Scale and the Illinois Test of Psycholinguistic Abilities When Administered to a Population of Cerebral-Palsied Children," master's thesis, University of Southern California, 1974.
5. Kassoff, N. "A Comparison of Various Preschool Scales," master's thesis, University of Southern California, 1972.
6. Kinsler, E. Language development in the normal child. *The Voice* 16 : 8, 1966.
7. Mauer, E. F. "An Investigation of the Validity and Reliability of the Preschool Language Scale," master's thesis, Illinois State University, 1973.
8. McCarthy, D. *McCarthy Scales of Children's Abilities.* New York: Psychological Corporation, 1972.
9. Roston, A. "Peabody Picture Vocabulary Test and Preschool Language Scale: Results for Preschool and Kindergarten Children," unpublished paper, 1977.
10. Scott, G. H. "A Comparison of the Utah Test of Language Development and the Preschool Language Scale," master's thesis, Illinois State University, 1973.
11. Steiner, V. G., and Evatt, R. L. "Diagnostic Curriculum Planning for the Preschool Child," unpublished paper, 1970.

12. Steiner, V. G., and Evatt, R. L. "PLS Item Analysis of Head Start, Early Childhood Education and Nursery School Children," unpublished paper, 1978.

13. Termin, L. M., and Merrill, M. A. *Manual to the Stanford-Binet Intelligence Scale* (Third Revised Edition, Form L-M). Boston: Houghton Mifflin, 1960.

14. Termin, L. M., and Merrill, M. A. *Stanford-Binet Intelligence Scale.* Boston: Houghton Mifflin, 1973.

15. Wechsler, D. *Manual to the Wechsler Intelligence Scale for Children* (Revised Edition). New York: Psychological Corporation, 1974.

16. Zimmerman, I. L., and Steiner, V. G. Validity and evaluation of the Preschool Language Scale. *Am. Psychol.* 25 : 1125, 1970.

17. Zimmerman, I. L., and Steiner, V. G. "An Item Analysis of the Spanish and English Versions of the Preschool Language Scale Administered to Bilingual Children," unpublished paper, 1972.

18. Zimmerman, I. L., and Steiner, V. G. The relationship between preschool language status of bilingual children and later school success. *Am. Psychol.* 28 : 740, 1973.

19. Zimmerman, I. L., Steiner, V. G., and Pond, R. E. *Manual to the Preschool Language Scale* (Revised Edition). Columbus, Oh.: Merrill, 1979.

SEQUENCED INVENTORY OF COMMUNICATION DEVELOPMENT

Descriptive Information

Test Identification

The title of this test is *Sequenced Inventory of Communication Development* (SICD), 1975. Its authors are Dona Lea Hedrick, Elizabeth M. Prather, and Annette R. Tobin. All three authors are speech and language pathologists. University of Washington Press (Seattle, Washington 98105) publishes the test at a cost of approximately $100–$120.

Age and Type of Client

This test is designed for children whose chronological age is between 4 months and 4 years or for persons who are developmentally delayed.

Purpose

The authors have designed receptive and expressive scales along a developmental sequence for the purpose of assessing children under the age of 3 years. At the time of development of the SICD, there were no reliable measurement devices for these children. The success and failure patterns on this instrument suggest possible avenues for remediation.

Time Required to Administer and Score Test

Approximately 30 minutes is needed to administer this test to infants and up to 75 minutes for 2 year olds and older, with 15 to 20 minutes needed for scoring.

Evaluator

No specific professional credentials are listed as requisite for the administration of this test, but because of the manipulation of many objects and pictures and specificity of questioning techniques, the examiner must be extremely familiar with the test. This test is not appropriate for administration by a nonprofessional.

Historical Perspective of Test Construction

Development and Source of Test Items

Information was collected from many sources on the progressive steps in communication development of the preschool-aged child. Sources included items from the Receptive-Expressive-Phonetic Scale [1], the Denver Developmental Screening Test [3], and the Illinois Test of Psycholinguistic Abilities [5]. Thus, the SICD is criterion-referenced in nature. The authors present these developmental tasks on a receptive and an expressive scale; through observation of the child and interview of the parents, the examiner identifies the child's capability on these small developmental segments.

Content and Test Administration

Content

On the receptive scale, areas of speech awareness and sound awareness, speech discrimination and sound discrimination, and understanding of words and words plus nonspeech and situation cues are evaluated. On the expressive scale, motor, vocal, and verbal imitation; motor, vocal (nonspeech sound, e.g., cough, motor sound) and verbal initiation; and vocal and verbal responding are assessed. In addition, quantitative and descriptive elements of verbal output and speech articulation are assessed.

Setting and Equipment

A comfortable, quiet setting is recommended. A parent may be present in the test room but should be seated outside of the child's vision. No additional equipment is required other than that included in the test kit. A tape recorder is recommended.

Administration Procedures

There are specific instructions for each test item in the test manual. Both direct observation of the child's behavior following stimulation by the examiner and interview of the parents are included in both the receptive and the expressive scale. Directions are straightforward and clear to follow. In some instances, the examiner is asked to manipulate the equipment, provide the stimuli for the child's response, assess the response, and score it. This procedure is complex, especially for an inexperienced examiner. The authors recognize this difficulty and suggest that test administration would proceed more smoothly if there were two examiners, one to present the materials and a second one to score.

Scoring

Items are scored "yes" or "no" indicating whether the child exhibited a certain characteristic sought in the items. The items are then transferred to the profile form indicated by a circle (for those items produced correctly) or an underline (for those incorrect). The examiner then computes the percentage of correct responses for each age level (the numerator is the number of items passed, the denominator is the number of total items for that section). The expressive section includes a language sample. Mean length of response is computed within this section. These scores are then transferred to the profile sheet. The highest age level at which the child has at least 70 percent correct is considered the child's age equivalent score. The authors provide information regarding interpretation of widely scattered scores in the test manual. Final scores are presented as receptive communication and expressive communication age equivalents.

Psychometric Properties

Standardization

A total of 252 children, 21 at each of 12 age levels at 4-month intervals, were used as the normative population. Subjects were representative of the general population of greater Seattle, Washington. Socioeconomic status of this population included seven per group from each of three socioeconomic status levels computed by occupation and educational level of the parents. The normal population consisted of Caucasians only, with both males and females distributed equally across groups. A child was excluded from the normal population if language development was judged abnormal by the parents or if he or she were from a home where a language in addition to English was spoken. Children were also excluded if they possessed a known ear pathology within the previous 6 weeks or if he or she appeared to possess any abnormal physical or mental health conditions as assessed by the examiner. All of the children were assessed as having normal hearing acuity.

Reliability

The authors [4] report several measures of reliability. To study interexaminer reliability, 16 subjects, two or three at each of six age levels were randomly selected. These subjects were independently but simultaneously scored by two examiners. The mean percent of agreement on pass/fail of each item tested was 96. The range was 90.3 to 100.0. Test-retest reliability was evaluated by testing 60 youngsters, 10 from each of six age groups, once, then again 1 week later. The mean percent of agreement across the subjects was 92.8 percent. The authors tested the reliability of the assignment of Receptive Communication Age (RCA) and Expressive Communication Age (ECA) for individual subjects. Following the compilation of normative data, two of the authors independently assigned RCAs and ECAs to 21 subjects at 32 months of age. There was agreement on 38 of the 42 age assignments, with the other four being different by only one age level.

Validity

The authors tested the validity of the SICD by comparing test scores with those obtained on other well-established measures purporting to test similar areas. Pearson product-moment correlation coefficients were determined between the SICD Receptive Communication Age and the Peabody Picture Vocabulary Test [2], mean length of response, and structural complexity scores. Correlations ranged from .75 to .80. The authors note that the PPVT, mean length of response, and structural complexity score "tap only a segment of the expected skills in the SICD" [4].

The correlation between the RCA and ECA was .9477 and the mean of both the RCAs and ECAs was very close to the chronological ages of the 259 subjects in the normal groups.

Additional measures of test validity were not included in the test manual.

Guidelines for Use in a Clinical Setting

This test uses both auditory and visual channels as the stimulus mode and requires verbal, localization, and pointing responses. Items that are biased against physically and sensorially handicapped children can be omitted in administration and in the final scoring. While the test was not standardized on this population, it can be used to compute approximate RCA and ECA for these children.

Because various components of receptive language and expressive language are categorized in the scoring procedure, patterns of weakness and strength are easily determined. This information is readily available for use in program planning.

Review

The normative sample used for standardization of the SICD was weak, reliability fair, and validity underinvestigated. Procedures for administration of the test are complex. A wide range of skill development is assessed by this test. Results can be compiled in a compact profile of the child's language abilities. The combination of direct observation of the child and input from parental interview strengthens the information obtained on this instrument. While many items are required for administration of this test, in some instances, there are only one or two items to represent a child's performance of a certain skill. In examination of test-retest reliability, the authors note that on second testing, children passed more items and scored somewhat higher than on the first testing. This increase may have resulted, as the authors suggest, from increased familiarity with the setting, a learning factor from first administration, or teaching by the parent who observed the testing. Clinicians may want to use the SICD as a measure of true progress with some caution.

REFERENCES

1. D'asaro, M. J., and John, V. A rating scale for evaluation of receptive, expressive, and phonetic development of the young child. *Cerebral Palsy Rev.* 22 : 5, 1961.
2. Dunn, L. M. *Peabody Picture Vocabulary Test.*

Circle Pines, Minn.: American Guidance Service, 1959.

3. Frankenberg, W. K., and Dobbs, J. B. Denver Developmental Screening Test. *J. Pediatr.* 71 : 181, 1967.
4. Hedrick, D. L., Prather, E. M., and Tobin, A. R. *Sequenced Inventory of Communication Development: Examiner's Manual.* Seattle: University of Washington Press, 1975.
5. Kirk, S., McCarthy, J. J., and Kirk, W. D. *Illinois Test of Psycholinguistic Abilities, Revised Edition.* Champaign, Ill.: University of Illinois Press, 1968.

TEST FOR AUDITORY COMPREHENSION OF LANGUAGE

Descriptive Information

Test Identification

The title of this test is *Test for Auditory Comprehension of Language* (TACL), 1973. Its author is Elizabeth Carrow-Woolfolk, Ph.D. Dr. Carrow-Woolfolk is a speech and language pathologist currently on the faculty of the University of Texas at Austin. Teaching Resources Corporation (50 Pond Park Rd., Hingham, Massachusetts 02043) publishes the test at a cost of $50–$60.

Age and Type of Client

The test is for children 3 years to 6 years of age or children or adults with language disorder, severe hearing impairment, mental retardation or aphasia; no verbal response is required.

Purpose

The TACL measures the areas of receptive language of vocabulary, morphology, and syntax.

Time Required to Administer and Score Test

Approximately 30 minutes is needed to administer and score this test.

EDITORS' NOTE: The extensively revised TACL-R, copyright 1985, is available from DLM Teaching Resources, One DLM Park, Allen, Texas 75002 at a cost of $99–$115.

Evaluator

The author suggests that the examiner should hold a bachelor's degree in education, psychology, or sociology and have significant testing experience. The examiner should be thoroughly familiar with the test items and manual before administering the TACL.

Historical Perspective of Test Construction

Development and Source of Test Items

The first version of the TACL was developed in 1965. Forty children between the ages of 2 years 6 months and 6 years 6 months were given the test in order to standardize the procedure, revise some of the items, and determine the order of presentation. The author then administered the test to 159 children, ages 2 years 10 months through 7 years 9 months. She made further modifications to the test and reported her preliminary findings [6]. A Spanish translation of the test was made in 1968, and the TACL was revised by the author in 1969, 1970, and 1971. From 1968 to 1972 the test was used by Southwest Educational Development Laboratory as a tool to evaluate the laboratory's early childhood education curriculum. The author estimates that thousands of children were administered the test during that time. None of these data were computed into the normative sample. However, Carrow-Woolfolk examined reliability of the test on a sample of 51 of these children. She notes that measurement of auditory comprehension, prior to the development of the TACL, involved only the *understanding* of vocabulary. The development of the TACL was her effort to focus the comprehension of the meaning of language on two aspects of utterances, namely the lexicon (semantics) and the structure (syntax). The TACL has two functions: (1) to measure the auditory comprehension of language structure, allowing the assignment of the child to a developmental level of comprehension; and (2) to determine the areas of linguistic difficulty.

Content and Test Administration

Content

The TACL consists of 101 plates of line drawings. The plates each provide three pictures, one of which represents the referent or choice for the linguistic form being tested. The pictures consist of black-and-white line drawings. Several of the pictures use primary color.

Setting and Equipment

The testing environment should be quiet, free from outside disturbances and visual distractions, and well lighted. The room should have a table or desk at which the examiner and child can sit facing each other.

Equipment necessary for administration of the TACL includes the test booklet, which contains the picture plates, and a scoring sheet. No other materials are needed.

Administration Procedures

The test booklet is placed on the table in front of the child. The examiner tells the child that he or she will be looking at some pictures, and that he or she is to point to the picture that matches what the examiner says. The examiner then presents the first example picture plate to the child. If the child successfully points to the appropriate picture as directed by the examiner, the examiner then moves to item one of the test. If the child has difficulty following directions on the example items, the examiner is directed to proceed through several example items until the child clearly understands the instructions. The examiner must not elaborate on the pictures of test items or encourage or discourage the child during the test administration. No stimulus item is to be repeated unless the examiner has not provided it correctly.

Scoring

Each of the child's responses is recorded on the scoring sheet by writing in the appropriate blank the number of the picture the child selects in response to each stimulus. Each correct response is given 1 point, and the total raw score is the sum of these points. The test items are sequenced by a grammatical category and not by difficulty. The author notes that the entire test must be administered in order to use the normative data. The raw scores can be converted to age scores by using the table in the manual that has raw score equivalency norms. The examiner may compare a child's performance with that of other children by using measures of central tendency. Means and median performance scores of each age group and the respective measures of variability are listed in the test manual. The examiner can determine percentile rank equivalents for the total raw score by age group, again, by referring to the appropriate table in the test manual. Scoring and interpretation of scores is an easy and straightforward process.

Psychometric Properties

Standardization

Normative data as well as reliability and validity information were determined on the population of children described in the section on Historical Perspective of Test Instruction.

Reliability

Reliability data on the TACL were obtained in the 1971 English and Spanish revisions. Fifty-one children, 28 males and 23 females with a mean age of 82.43 months, were administered the English version of the test. Half of this group were Mexican-American children. Thirty-two Mexican-American children, 12 males and 20 females with a mean age of 85.71 months, were administered the Spanish version of the test. All of these children were then retested within a 2-week interval. The author reports a high test-retest reliability for total score on both the English (.94) and the Spanish test (.93) [3]. Marquardt and Saxman [9] investigated test-retest reliability by examining five subjects with poor articulation and five with good articulation 4 weeks after an initial testing. The rank order correlation between error scores for the first and second test administration was .92. Jones [8] examined consistency of performance on items within the TACL in a study of middle- and lower-class black and Anglo children. The Kuder-Richardson Reliability Test was used, with a total test reliability for these groups of .77.

Validity

The author suggests that the TACL has content validity because increase in chronological age is paralleled by increase in score on the test. She points to results of her initial evaluation used in the development of the TACL as well as to the study by Jones [8] described in the section on Test Reliability. The second support of test validity found in the TACL manual contains citations of various pieces of research which Carrow-Woolfolk indicates have shown a statistically significant difference between the performance of children having known disorders of language comprehension and those who do not [1, 3, 4, 7, 9, 12]. The author suggests that the TACL reflects the improvement that occurs in language function. Dr. Carrow-Woolfolk notes that in the study performed by Weiner [12], the TACL had "high predictive ability for the performance of dysphasic children tested at one-year intervals" [5]. In a review of 30 language and articulation tests developed for use with preschool children, McCauley and Swisher [10] looked at 10 psychometric criteria appropriate to norm reference tests. They indicate in this review that the TACL does not meet these criteria in areas of concurrent validity, predictive validity, test-retest reliability, or interexaminer reliability.

Guidelines for Use in a Clinical Setting

Information obtained from results of the administration of the TACL can provide for the clini-

cian information about a child's understanding of vocabulary, grammar, and syntax. A limited profile of a child's strengths and weaknesses in these areas can be determined and may be useful in development and implementation of an individual treatment program. Because the test relies solely on the child's choice of a picture in response to the examiner's verbal stimuli, it can be used in testing nonverbal physically handicapped. The test is not appropriate for use, by itself, as a basis on which to make a language diagnosis.

Review

The black-and-white line drawings used as stimulus pictures for administration of the TACL are not engaging for young children. In a comparison of the results of two norm-referenced tests, the TACL and the Preschool Language Scale [13] to one criterion-referenced task, namely the Basic Two Choice Object Discrimination Task [2], Pecyna and Sommers [11] evaluated nine children identified as severely handicapped. Subjects were found to respond most accurately to items on the Two Choice Task and least accurately to items on the TACL. Further, subjective ratings of each subject's testing behavior were most favorable for the Two Choice Task and least favorable for the TACL. The authors noted that the poor performance of these subjects on the TACL relative to the other two measures may have had to do with the response choices available on the TACL. They observed that the children performed better on tests that allowed them to manipulate objects. While the author has developed a Screening Test for Auditory Comprehension of Language, administration of the full TACL requires that a child complete responses to the full 101 items. This process can be tedious and boring. In the test's favor is its adaptability for use with nonverbal, physically handicapped children. The test can be modified by allowing these children to use eye gaze or scanning as an appropriate response. The normative sample used in the standardization of the TACL is small. No clear information is given on the racial, geographical, and socioeconomic distributions in the sample.

REFERENCES

1. Bartel, N. R., Bryan, D., and Keehn, S. Language comprehension in the moderately retarded child. *Except. Child.* 1973.
2. Bricker, W., and Campbell, P. *Basic Two-Choice Object Discrimination Task,* unpublished test, 1978.
3. Carrow, E. Comprehension of English and Spanish by preschool Mexican-American children. *Mod. Lang. J.* 55 : 299, 1971.
4. Carrow, E. Auditory comprehension of English by monolingual and bilingual preschool children. *J. Speech Hear. Res.* 2 : 407, 1972.
5. Carrow, E. *Test for Auditory Comprehension of Language.* Austin, Tex.: Urban Research Group, 1973.
6. Carrow, Sister Mary. The development of auditory comprehension of language structure in children. *J. Speech Hear. Dis.* 2 : 99, 1968.
7. Carrow, E., and Lynch, J. "Comparison of Semantics Versus Syntactic Comprehension in Three Groups of Linguistically Deviant Children," unpublished manuscript, 1973.
8. Jones, B. J. "A Study of Oral Language Comprehension of Black and White, Middle and Lower Class, Preschool Children Using Standard English and Black Dialect in Houston, Texas, 1972," doctoral dissertation, University of Houston, 1972.
9. Marquardt, T. P., and Saxman, J. H. Language comprehension and auditory discrimination in articulation-deficient kindergarten children. *J. Speech Hear. Res.* 2 : 382, 1972.
10. McCauley, R. J., and Swisher, L. Psychometric review of language and articulation tests for preschool. *J. Speech Hear. Dis.* 49 : 34, 1984.
11. Pecyna, P. M., and Sommers, R. K. Testing the receptive language skills of severely handicapped preschool children. *Lang. Speech Hear. Serv. Schools* 16 : 41 (January), 1985.
12. Weiner, P. S. The perceptual level functioning of dysphasic children: A follow-up study. *J. Speech Hear. Res.* 2 : 423, 1972.
13. Zimmerman, I., Steiner, V., and Pond, R. *Preschool Language Scale.* Columbus, Oh.: Merrill, 1979.

TEST OF LANGUAGE DEVELOPMENT—PRIMARY

Descriptive Information

Test Identification

The title of this test is *Test of Language Development–Primary* (TOLD-P), 1982. Its authors are Phyllis L. Newcomer and Donald D. Hammill. Both Newcomer and Hammill are Special Educators. Dr. Newcomer is Professor of Education at Beaver College in Glenside, Pennsylvania. Dr. Hammill is President of PRO-ED, Inc. PRO-ED, Inc. (5341 Industrial Oaks Blvd., Austin, Texas 78735) publishes the test at a cost of $60–$75.

Age and Type of Client

The test is designed for children ages 4 years to 8 years 11 months who can hear and who speak English.

Purpose

The TOLD-P has seven subtests, each measuring different components of language. The TOLD-P can be used to identify children who are functioning below their peers in language proficiency, determine specific strengths and weaknesses, document progress, and serve as a measurement device in research on language.

Time Required to Administer and Score Test

Between 45 and 60 minutes is usually required to administer and score this test.

Evaluator

The TOLD-P may be used by teachers, counselors, psychologists, language therapists, or other professionals who have experience in test administration. The examiner must be thoroughly familiar with the test manual, especially with those sections relating to the use of norms and to the interpretation and recording of the scores.

Historical Perspective of Test Construction

Development and Source of Test Items

The TOLD-P is a modification of the original Test of Language Development (Newcomer and Hammill, 1977). An additional Test of Language Development entitled the *Test of Language Development-Intermediate* has been developed in conjunction with the primary edition. The intermediate edition was designed to be administered to children ages 8 years 6 months to 12 years 11 months. The TOLD-P is developed on a linguistic model of language and measures selective listening and speaking aspects of semantics, syntax, and phonology.

Content and Test Administration

Content

The TOLD-P has five subtests measuring language: Picture Vocabulary, Oral Vocabulary, Grammatic Understanding, Sentence Imitation, and Grammatic Completion. Word Articulation and Word Discrimination subtests are included on a supplemental basis. These supplemental subtests measure the ability to say words correctly and to distinguish between words that sound similar.

Setting and Equipment

The authors direct that the test should be administered in an environment that is free from distractions, well ventilated, well lighted, quiet, private, and comfortable. The examiner should be alert to the child's level of fatigue and cease testing if the child shows signs of tiring. The examiner should praise and encourage the child but avoid prompting.

The necessary equipment for administration of the TOLD-P are the manual, the picture book (which contains pictures for the Picture Vocabulary, Grammatic Understanding and Word Articulation subtests), and answer sheets, all included in the test kits.

Administration Procedures

The TOLD-P subtests should be administered in the same order that was used when the test was standardized. This order is Picture Vocabulary, Oral Vocabulary, Grammatic Understanding, Sentence Imitation, and Grammatic Completion. There are no time limits on the TOLD-P subtests. Usually, the TOLD-P can be completed in one testing session. However, for young or inattentive children, the authors direct that testing may be extended over several sessions. The administration procedures for the various subtests are as follows:

Picture Vocabulary: The child is shown a page with an array of four pictures on it. The examiner directs the child to "show me" or "point to" the stimulus item.

Oral Vocabulary: The examiner is directed to say to the child "I am going to say some words. Will you tell me what each word means? For example, if I said 'what's a dog,' you might say 'It's an animal, it barks, it wears a collar.' Now you do one. 'Tell me, what's a bird?'" The examiner then proceeds with a list of words. The child may be stimulated to produce more information by the examiner's request "Tell me more about it."

Grammatic Understanding: The child is shown a page with an array of three pictures. The child is then directed to point to the picture that matches what the examiner says.

Sentence Imitation: The child is directed to say the sentence after the examiner.

Grammatic Completion: The examiner says "I'm going to say some sentences now. In each sentence one word is missing. See if you can tell me the missing word in each sentence. Try this one." "Bill is a boy and

John is a _____.'' The examiner then reads each item, providing sufficient time for the child to respond.

Scoring

The examiner is directed to begin each subtest with the first item. For each of the subtests, testing is terminated when the child misses five items in succession. All items on all subtests are scored either as correct or incorrect. Correct responses earn 1 point, while incorrect responses are designated with a 0. The points are summed, and this value is called the *raw score*. The raw scores for each subtest can be converted to language ages, percentiles, standard scores for the subtests, and quotients for the composites. The authors indicate that the clearest indication of a student's performance on the TOLD-P subtest is provided by standard scores. Standard scores are transformations of raw scores that establish a common subtest mean score and standard deviation. For each of the subtests at each age level, the mean score is set at 10 and the standard deviation is fixed at 3. Scores are summarized on the front page of the answer form. In addition to numerical scores, the summary sheet includes a profile chart that may be used to graph the standard scores and quotients that the child has obtained.

Psychometric Properties

Standardization

The TOLD-P was standardized on a sample of 1836 children residing in 19 states and one Canadian province. Of these children, 47 percent were tested by special education teachers, 22 percent by speech therapists, 5 percent by regular classroom teachers, 2 percent by psychologists, and 24 percent by educational diagnosticians, supervisors, administrators, and others. Characteristics of the subjects relative to sex, place of residence, race, geographic distribution, and occupation of parents were compared in

terms of percentages to the standardization sample of the United States population that were reported in the Statistical Abstract of the United States [8].

Reliability

Three studies were used by the test instructors who estimated the internal consistency of the TOLD-P. The first study was a split-half procedure using 250 children from the standardization population. Fifty children were drawn randomly from each of the five age levels for which the TOLD-P is appropriate. The Sentence Imitation, Word Discrimination, and Word Articulation Subtests have internal consistency coefficients at all age levels that equal or exceed .80. The Grammatic Completion Subtest was found to be reliable for use with all children except 4 year olds. The internal consistency of the Oral Vocabulary items was found to be relatively weak at the 4-year (.70) and the 8-year (.67) level. Reliability coefficients for internal consistency associated with Picture Vocabulary and Grammatic Understanding subtests failed to reach the .80 criterion at any age level. A second split-half procedure was conducted by the authors of the test. Using a different population, this study showed that the internal consistency of the TOLD-P subtests were adequate at all ages studied. The third study of internal consistency was conducted by Wong and Roadhouse [13]. They reported coefficients ranging from .67 for Grammatic Understanding to .98 for Grammatic Completion.

In a measure of test-retest reliability, reliability coefficients exceeded .80 for every subtest at every age.

Validity

The authors measured three types of validity: content validity, criterion-related validity, and construct validity. In the authors' fairly subjective measurement of content validity, they cite their careful selection of items for each subtest. In addition, Newcomer and Hammill submitted

Table 7-2. Criterion-related validity

TOLD-P values	Criterion tests
Picture Vocabulary	Peabody Picture Vocabulary Test
Oral Vocabulary	Wechsler Intelligence Scale for Children (Vocabulary)
Grammatic Understanding	Northwestern Syntax Screening Test (Receptive)
Sentence Imitation	Northwestern Syntax Screening Test (Expressive); Detroit Tests of Learning Aptitude (Related Syllables)
Grammatic Completion	Illinois Test of Psycholinguistic Abilities (Grammatic Closure)
Word Discrimination	Auditory Discrimination Test
Word Articulation	Templin-Darley Tests of Articulation
Total Raw Score	Test of Auditory Comprehension of Language

descriptions of the formats of the five principal TOLD-P subtests to a group of 100 professionals and asked them to rate them according to the degree to which they measured aspects of two dimensions of language: semantics or syntax and listening or speaking. The authors concluded that the professionals rated the TOLD-P subtest in a manner that was consistent with the linguistic model used as the theoretical basis in the construction of the test.

Criterion-related validity was assessed for each TOLD-P subtest. Correlation coefficients were determined showing the relationship of each TOLD-P subtest with appropriate criterion tests at ages 4, 6, and 8 years (Table 7-2). The authors determined coefficients by using the Pearson product-moment method, with correction for attenuation showing the relationship existing between the subtest and criterion test after the criterion tests' reliability has been "accounted for" [7]. The authors, using .35 as a minimum criterion for validity coefficients, suggest that the validity of the TOLD-P values is supported in all cases except for the Grammatic Understanding Subtest. Newcomer and Hammill report on several additional validity studies in the TOLD-P test manual [7].

Construct validity is examined thoroughly by the authors [7]. They support the hypothesis that because the abilities measured by the TOLD-P are developmental, performance on the subtest

should be related to chronological age. In addition, because the abilities measured by the TOLD-P subtests all measure aspects of spoken language, the authors prove the hypothesis that the subtests are intercorrelated. They show that the TOLD-P scores relate strongly with tests of intelligence and correlate well with tests of academic achievement and school readiness. Newcomer and Hammill further demonstrate that the TOLD-P results differentiate between groups of children known to be normal in spoken language and those known to be poor in spoken language.

Guidelines for Use in a Clinical Setting

The TOLD-P is a comprehensive procedure useful in assessment of components of both receptive and expressive language. The authors note, however, that the test results should not be regarded as providing definitive information about a child's competence in the area being assessed but, rather, as hypotheses to be further investigated and either validated or invalidated. The results do not provide specific or detailed information about a child's specific ability; therefore, they are not sufficient for planning instructional programs. The TOLD-P provides a broad, global look at the child's strengths and weaknesses. Results are best used to focus attention on particular areas of deficiency for additional diagnostic testing.

Review

The black-and-white pictures used as stimuli in various areas of the subtest are not particularly engaging for young children. The fact that each of the subtests examines very different skills allows the child to move to a new task before becoming bored with the task at hand. Much information can be gathered in a relatively short period of time. While the psychometrics of the TOLD-P are adequate, the examiner should resist the urge to overinterpret the results of the test. Reliability and validity measures vary across subtests and across age levels.

REFERENCES

1. Ammons, R., and Ammons, H. *Full Range Picture Vocabulary Test.* Missoula, Mont.: Psychological Test Specialist, 1958.
2. Baker, H. J., and Leland, B. *Detroit Test of Learning Aptitude.* Indianapolis: Test Division of Bobbs-Merrill, 1967.
3. Carrow, E. *Test of Auditory Comprehension of Language.* Austin, Tex.: Learning Concepts, 1973.
4. Dunn, L. M. *The Peabody Picture Vocabulary Test.* Circle Pines, Minn.: American Guidance Service, 1965, 1981.
5. Kirk, S., McCarthy, J., and Kirk, W. *The Illinois Test of Psycholinguistic Abilities.* Chicago: University of Illinois Press, 1968.
6. Lee, L. *Northwestern Syntax Screening Test.* Evanston, Ill.: Northwestern University Press, 1971.
7. Newcomer, P. L., and Hammill, D. D. *Test of Language Development-Primary.* Austin, Tex.: PRO-ED, 1982.
8. Statistical Abstract of the United States: 1980. Washington, D.C.: U.S. Bureau of Census, 1980.
9. Templin, M., and Darley, S. *The Templin-Darley Test of Articulation.* Iowa City, Io.: Bureau of Educational Research and Service, University of Iowa, 1980.
10. Termin, L. M., and Merrill, M. A. *Stanford-Binet Intelligence Scale.* Boston: Houghton Mifflin, 1960.
11. Wechsler, D. *Wechsler Intelligence Scale for Children-Revised.* New York: Psychological Corporation, 1974.
12. Wepman, D. *Auditory Discrimination Test.* Chicago: Language Research Assoc., 1968.
13. Wong, B. Y. L., and Roadhouse, A. The Test of Language Development: A validation study. *Learn. Disabil. Q.* 1 : 48, 1978.

TEST OF LANGUAGE DEVELOPMENT-INTERMEDIATE

Descriptive Information

Test Identification

The title of this test is *Test of Language Development-Intermediate* (TOLD-I), 1982. Its authors are Donald D. Hammill, Ph.D., and Phyllis L. Newcomer, Ph.D. Both Newcomer and Hammill are Special Educators. Dr. Newcomer is Professor of Education at Beaver College in Glenside, Pennsylvania. Dr. Hammill is President of PRO-ED, Inc. PRO-ED, Inc. (5341 Industrial Oaks Blvd., Austin, Texas 78735) publishes this test at a cost of $34–$40.

Age and Type of Client

This test is designed to be used with children ages 8 years 6 months to 12 years 11 months who can hear and who speak English.

Purpose

The TOLD-I has five subtests that measure various components of spoken language.

Time Required to Administer and Score Test

Approximately 40 to 60 minutes is needed to administer and score the TOLD-I.

Evaluator

The TOLD-I can be used by teachers, counselors, psychologists, language therapists, or other professionals who have experience in test administration.

Historical Perspective of Test Construction

Development and Source of Test Items

The TOLD-I, like the TOLD-P discussed previously, uses the linguistic model as its theoretical base. Accordingly, the major components tested by this instrument are the linguistic features of phonology, syntax, morphology, and semantics. The TOLD-I is essentially an expansion of the initial Test of Language Development [4]. Much of the structure of the test is identical to the TOLD-Primary edition (TOLD-P).

Content and Test Administration

Content

The TOLD-I consists of five subtests: Sentence Combining, Characteristics, Word Ordering, General, and Grammatic Comprehension.

Setting and Equipment

The test should be administered in an environment that is free from distractions, well ventilated, well lighted, quiet, private, and comfortable. The necessary materials for administration of the TOLD-I are the manual and answer sheets, which are included in the test kit.

Administration Procedures

The authors direct that the TOLD-I subtest should be administered in the same order that was used when the test was standardized. That order is listed above. Specific subtest instructions are as follows:

Sentence Combining: The examiner says, "I am going to say some sentences. I want you to listen carefully, then put the sentences together. Make one sentence out of the sentences. Make your sentences as short as you can. For example, if I say, I am big, I am tall, you should say, I am big and tall. You should make one sentence and you should make it as short as you can."

Characteristics: The examiner reads a list of sentences and the child's task is to indicate whether the information in the sentence is true or false. For example, the child might hear "All birds are blue" or "All birds have wings." He or she then responds "True" or "False."

Word Ordering: The examiner presents to the child a list of words and asks the child to put these words together in a sentence.

General: The examiner presents three words to the child. The child is directed to say how these words are all alike.

Grammatic Comprehension: The examiner reads a list of sentences one at a time. The child is told that some of the sentences are correct and some are incorrect. The child's task is to say whether the sentence is correct or incorrect. For example, the examiner would read "Me play ball." The child would then indicate whether that sentence was correct or incorrect.

Scoring

The authors of this test have indicated places on the score sheet as points for initiation of testing according to chronological age. The examiner is directed to begin at the proper chronological age, test downward until a basal has been obtained, and then test upward until a child reaches his or her ceiling. On all subtests except Characteristics and Grammatic Comprehension, testing is terminated when the child misses five items in succession. On Characteristics and Grammatic Comprehension, the ceiling is that point at which the child misses three out of five consecutive items. All items on all subtests are scored either correct or incorrect. Raw scores are simply the number of items scored correct on each subtest. Additional test score computation interpretation information in the TOLD-I manual is much the same as that in the manual for the TOLD-P.

Psychometric Properties

Standardization

The TOLD-I was standardized on a sample of 851 children residing in 13 states. Characteristics of children in the standardization sample were equal in percentage to those reported for the population of the United States [5]. The authors discuss standard score norms, percentile ranks, grade and age equivalence, and relationship of TOLD-I scores to other deviation standard scores in the manual.

Reliability

The authors estimated the internal consistency of the TOLD-I subtest and composite scores by analyzing the test performance of 200 randomly selected children who were used as subjects in an item analysis. According to this analysis, the scores associated with the composites were found to have "more than adequate internal consistency at all age levels studied" by the authors [2]. The coefficients for the subtests ranged from .78 to .90 across age levels. The test authors examined test-retest reliability by administering the TOLD-I to 30 normal fifth and sixth grade children twice, with 1 week intervening. The reliability coefficients were all statistically significant at beyond the .01 level of confidence.

Validity

Content validity was examined by obtaining ratings of TOLD-I subtests by 100 professionals. The professionals were directed to read the descriptions of the formats of the five subtests and rate them according to the degree to which they measured aspects of two dimensions of language: semantics or syntax and listening or speaking. The professionals rated the TOLD-I subtests in a manner that was consistent with the model presented by the authors. Criterion related validity was measured by correlating the scores derived from the TOLD-I with those derived from the Test of Adolescent Language (TOAL) [1]. The TOLD-I and the TOAL were administered to a group of 30 normal children enrolled in either the fifth or sixth grades. The resulting coefficients, computed using an elaborate and complex process, yielded 70 corrections. The authors note fairly weak validity in that just 61 of these correlations were statistically significant and above .35 in magnitude.

The authors support the construct validity of the TOLD-I in much the same manner as was done for the TOLD-P [3]. That is, several constructs presumed to account for test performance were identified. Second, hypotheses were generated that were based on the identified constructs; and third, the hypotheses were verified by logical or empirical methods. Relationship of the TOLD-I to tests of school achievement was made by measuring results of the TOLD-I with the TOAL subtest and composite scores that tap written language.

Guidelines for Use in a Clinical Setting

The authors note that the TOLD-I is a tool developed to measure only certain aspects of an incredibly complex topic, that is, spoken language. The items assess only a few selected aspects of each major linguistic construct. The results of the test can show areas, represented by those in the test, in which a child is having particular difficulty. It would be inappropriate to identify a child as language-disordered, aphasic, or even communication-disordered based on the results of this testing. The test would be appropriately used in conjunction with another test that measures receptive language and other elements of expressive language.

Review

It is curious that the authors have selected to measure criterion-related validity against only one test, the *Test of Adolescent Language*. There are many other measures against which the TOLD-I could have been more appropriately measured. There is an excellent section included in the test manual on the importance of determination of local norms and the means to construct such norms. Few test instruments are designed to measure the spoken language of children in this age range. The TOLD-I is successful in filling this void.

REFERENCES

1. Hammill, D. D., et al. *Test of Adolescent Language.* Austin, Tex.: PRO-ED, Inc. 1980.
2. Hammill, D. D., and Newcomer, P. L. *The Test of Language Development-Intermediate.* Austin, Tex.: PRO-ED, Inc. 1982.
3. Newcomer, P. L., and Hammill, D. D. *Test of Language Development-Primary.* Austin, Tex.: PRO-ED, Inc. 1982.
4. Newcomer, P. L., and Hammill, D. D. *Test of Language Development.* Austin, Tex.: PRO-ED, Inc. 1977.
5. Statistical Abstract of the United States: 1980. Washington, D.C.: U.S. Bureau of Census, 1980.

THE TOKEN TEST FOR CHILDREN

Descriptive Information

Test Identification

The title of this test is *The Token Test for Children,* 1978. Its author is Frank G. DiSimoni. Dr. DiSimoni is a speech and language pathologist and Clinical Director of Logopedic Associates, Delaware, Pennsylvania. Teaching Resources Corporation (50 Pond Park Rd., Hingham, Massachusetts 02043) publishes this test at a cost of $22–$30.

Age and Type of Client

This test is designed to be used with individuals between 1 and 15 years of age who know primary colors, big and little, and three shapes.

Purpose

The Token Test for Children assesses receptive language function. The test is divided into five parts, each part presenting progressively longer and more complex commands.

Time Required to Administer and Score Test

Between 20 and 30 minutes is required to administer and score this test.

Evaluator

No specific professional qualifications are listed as requisite for administration of the Token Test for Children. The author reports, however, that most of the examiners who collected the normative data on the test were practicing speech pathologists or supervised students in advanced undergraduate or graduate classes. All of the examiners were supplied with training sessions on how to administer the test and detailed written instructions in booklet form for practice use.

Historical Perspective of Test Construction

Development and Source of Test Items

Dr. DiSimoni presents information in the manual for the Token Test for Children in the form of a study. He states in the preface to the manual that neither he nor Dr. Noll [5] (the person who developed the test format used in the Token Test for Children) are, in fact, the test authors. Rather, the Token Test for Children is based on the work by DeRenzi and Vignola [2] who developed the Token Test for Adults. Dr. DiSimoni cites many studies validating the Token Test used clinically with language-impaired adults. In addition, several studies applying the Token Test for use with children are listed [3]. The author notes that the widespread use of the Token Test with children has been hampered by several factors, including no completely adequate norms for children and norms reported simply as means or standard deviations for the various age groups.

Dr. DiSimoni describes the Token Test for Children as an attempt to generate more adequate normative data employing one of the more widely used, standardized long forms of the Token Test [5].

Content and Test Administration

Content

The test consists of elicited commands given orally by the examiner and carried out by the child using small and large circles and square tokens colored green, blue, red, yellow, and white. A specified pattern of tokens is placed in front of the child. The test items progress in complexity and include such commands as "touch the red circle"; then on Part II, "touch the small red circle"; Part III, "touch the yellow circle and the red square"; Part IV, "touch the small yellow circle and the large red square"; and then "after picking up the green square, touch the white circle."

Setting and Equipment

Twenty tokens are used: five large circles, five small circles, five large squares, and five small squares each in five colors. These are supplied in the test kit. The tokens are placed before the child in a standard manner. The examiner is seated behind and to the right of the child. The child's behavioral response to the direction given by the examiner is recorded on a score sheet.

Administration Procedures

Before starting the test, the examiner is instructed to formally test the child to be certain that the child understands the meaning of the words circle, square, large, and small and that he or she can identify all five colors of the tokens. The examiner presents instructions in a clear voice and each item is presented only once. After the children perform each command, the tokens are returned to their standard positions.

Scoring

The child's individual responses are scored as either correct or incorrect, and the score on each subtest is the total number of correct responses. In the case of multistep commands, the entire command must be performed correctly for it to be scored as correct. All subtest raw scores are summed to obtain the overall raw score. The examiner is then directed to obtain standard scores by consulting two different sets of tables: one appropriate to the child's chronological age and the other, to grade placement. The examiner converts raw scores to standard scores using these tables. The mean standard score and standard deviation selected for this test are 500 and 5, respectively. Therefore, average performance is viewed as raw scores in any category that are equal to standard scores in the range of 495 to 505.

Psychometric Properties

Standardization

The Noll [5] form of the Token Test was administered to 1304 children ranging in age from 3 to 12½ years. All were native speakers of English and spoke a general American dialect. The author points out that most children in the study were living in small towns near urban centers. In addition, he notes that there was a high mobility rate in the population. Forty-eight percent of the children were male, and 52 percent were female. The majority of children (68%) were from middle-class backgrounds. Children were not included who had a known language problem, who had failed a grade in school, or who were suspected of having any learning problem. Most of the preschool children were enrolled in preschool classes. No sophisticated sampling procedure was used in the selection of children.

Reliability and Validity

Dr. DiSimoni lists neither reliability nor validity data obtained for this test development. Various measures of validity and reliability are, however, listed from previous studies with children and adults [1, 4, 5, 7].

Guidelines for Use in a Clinical Setting

The Token Test for Children is easily administered with very little equipment necessary. Results of the Token Test reveal subtle difficulties in a child's receptive language. This information can be used, in coordination with other test results, in comprehensive planning of a therapeutic program.

Review

The author states that the data presented in the Token Test for Children is intended to stimulate further interest in research in the use of this procedure. Given the ease of administration, and the broad body of literature available on the adult version of the Token Test, additional research would be well worth the effort. Currently, it is impossible to generalize any diagnoses from the results of the test.

REFERENCES

1. Cartwright, L., and Lass, N. A. Comparative study of children's performance on the Token Test, Northwestern Syntax Screening Test, and Peabody Picture Vocabulary Test. *Acta Symbol.* 5 : 19, 1974.
2. DeRenzi, E., and Vignola, L. The Token Test: A sensitive test to detect receptive disturbances in aphasics. *Brain* 85 : 665, 1962.
3. DiSimoni, F. *The Token Test for Children.* Hingham, Mass.: Teaching Resources, 1978.
4. Fusilier, F., and Lass, N. "A Comparative Study of Children's Performance on the Illinois Test of Psycholinguistic Abilities and the Token Test," unpublished manuscript, West Virginia University, 1973.
5. Noll, J. D. "The Use of the Token Test with Children." Paper presented at the Annual Convention of the American Speech and Hearing Association, New York. November 1970.
6. Orgass, B., and Poeck, K. Clinical validation of a

new test for aphasia: An experimental study of the Token Test. *Cortex* 2 : 222, 1966.
7. Robb, E., and Lass, N. A. Correlational investigation of children's performance on the Token Test, the Brenner Developmental Gestalt Test of School Readiness and a Basic Grammatical Concept Test. *J. Aud. Res.* 16 : 64, 1976.

THE UTAH TEST OF LANGUAGE DEVELOPMENT

Descriptive Information

Test Identification

The title of this test is *The Utah Test of Language Development, Revised* (UTLD-R), 1977. Its authors are Merlin J. Meacham, J. Lorin Jex, and J. Dean Jones. The authors are speech and language pathologists and Dr. Jones is a principal of a state training school. Communication Research Associates (BH11012, Salt Lake City, Utah 84147) publishes the test at a cost of $45–$50.

Age and Type of Clients

Test sections are presented for ages 1 through 15 years of age for computation of language age equivalents from 9 months to 16 years.

Purpose

The purpose of this test is to objectively measure both expressive and receptive verbal language skills for both normal and handicapped children, using a developmental approach to the evaluation of language readiness. The authors also state that this test is useful with aphasics and hyperactive brain-injured individuals, although no rationale is given for this.

Time Required to Administer and Score Test

The UTLD takes approximately 15 minutes to administer; language sampling and analysis, 45 minutes.

Evaluator

The authors do not list any specific professional group as being specially trained to administer this test. No special training is listed as necessary either.

Historical Perspective of Test Construction

Development and Source of Test Items

All items on the test were selected from "various standard sources" and put together in normal developmental sequence. The authors suggest that the test should be seen as a screening instrument rather than a diagnostic tool.

Content and Test Administration

Content

The test is divided by age levels, with one to eight items representing each of those age levels.

Setting and Equipment

The authors suggest that there be a table, a chair for the examiner, and one for the child. Equipment required includes objects, test manual, and test plates (contained in the test kit), and the record form.

Administration Procedures

Instructions are provided to the examiner within the test manual, and the authors suggest that they should be read exactly as written. Directions are clear and simple. This test is very easily administered. The authors suggest that if the child becomes too restless to complete testing, testing can be continued a few minutes or even a few days later.

Scoring

Items are scored either plus (correct) or minus (incorrect). Each plus counts as 1 point, and minuses receive no points. A basal score is established by obtaining eight consecutive plus responses. The test is completed when eight consecutive minus responses are scored. The total number of plus responses yield a raw score, which can be converted into a language age equivalent (there is a conversion table contained in the test manual). The language age quotient can be calculated by dividing the language age by the child's chronological age.

Psychometric Properties

Standardization

The first edition of this test (1958) contained a statement of recognition by the authors that standardization was questionable because of the small size and limited geographical distribution of the normative sample. The 1969 test was calibrated on 273 normal white children in Utah, 10 boys and 10 girls at each age. The authors have gathered together a more representative normative sample for the 1977 edition, however, but they still suggest that the test be used for screening rather than diagnostic purposes. Elaboration of the normative sample is not included in the test manual.

Reliability

Correlation between two test versions—direct test version and informant interview version—was .976. Test-retest reliability was .96, and split-half odd versus even was .93.

Validity

The authors suggest that since all items of this scale had been selected previously from standardization sources, it was felt that items had good "face validity" [1].

Guidelines for Use in a Clinical Setting

This test is suitable only as a screening test for children who present with delayed language. It is not an appropriate instrument to be used in assessment for children with physical or sensory handicaps because most items require auditory-visual input, manipulation of objects, and verbal response.

Review

This test has value only as a screening instrument. It serves no clinical use in description of specific language deficits or in clinical programming. It may serve to provide the examiner with a broad idea as to the type and extent of diagnostic testing that will be required. It is easily administered, and all objects necessary for test administration are included in the test kit.

REFERENCE

1. Meacham, M., Jex, L. and Jones, J. D. *The Utah Test of Language Development-Revised.* Salt Lake City: Communication Research Associates, 1977.

LANGUAGE SAMPLING TECHNIQUES

The recent emphasis on pragmatic or situational use of language has placed renewed focus on the systematic analysis of a sample of a child's language. Numerous authors have suggested a variety of strategies to obtain a language sample and a variety of methods for its analysis [2–4]. The assessment concept, however, is very basic. Using a tape recorder, the examiner first collects a sample of the child's expressive language. The child's spontaneous discourse should be recorded in a variety of situations. A sample can be taken while the child engages in free play, during picture description task, and while retelling a sequenced story or event. These three contexts can provide a representative sample of the child's expressive language abilities. As the child participates in these activities, the examiner should ask open-ended questions to elicit expressive language. It has proved helpful to repeat the child's utterances *exactly* during the sample to improve transcription reliability. Transcription of the taped sample should take place as soon after the session as possible.

Analysis of transcribed samples are tedious and time-consuming, but such analysis can serve to provide the richest information possible on a child's natural language performance. Analysis can yield information on the child's syntax (structure of sentences), semantics (word meaning), morphology (structure of words), phonology (speech sounds), and pragmatics (functional use of language). There are a variety of language sample analysis programs available that assist in providing a thorough description of the child's expressive language. These programs can take the form of computer programs, handbooks, and/or checklists. Analysis of language samples does have limitations, however, of which the examiner should be aware. Barrie-Blackley, Musselwhite, and Rogister [1] have noted in their handbook that "of all issues in oral language sampling, the reliability is one of the greatest concerns." This is due, in large measure, to the exacting detail necessary in duplication of the process. Interpretation of language sample analyses are widely reported in the speech and language literature. Rarely, however, are the authors of these reports precise in their notation of the sample itself. Barrie-Blackley, Musselwhite, and Rogister [1] suggest that in language sample analysis it may be more appropriate to "judge reliability with regard to descriptive consistency rather than quantitative consistency."

Language sampling is an important component of a diagnostic battery. Results have straightforward application to the planning of an intervention program. These techniques should not, however, be undertaken by the inexperienced examiner since their use requires *thorough* knowledge of all language components.

REFERENCES

1. Barrie-Blackley, S., Musselwhite, C. R., and Rogister, S. H. *Clinical Oral Language Sampling: A Handbook for Clinicians.* In S. Hadjian (ed.), *NSSHA Clinical Series* (Vol. 5). Danville, Ill.: Interstate Publishers, 1978.
2. Crystal, D., Fletcher, P., and Garman, M. *The Grammatical Analysis of Language Disability.* New York: Elsevier, 1976.
3. Lee, L. L. *Developmental Sentence Analysis.* Evanston, Ill.: Northwestern University Press, 1974.
4. Tyack, D., and Gottsleben, R. *Language Sampling, Analyses and Training.* Palo Alto, Calif.: Consulting Psychologists Press, 1974.

CHAPTER REVIEW

This chapter has presented tests and individual assessment methods to help identify and describe language disorders in children. The tests presented assess language across three basic dimensions: semantics, syntax, and pragmatics. The usefulness of each of these instruments varies. Some are especially efficient for generating samples of behavior that can be compared with normal language development. Others were found to be more helpful in determining patterns of language difficulty, thereby providing a clear foundation for language therapy. Some tests have fair to good normative studies and reliability and validity research, while others have very poor psychometric properties. Table 7-3 summarizes the tests reviewed in the chapter according to the areas of language and speech evaluated, the age range of the test, the normative sample, and available reliability and validity studies. When a diagnostician selects a language test, he or she selects more than a test kit, a test form, and a set of procedures. Rather, the diagnostician selects a particular test author's theory of language. Every test reflects the author's biases about the nature of language and its development, and these biases affect the content, construction, and suggested use of that instrument. Test data provide one source of information about the state of a child's language comprehension and use. A knowledgeable clinician will also draw on other assessment information (e.g., cognitive, motor, academic), historical data about the child, and information about the physical status of the youngster before planning a therapeutic course.

REFERENCES

1. Bangs, T. *Language and Learning Disorders of the Pre-Academic Child* (2nd ed.). Englewood Cliffs, N.J.: Prentice-Hall, 1982.
2. Bloom, L., and Lahey, M. *Language Development and Language Disorders.* New York: Wiley, 1979.
3. Carrow, E. Assessment of Speech and Language in Children. In J. E. McLean, D. E. Yoder, and R. L. Schiefelbusch (eds.), *Language Intervention in the Retarded.* Baltimore: University Park Press, 1972.
4. Darley, F. (ed.). *Evaluation of Appraisal Techniques in Speech and Language Pathology.* Reading, Mass.: Addison and Wesley, 1979.
5. Leonard, L. Early Language Development and Language Disorders. In G. H. Shames and E. Wiig (eds.), *Human Communication Disorders: An Introduction.* Columbus, Oh.: Merrill, 1982.
6. Lloyd, L. L. (ed.). *Communication Assessment and Intervention Strategies.* Baltimore: University Park Press, 1976.
7. MacDonald, J., and Blott, J. Environmental language intervention: A rationale for a diagnostic and training strategy through rules, context and generalization. *J. Speech Hear. Dis.* 39 : 244, 1974.
8. McCauley, R. J., and Swisher, L. Use and misuse of norm-referenced tests in clinical assessment: A hypothetical case. *J. Speech Hear. Dis.* 49 : 338, 1984.
9. Rees, N. S. Pragmatics of language application to normal and disordered language development. In R. L. Schiefelbusch (ed.), *Bases of Language Intervention.* Baltimore: University Park Press, 1978.
10. Thorum, A. R. *Language Assessment Instruments: Infancy Through Adulthood.* Springfield, Ill.: Thomas, 1981.
11. Weiner, P. S., and Hoock, W. C. The standardization of tests. *J. Speech Hear. Res.* 16 : 616, 1973.
12. Wiig, E. H. Language Disabilities in the School-Aged Child. In G. H. Shames and E. H. Wiig (eds.), *Human Communication Disorders: An Introduction.* Columbus, Oh.: Merrill, 1982.

Table 7-3. Summary of language tests

Test	Areas Evaluated	Age Range	Normative Sampling	Reliability	Validity*
Assessment of Children's Language Comprehension (ACLC)	Understanding of critical elements of language; no speech required	3–6 yr	N = 311; subjects from Tallahassee, FL and rural VT; mixed SES, 38% black	Odd-even reliability: .86 and .80, respectively	No validity data
Bankson Language Screening Test (BLST)	Expressive language	4 yr 1 mo to 8 yr 0 mo	N = 637; subjects from semirural county near Washington, D.C.; majority were middle-class	Test-retest reliability: .94 Kuder-Richardson formula 20: .96	Concurrent validity with 3 tests: range, .54–.64
Boehm Test of Basic Concepts (BTBC)	Assesses 50 language concepts needed to understand instructions and communicate; no speech required	4–7 yr	2 revisions of test; more than 10,000 subjects used to standardize over 3 data collection times; subjects from 2 large northeastern cities	Split-half reliability Form A: range, .68–.90 Form B: range, .12–.94 Alternate form reliability combined Forms A and B: median, .76	Content validity
Carrow Elicited Language Inventory (CELI)	Measures syntax (grammatical structure)	3 yr 0 mo to 7 yr 11 mo	N = 475; white middle-class children from Houston, TX	Test-retest reliability: .98 Interexaminer reliability: .98 and .99	Concurrent validity: range, .42–.94
Clinical Evaluation of Language Function (CELF)	Language function: phonology, syntax, semantics, memory, and word finding and retrieval	4–18 yr	N = 1405; normative population reflected 1970 U.S. census data for CELF Screening Test CELF Diagnostic Battery: N = 159; 70% with suspected problems, 30 normal 1982 update: N = 1378	Test-retest reliability: .56–.98 Combined subtests: .96	Concurrent validity: range, .42–.94
Environmental Language Inventory (ELI)	Expressive language; pragmatics	Young child or developmentally delayed child	Not formally normed; data on test performance available on limited graph of	Test-retest reliability Mean length utterance: free play not different from data of	Content validity

				than test	
Illinois Test of Psycholinguistic Abilities (ITPA)	Receptive and expressive language abilities	2–10 yr	opmentally delayed children N = 932; middle-class children from suburban Chicago	Test-retest reliability Subtest: .42–.87 Entire test: .81–.91 Internal consistency above .87 Interrater reliability for verbal expression: .98	Authors' study: no validity Other studies: construct validity
Peabody Picture Vocabulary Test–Revised (PPVT-R)	Receptive vocabulary; no speech required	2½–40 yr	Pediatric sampling; N = 4200; ages 2½–18 yr, sample based on 1970 census	Split-half reliability Form L: .67–.88 Form M: .61–.86	Content validity Construct validity
Porch Index of Communicative Ability in Children (PICAC)	Verbal, gestural, graphic abilities	4–12 yr	Basic Battery, N = 189 Advanced Battery, N = 426 Subjects from private and parochial schools in CA, NM, and OH	Interrater reliability: score differences were very small; no coefficient given Split-half: range, .86–.98 Test-retest Basic Battery Gestural: .86 All other: .90 Advanced Battery: .94 or higher for subtests	Content validity
Preschool Language Scale (PLS)	Receptive and expressive language (better used as a screening test)	1–7 yr	Criterion-referenced test	Split-half reliability: range, .75–.92	Content validity (descriptive) Concurrent validity Predictive validity (functional)
Sequenced Inventory of Communication Development (SICD)	Receptive and expressive language	4 mo to 4 yr CA or MA	N = 252; SES representative of low-, middle-, or high-income levels; greater Seattle area; white only	Interrater reliability: mean % of agreement, 96% Test-retest reliability: mean % of agreement, 92.8%	Concurrent validity: range, .75–.80

Table 7-3 (continued)

Test	Areas Evaluated	Age Range	Normative Sampling	Reliability	Validity*
Test for Auditory Comprehension of Language (TACL)	Auditory comprehension of semantics and syntax; no speech required; Spanish version available	3–6 yr	N = 159; ages 2 yr, 10 mo to 7 yr, 9 mo (earlier version); no other information available about normative sample	Test-retest reliability English: .94 Spanish: .93 Kuder-Richardson reliability: .77	Content validity
Test of Language Development-Primary (TOLD-P)	Expressive and receptive language	4 yr 0 mo to 8 yr 11 mo	N = 1836; subjects characteristics of children were equal in percentage to those reported in the 1980 U.S. census	Internal consistency Split-half: subtests vary according to subtest and age range: .67–.98 Test-retest: >.80	Content validity Criterion-related validity Construct validity
Test of Language Development-Intermediate (TOLD-I)	Spoken language	8 yr 6 mo to 12 yr 11 mo	N = 851; subjects characteristics of children were equal in percentage to those reported in the 1980 U.S. census	Internal consistency: range, .78–.90 across all age levels Test-retest: significant .01 level	Content validity Criterion-related validity Construct validity
Token Test for Children	Receptive language; following instructions; no speech required	1–15 yr	Noll form of Token: N = 1304; ages 3 yr to 12 yr, 5 mo; majority from middle class, living in small towns near urban center	Author reported no studies, but studies are available	Author reported no studies, but studies are available
Utah Test of Language Development-Revised (UTLD-R)	Expressive and receptive language	1–15 yr	N = 273; white children in Utah-1969 normative sample 1977 sample not reported in test manual	Test-retest reliability: .96 Split-half reliability: .93	Content validity

SES = socioeconomic status; CA = chronological age; MA = mental age.
*Available validity studies are reported, but generally results are not indicated.

Psychological and Cognitive Tests

Victoria Shea
Patricia O'Brien Towle
Betty N. Gordon

Psychological assessment has many facets, partly because the field is so old and partly because there are so many human abilities, attributes, and behaviors that can be measured. The assessment of children was one of the first activities of modern psychologists, beginning with the work of Seguin, Cattell, Binet, and others in the nineteenth century. Today all psychologists in the specialty areas of clinical, school, or counseling psychology are trained in the use of intelligence and cognitive tests. In addition, psychologists also administer tests of emotional and behavioral status and personality characteristics, and are trained in interviewing skills and techniques of behavioral observation. Rather than attempting to cover all of these areas of psychological assessment, this chapter focuses on the tests of intelligence or cognitive skills that are most useful in pediatric assessment today. The reader should be advised that relatively few psychologists are familiar with all of the tests covered in this chapter, since many are highly specialized.

None of the various psychological tests are perfectly reliable and valid; consequently, all test findings must be regarded with some skepticism. The best tests allow us to measure some abilities of many people much of the time with fairly good accuracy—by no means a precise science! Most tests have shortcomings, and very few have had the extensive research and development support that would allow all of their psychometric characteristics to be studied. As long as test results are considered only sugges-

tive and are integrated with other sources of information about the child, little harm will come from using a test that has some imperfections. On the other hand, some tests are so poorly constructed or normed that the results obtained are meaningless; these tests should not be purchased or used.

Many excellent books on psychological testing provide more extensive literature reviews and discussions of psychometric issues than is practical here. These works include *Psychological Testing* [2], *Assessment of Children's Intelligence and Special Abilities* [5], and the *Mental Measurements Yearbook* series [3]. These three are the standard references used by pediatric psychologists when they want expert opinions about the construction, reliability, validity, and clinical usefulness of a particular test. Rather than attempting to duplicate the extensive information contained in these works, we have chosen to consult these sources and others, add our own clinical experience with handicapped children, and provide evaluative essays about the various tests we have reviewed. This format should enable readers in other fields to evaluate psychological test reports they receive, and to collaborate more effectively with their psychologist colleagues.

Several important issues are relevant to the selection and administration of the tests presented in this chapter. First, the subject of who should administer psychological tests is often a source of confusion among child development professionals. Guidelines for user qualifications are available from several sources. For example, the major textbooks on psychological assess-

Supported in part by U.S. Public Health Service, Maternal and Child Health Project No. 916 and Grant HD-03110.

ment [2, 5] devote extensive discussions to the appropriate training of test administrators, and to the areas of background knowledge necessary for responsible use and interpretation of psychological tests. The publishers of psychological and educational tests also provide guidelines as to who may actually purchase the tests. Different qualifications for training and educational degree apply to different classes of tests, with the most stringent standards applying to purchasers of the major intelligence and personality tests. Most of these tests are available to what we will call "fully qualified psychologists," that is, members of the American Psychological Association who are in good standing, holders of doctorates in some area of psychology, master's level psychologists having taken advanced assessment courses, or psychology graduate students sponsored by a professor. Of course, various states' licensing laws for practicing psychologists provide further restrictions and guidelines for who may use such tests and for what purposes. In any event, the set of guidelines to which all sources ultimately refer is the Ethical Principles of Psychologists, published by the American Psychological Association [1]. This document sets forth a code of ethics for psychologists and enumerates a series of principles relevant to the training of testers and the use of tests, including the principles labeled Responsibility, Competence, Moral and Legal Standards, Confidentiality, Welfare of the Consumer, and Assessment Techniques. The reader is referred to this document and to Anastasi [2] for further details on this very important subject. Nonpsychologists who are interested in their qualifications to administer and interpret a given test should consult the publisher's catalogue for initial guidelines.

Standardized administration and scoring are common features of virtually all psychological tests, the only exceptions being a few projective personality instruments. The underlying assumption is that an individual's performance can be meaningfully compared with a normative group only if the conditions of administra-

tion and scoring are as similar as possible, so that sources of error or bias are minimized. All of the tests reviewed should be individually administered to a child who is comfortably seated at a table of appropriate height. The room should be well lighted and ventilated, quiet, and free of distractions. This setting is referred to as the *standard testing environment* in the test reviews that follow.

Most of the instruments reviewed in this chapter are tests of intelligence that yield a summary score, usually called an *intelligence quotient* (IQ). A full discussion of theories of intelligence and its measurement is beyond the scope of this chapter. Briefly, although almost everyone would agree that there is a great deal of variability among humans in cognitive skills (such as perception, learning memory, and expression of ideas), there is much disagreement about the relative importance of these skills in determining overall intellectual functioning. Different theorists have focused on different clusters of skills in defining intelligence. For example, Alfred Binet, the forefather of the Stanford-Binet Intelligence Scale (reviewed in this chapter) considered intelligence to be "a collection of faculties: judgment, practical sense, initiative, and the ability to adapt oneself to circumstances" [5]. David Wechsler, author of the Wechsler Adult Intelligence Scale-Revised (WAIS-R) for adults, Wechsler Intelligence Scale for Children-Revised (WISC-R) for school-age children (reviewed in this chapter) and Wechsler Preschool and Primary Scale of Intelligence (WPPSI) for preschool children (also reviewed in this chapter) defined intelligence as "the aggregate or global capacity of the individual to act purposefully, to think rationally, and to deal effectively with his environment" [6]. Alan and Nadeen Kaufman, who developed the Kaufman Assessment Battery for Children (reviewed in this chapter) considered intelligence in terms of both the style and the level of skill demonstrated in solving problems and processing new information [4]. Most psychologists agree that intelligence is a fairly stable trait across an individual's lifetime; however, since intelligence is determined both by inherited potential and by experiences in the environment, it can probably be affected to some degree by extreme deprivation or extraordinary enrichment. IQ scores may also vary because of the measurement tools, that is, the IQ tests themselves. To the extent that tests differ among themselves in content, and to the extent that error and chance influence results, the scores of different tests administered to the same individual may differ.

Since many of the tests reviewed in this chapter yield an IQ score, it is important that readers understand the difference between ratio and deviation IQs. The *ratio IQ,* which was first used in the early twentieth century, is the ratio of mental age divided by chronological age, then multiplied by 100. This type of IQ has many psychometric disadvantages; one disadvantage is that it does not take into account the uneven nature of development. For example, at 3 years of age there may be great variability in what normally developing children can do, so that a mental age of 2 years (which yields a ratio IQ of 67) is not seriously deviant. On the other hand, at age six normal development may be less variable, so that a child with a ratio IQ of 67 (mental age of 4 years) is quite seriously delayed. The IQ in both of these cases, however, is the same, and does not accurately reflect the child's status in relation to chronological age peers. This problem with the ratio IQ has been overcome through the use of a *deviation IQ,* in which the assigned IQ represents the child's deviation from average on a normal curve. The curve usually has a mean of 100 and a standard deviation of either 15 or 16, so that, for example, a child whose performance is at the eighty-fourth percentile (1 standard deviation above average) is assigned an IQ score of 115 or 116, depending on the test. Thus, deviation IQs are much more accurate and acceptable than ratio IQs.

Once tests have been administered and scored, the challenge to psychologists is to integrate test results with knowledge of test properties, behavioral observations, background information, and referral questions. Most psychological

reports will include information such as the child's degree of cooperation and motivation, and any sensory, motor, or health factors that seemed to affect the child's performance. It is vital that test scores be put into perspective in terms of their perceived validity and their practical implications for answering the referral questions.

REFERENCES

1. American Psychological Association. Ethical principles of psychologists. *Am. Psychol.* 36 : 633, 1981.
2. Anastasi, A. *Psychological Testing* (5th ed.). New York: Macmillan, 1982.
3. Buros, O. K. *The Ninth Mental Measurements Yearbook.* Lincoln, Nebr.: University of Nebraska Press, 1985.
4. Kaufman, A. S., and Kaufman, N. *Manual for the Kaufman Assessment Battery for Children.* Circle Pines, Minn.: American Guidance Service, 1983.
5. Sattler, J. M. *Assessment of Children's Intelligence and Special Abilities* (2nd ed.). Boston: Allyn & Bacon, 1982.
6. Wechsler, D. *The Measurement and Appraisal of Adult Intelligence* (4th ed.). Cleveland: The Psychological Corporation, 1958.

THE BENDER VISUAL MOTOR GESTALT TEST

Descriptive Information

Test Identification

The title of this test is the *Bender Visual Motor Gestalt Test* (BVMGT), 1938, 1946. Its author is Loretta Bender, M.D. Dr. Bender was a senior psychiatrist at Bellevue Hospital in New York City when the test was developed. The Psychological Corporation (555 Academic Court, San Antonio, Texas 78204-0952) publishes the test at a cost of $25–$35.

Age and Type of Client

The BVMGT is for children and adults aged 4 and older. The Developmental Scoring System of Koppitz [2] is the most popular scoring system used with children. It provides norms for children aged 5 years 0 months through 11 years 11 months.

Purpose

The purpose of the test as applied to children is to evaluate perceptual-motor skills and to detect developmental immaturities. In adults, the test is intended to be sensitive to brain damage of various etiologies.

Time Required to Administer and Score Test

Administration usually requires no more than 5 minutes, with another 5 minutes needed for scoring. Occasionally, a child takes up to 15 minutes because of excessive erasing, slowness, or other noteworthy response styles.

Evaluator

Although almost any professional adult could master the administration procedures, which are straightforward, the results of the test should be interpreted only by a fully qualified psychologist.

Historical Perspective of Test Construction

Development and Source of Test Items

The test stimuli were adopted from the research materials of Wertheimer, a psychologist noted for studies of perception ("gestalt psychology") in the 1920s.

Review of Literature in Terms of Test Use

Loretta Bender devised the BVMGT as an index of brain damage in psychiatric inpatient adults, and as a developmental test for use with children. Her approach to test use was qualitative and clinical rather than quantitative. She evaluated whether or not the examinee was able to perceive and copy the "gestalt", or main configural features, of each design without distortion or fragmentation. A number of scoring systems were subsequently developed to evaluate performance quality. Most scoring systems are for the adult test, but the Koppitz Developmental Scoring System [2] is available for children's productions.

Since its development, the BVMGT has been one of the most widely used psychological tests. It is commonly included in the standard test battery for children in evaluations done, for example, at outpatient mental health centers and in public schools. Although Bender intended the test to be a measure of perceptual maturity and a sensitive indicator of developmental lags in maturation, the most common use with children for many years was as a screening instrument for "organicity" or brain damage [1]. The difficulty in establishing validity based on this use, however, results from the diffuse meaning of the term *brain damage* and the inexact methods available for diagnosing brain damage in children so that an accurate criterion measure could be used. Currently, the BVMGT is used by most clinicians at face value, i.e., as a test of visual-motor or perceptual-motor functioning. The results are then integrated with other psychological test results in terms of an overall profile of abilities.

In addition to its use as a perceptual-motor test, the BVMGT has been used to evaluate emotional functioning (e.g., Koppitz describes 11 "emotional indicators") and as a projective test. These uses of the test, however, currently are less common than its use as a visual-motor performance sample.

Theoretical Constructs and Implications for Intervention

The BVMGT provides a demonstration of the child's visual perception, motor coordination, and visual-motor integration [3]. Thus, results can be used, in combination with results from intelligence and other tests, to pinpoint weaknesses that affect academic functioning. Remediation planning should be based on the integration of many pieces of information, including the BVMGT results.

Content and Administration

Content

The test stimuli consist of nine designs printed on 4- by 6-in. white cards.

Setting and Equipment

The standard testing environment is required. The child is given a lead pencil and one sheet of plain white paper, but extra sheets are kept in view in case the child spontaneously asks for them.

Administration Procedures

Administration of the BVMGT is straightforward. Koppitz supplies an introductory paragraph for the examiner to use in which the child is briefly informed that there are nine designs to copy and that his or her designs should be made just like them. The cards are presented one by one, and no timing is involved.

Scoring

Each design is scored for a number of possible errors falling into four categories: distortion, rotation, integration, and perseveration. Each error earns 1 point, the total score being the sum of all errors. An individual child's score is then compared with the norms tables of school-aged children. What is usually presented in test reports is the age at which children typically achieve the score that the child currently being tested has obtained.

If the Koppitz system is used for emotional assessment, the examiner will note behaviors such as drawing sketchy lines and then going over them repeatedly, drawing excessively large or small designs, or substituting dashes for circles. There is no quantitative system for interpreting the emotional indicators, however.

Psychometric Properties

Standardization

The standardization of the Koppitz norms was based on the performance of 975 school children from 5 to 11 years of age. Although the sample was large and drawn from rural, suburban, and metropolitan areas, it was not representative of the country with respect to geographic location. Additionally, its socioeconomic status distribution was not described.

Reliability

Test-retest reliability coefficient, based on intervals ranging from the same day to 8 months, are adequate (median of .77). Interrater reliabilities are quite high and range from .77 to .91 [3].

Validity

The concurrent validity of the BVMGT as a perceptual-motor task is supported by moderate to high correlations with other tests of the same construct [3]. For example, a correlation of .82 with the Beery-Buktenica Developmental Test of Visual-Motor Integration (VMI) has been obtained. Concurrent and predictive validity research, based on correlations with school achievement indices, has produced low to moderate coefficients. Arithmetic abilities appear to be better predicted by BVMGT scores than reading abilities. Sattler [3] concludes that the validity of the Koppitz scoring system depends on what the test is being used to evaluate, and that its most valid use is as a perceptual-motor test.

Guidelines for Use in a Clinical Setting

The BVMGT is often used as the first test in an evaluation session because it is nonverbal, quick, and generally nonthreatening. Along with the developmental scoring, observations of the child's approach to the task are frequently useful. The child's ability to organize his or her paper, tendencies toward impulsivity or perfectionism, and ease or difficulty with the task in general are observable and provide clinically useful information. The test is virtually never used in isolation and is no longer considered a reliable diagnostic tool for "brain damage" or emotional disturbance when used alone. Instead, it should be considered a test of perceptual-motor functioning to be used in conjunction with other tests. The most popular alternative to this test is the Beery-Buktenica Developmental Test of VMI (see Chap. 5).

Review

The BVMGT is a test of perceptual-motor functioning. It has a long history of clinical use and has been extremely popular. Its advantages are that it is a quick, nonthreatening test. In combination with other tests, it provides a sample of behavior having relevance to academic functioning. The test should not be used in isolation, as validity research has not supported it to be a highly reliable tool for diagnosis of brain damage or for prediction of school achievement when used alone.

REFERENCES

1. Eno, L., and Deichmann, J. A review of the Bender Gestalt test as a screening instrument for brain damage with school-aged children of normal intelligence since 1970. *J. Spec. Ed.* 14 : 37, 1980.
2. Koppitz, E. M. *The Bender Gestalt Test for Young Children.* New York: Grune & Stratton, 1964.
3. Sattler, J. M. *Assessment of Children's Intelligence and Special Abilities.* Boston: Allyn & Bacon, 1982.

COLUMBIA MENTAL MATURITY SCALE

Descriptive Information

Test Identification

The title of this test is *Columbia Mental Maturity Scale* (CMMS), 1972. Its authors are Bessie B. Burgmeister, Lucille H. Blum, and Irving Lorge. All three authors were psychologists and educators at Columbia University in the 1940s, and each was concerned with the problem of measuring mental abilities in children with cerebral palsy and other handicapping conditions that limit verbal or motor skills. The Psychological Corporation (555 Academic Court, San Antonio, Texas 78204-0952) publishes the test at a cost of $200–$250.

Age and Type of Client

The CMMS was designed for use with children aged 3 years 6 months through 9 years 11 months.

Purpose

According to the manual, the CMMS is a nonverbal test of "general reasoning ability" using pictorial and geometric symbols. The authors state that the test results may be helpful for making decisions about curriculum materials and learning tasks.

Time Required to Administer and Score Test

Administration time is 15 to 20 minutes, with 5 to 10 additional minutes needed for scoring.

Evaluator

Because this test is extremely simple to administer, no specific professional credentials are required. However, all administrators should be familiar with the principles and techniques of individual testing, and with the special difficulties involved in evaluating young and handicapped children.

Historical Perspective of Test Construction

Development and Source of Test Items

The first edition was published in 1954, with a revision published in 1959. The current edition, published in 1972, was extensively revised and nationally standardized in 1970. The source of items and theory underlying their selection are not described in the 1972 manual.

Review of Literature in Terms of Test Use

The CMMS is not widely used and is generally thought of as a minor instrument that is occasionally useful when other, more popular tests are unsuitable. This view is somewhat surprising, given the instrument's good standardization and simple format.

Theoretical Constructs and Implications for Intervention

The CMMS is not a theoretically based test. Its primary feature is that it assesses reasoning abilities without requiring extensive speech or motor abilities. The rationale for the types of reasoning assessed, however, is not described in the test manual. Test users are therefore left to draw their own conclusions based on the child's pattern of successes and failures.

Content and Test Administration

Content

The CMMS test kit consists of 92 large cards (6 by 19 in.); each card contains three to five pictures (3 by 4 in. in size). The child's task, for each card, is to indicate which picture does not belong with the others, so that the child must understand the concept of same/different. At early levels, items involve simple visual discrimination among pictures (e.g., two cars, one cat). Later items require recognition of concepts such as orientation in space, number, and categories (e.g., fences, trees). Some reviewers [1, 2] have criticized the limited range of item content, and questioned how complete a measure of "general reasoning ability" the CMMS really is.

Setting and Equipment

The standard test environment is required. No special equipment is needed.

Administration Procedures

The examiner is allowed to explain the task in a variety of ways (e.g., find the picture that is "different," "not the same," "does not have a partner"). Testing begins at one of eight levels, depending on the child's age. The levels contain between 51 and 65 items. Three sample items are used to teach the test task to all children.

Scoring

The test protocol provides a slightly confusing format for circling the child's selection of a response, and adequate space for recording notes about the child's behavior. Based on the child's raw score of number correct, the manual provides an "age deviation score" (mean = 100, standard deviation = 16), percentile ranking, and stanine. Also provided for each raw score is a "maturity index," which is less precise than an age equivalent, but can provide a useful representation of the child's developmental level. Thus, the administration and scoring procedures are straightforward. However, because the test requires the child to indicate only a choice of response, examiners must be alert for children who may be merely guessing, answering based on a positional response set (e.g., always picking the far left picture), or selecting responses based on unintentional cues from the examiner's facial expression or eye gaze [1].

Psychometric Properties

Standardization

The CMMS was standardized on 2600 children stratified on the variables of geographic region, parental occupation, age, and sex, based on the 1960 census. There were 200 children at each of thirteen 6-month age levels (e.g., 3 years 6 months–3 years 11 months; 4 years 0 months–4 years 5 months).

Reliability

Reliability data reported in the test manual are test-retest and split-half, both of which are in the high .80s. Interexaminer reliability is not reported, but would almost certainly be acceptable, because the child's selection of a response is rarely ambiguous.

Validity

Concurrent validity of the CMMS, using the Stanford-Binet as a criterion, was described by Sattler [4] as satisfactory ($r = .74$), and the manual describes several studies that indicate a moderate (.50s–.60s) relationship with school achievement. Egeland [1] characterized these results as lower than those obtained by longer tests of cognitive abilities with a greater variety of item content.

Guidelines for Use in a Clinical Setting

The CMMS provides a mechanism for evaluating cognitive skills in young children without requiring expressive language. Thus, the test may be useful for children with speech, language, or hearing impairments. However, it is sometimes difficult for the examiner to communicate the directions (i.e., different/not the same/does not belong) so that young language- or hearing-impaired children understand the task. Because the pictures are large, visually impaired children with some usable vision may be able to respond to the CMMS materials when the Stanford-Binet, Wechsler Preschool and Primary Scale of Intelligence (WPPSI), or Wechsler Intelligence Scale for Children-Revised (WISC-R) materials are too small. In addition, motorically impaired children can often communicate their answers by touching a picture, focusing their gaze on it, or indicating their choice as the examiner points to each picture in turn. Thus, the CMMS may be a useful test with several categories of exceptionality. However, the norms compare these children only with normally developing children, so that the validity of results for handicapped children is undocumented [3].

Another limitation of the CMMS is that it measures a very limited cluster of cognitive skills (i.e., the ability to discriminate visually among pictures, with little reasoning involved), especially at lower levels. For some children, especially the mentally retarded and autistic, scores based on these skills may be spuriously high and may overestimate the child's general cognitive abilities. Conversely, for youngsters with specific deficits in visual-perceptual skills, the CMMS may underestimate cognitive abilities. In order to obtain a balanced estimate of an exceptional child's functioning, it would be important to supplement the CMMS with measures of adaptive behavior and language.

Review

The CMMS is a nonverbal test of reasoning that requires the child to identify the picture that does not belong in a set of pictures or symbols. The test is well standardized, but studies of its concurrent and predictive validity, especially with handicapped children, are scarce. It can be a useful measure of mental ability for several categories of exceptional children, but should always be supplemented with measures of language development and adaptive skills.

REFERENCES

1. Egeland, B. R. Review of the Columbia Mental Maturity Scale. In O. K. Buros (ed.), *The Eighth Mental Measurements Yearbook*. Highland Park, N.J.: Gryphon Press, 1978.
2. Kaufman, A. S. Review of the Columbia Mental Maturity Scale. In O. K. Buros (ed.), *The Eighth Mental Measurements Yearbook*. Highland Park, N.J.: Gryphon Press, 1978.
3. Petrosko, J. M. Review of the Columbia Mental Maturity Scale. In O. K. Buros (ed.), *The Eighth Mental Measurements Yearbook*. Highland Park, N.J.: Gryphon Press, 1978.
4. Sattler, J. M. *Assessment of Children's Intelligence and Special Abilities* (2nd ed.). Boston: Allyn & Bacon, 1982.

GOODENOUGH-HARRIS DRAWING TEST

Descriptive Information

Test Identification

The title of this test is the *Goodenough-Harris Drawing Test,* 1963; it is also known as the *Draw-A-Man Test* (DAM). Dale B. Harris, a psychologist who is also co-author of the Piers-Harris Children's self-concept scale, is the author of this test. Western Psychological Services (12031 Wilshire Blvd., Los Angeles, California 90025) publishes this test at a cost of $38–$48.

Age and Type of Client

The test manual provides standard score norms for children aged 3 years 0 months to 15 years 11 months.

Purpose

The purpose of the test is to evaluate conceptual maturity in children based on their drawings of a human figure.

Time Required to Administer and Score Test

The DAM can be administered in the time it takes the child to draw one, two, or three persons, depending on the version of the task used. Scoring should take 3 to 5 minutes per drawing.

Evaluator

Although any professional adult can usually master the administration procedure, which is straightforward, the results of the test should be interpreted only by a fully qualified psychologist.

Historical Perspective of Test Construction

Development and Source of Test Items

In 1963, Harris revised Goodenough's [1] drawing test, which was similar to the current version in task, scoring approach, and objectives. The Goodenough version required the child to draw a man only, whereas Harris added the options of drawing a woman and the self as well. Harris also expanded the scoring system, extended the age range to 15 years 11 months, and standardized the scoring system, creating the current norms tables.

Review of Literature in Terms of Test Use

The DAM test was intended to measure "conceptual maturity." The scoring system of Harris provides a standard score that takes the same form as an intelligence quotient (IQ), and the test is in fact often used to obtain an estimate of intelligence. However, studies have not shown it to be a valid replacement for an intelligence test. The DAM appears to be most useful as a supplement to more extensive testing, as a sample of nonverbal conceptual development.

Harris added the self-drawing to the test with the intention of providing a vehicle for projective interpretation. There is no scoring system for this use of the drawing, however. Although the technique for asking a child to draw a person and then using the drawing as a basis for exploring self-concept has become popular, this use is not equivalent to administering the Goodenough-Harris Drawing Test.

Theoretical Constructs and Implications for Intervention

The DAM tests the degree to which the child has a differentiated, detailed, and integrated representation of a very familiar object—a person. This representation is considered by Harris to correlate with and reflect overall intellectual level; thus, the test may serve as a screening instrument for general cognitive ability. The drawing act itself also samples the child's perceptual-motor skills, which play an important part in academic skills. Finally, distortions or interpersonally symbolic aspects of the drawings that are unrelated to cognitive or perceptual-motor limitations may serve as indications of possible emotional maladjustment.

Content and Test Administration

Content

There are no formal test material, since the test task is simply to draw pictures on plain paper.

Setting and Equipment

The standard testing environment is required.

Administration Procedures

The DAM test is simple to administer. The child is provided with a lead pencil and plain white paper and is instructed to draw a man, to work carefully, to make all of him, and to do the best he or she can. Similar instructions are given for the Draw-A-Woman and the Drawing of the Self portions.

Scoring

The drawings are scored using Harris's Point Scale and/or Quality Scale. The *Point Scale* is based on 73 individual features; 1 point is earned for each feature present. Points are totaled for a raw score, which is converted to a standard score (mean of 100, standard deviation of 15) using the manual. Scoring sheets are available that have a large space for the drawing and places to note the presence or absence of each feature in columns beside the drawing.

The *Quality Scale* involves comparing the overall quality of the child's production with 12 examples of drawings printed in the book. The examples span the continuum in terms of excellence, and separate sets of examples are provided for the man and the woman drawing. Standard scores based on the number of the matching example and the chronological age of the child are provided in the manual.

Psychometric Properties

Standardizaton

Standardization for the test used 2975 children who were representative of the U.S. population based on the 1960 census statistics. Seventy-five children at each age level from 5 to 15 years were tested. Fewer were tested at the 3- and 4-year level, a limitation noted in the manual.

Reliability

Test-retest reliabilities are adequate (.50s–.70s), as are alternate-form reliability coefficients (.72–.90). Interrater agreement for the Point Scale is good (.80s–.90s) [5].

Validity

Validity of the DAM has involved mainly criterion-related studies. Correlations with a number of intellectual and achievement tests are quite variable, ranging from .05 to .92. Intelligence scores from the DAM tend to be lower than the Stanford-Binet and Wechsler Tests. Sattler [4] suggested that the validity of the test is less established than its reliability, and thus the test should not be used in isolation. Taylor [5] took a firmer stand, stating that the test is not a valid measure of intelligence.

Guidelines for Use in a Clinical Setting

Because of the nonverbal nature of the DAM, it has potential as a supplementary test where language or culture (such as bilingualism) may be a biasing factor for other tests. However, reviewers agree that the test should *not* be used as an intelligence test. It tends to underestimate IQs when longer tests are used as a criterion, and it is not useful in discriminating between children of average and superior intelligence [5]. Taylor [5] cited a study by Hartman [3] that concluded that the test was not appropriate for use with learning-disabled children. The cognitive and perceptual-motor components of the test must be considered as somewhat independent; for example, a child's fine motor coordination problems can result in a product that underestimates his or her intellectual capabilities. When using the test as an assessment instrument for emotional functioning, it should be viewed only as a screening or supplementary test. It can build rapport if the child enjoys drawing and talking about his or her pictures. Individual practitioners will make interpretations according to their training and predilections.

Review

The Goodenough-Harris Drawing Test, or Draw-A-Man Test, is a quick, easily administered test to be used as a screening measure for intellectual functioning and for observations of perceptual-motor skills, but not as an intelligence test, in spite of the fact that the standard score obtained looks like an IQ score. Its popularity is due to the ease of administration and the theory that the drawing can also be used as an assessment of emotional functioning. Although standardization procedures and reliability coefficients are acceptable, widely varying validity coefficients raise the question of what is actually being mea-

sured. The test should never be used in isolation, but should be integrated into a total picture of evaluation results.

REFERENCES

1. Goodenough, F. L. *Measurement of Intelligence by Drawings.* New York: World Book, 1926.
2. Harris, D. *Children's Drawings as Measures of Intellectual Maturity.* New York: Harcourt Brace Jovanovich, 1963.
3. Hartman, R. An investigation of the incremental validity of human figure drawings in the diagnosis of learning disabilities. *J. Sch. Psychol.* 10 : 9, 1972.
4. Sattler, J. M. *Assessment of Children's Intelligence and Special Abilities* (2nd ed.). Boston: Allyn & Bacon, 1982.
5. Taylor, R. L. *The Assessment of Exceptional Students.* Englewood Cliffs, N.J.: Prentice-Hall, 1984.

HISKEY-NEBRASKA TEST OF LEARNING APTITUDE

Descriptive Information

Test Identification

The title of this test is *Hiskey-Nebraska Test of Learning Aptitude* (Hiskey-Nebraska), 1966. Its author is Marshall S. Hiskey, Ph.D. Dr. Hiskey was a Professor of Educational Psychology and Special Education at the University of Nebraska at Lincoln when the test was developed. He stated [5] that the impetus for the development of this test was his encounter with a 10-year-old deaf boy who had been erroneously diagnosed as mentally retarded and confined to an institution. When Dr. Hiskey tested him on nonverbal tasks, the boy was found to be of average intelligence. He was eventually able to live and work independently, although he never fully recovered from his early lack of educational stimulation. This incident spurred Dr. Hiskey's interest in assessment of deaf youngsters. Dr. Hiskey (5640 Baldwin, Lincoln, Nebraska 68507) publishes this test at a cost of $68–$95.

Age and Type of Client

The Hiskey-Nebraska was designed for hearing-impaired or nonspeaking children aged 3 years 0 months through 16 years.

Purpose

This test was intended to be an individual ability test for deaf children.

Time Required to Administer and Score Test

Administration requires 45 to 50 minutes, with an additional 15 minutes needed for scoring.

Evaluator

The test should be administered only by a fully qualified psychologist. If it is administered to deaf students, the psychologist should be familiar with the developmental and behavioral characteristics of the deaf.

Historical Perspective of Test Construction

Development and Source of Test Items

The incident described above led Dr. Hiskey to develop the Nebraska Test of Learning Aptitude for Young Deaf Children (1941), which he subsequently revised and restandardized as the Hiskey-Nebraska Test of Learning Aptitude in 1966.

Review of Literature in Terms of Test Use

The Hiskey-Nebraska is the only intelligence test specifically designed for and standardized on deaf school-age children. It is frequently used with this population and is fairly well respected [1, 3], although according to Graham and Lilly [4] it is not used as commonly as the WISC or WISC-R Performance Scales.

Theoretical Constructs and Implications for Intervention

The Hiskey-Nebraska was not developed according to a theory of intelligence. Instead, items were designed to be similar to school tasks, correlated with learning ability, and useful in discriminating among ability levels.

Content and Test Administration

Content

The Hiskey-Nebraska materials are contained in a briefcase-sized kit. The test consists of 12 subtests (listed below). The first five subtests are administered only to children aged 3 to 10; the next four are administered only to children aged 11 and above; and the remaining three subtests are administered to all children. The subtests and brief descriptions are as follows:

> Bead Patterns: The child copies patterns with small beads of different shapes, either with a model or from memory.
> Memory for Color: The child recreates sequences of colored rectangles.
> Picture Identification: The child matches pictures to a model.
> Picture Association: The child chooses the picture that belongs in the category implied by the model.
> Paper Folding: The child recreates sequences of movements to fold paper.
> Memory for Digits: The child recreates sequences of numbers using plastic numerals.
> Puzzle Blocks: The child puts together parts of a block to make a whole.
> Picture Analogies: The child chooses which picture completes the analogy given in the model.
> Spatial Reasoning: The child chooses pictures of the parts which make up the model.
> Visual Attention Span: The child recreates sequences of pictures.

Block Patterns: The child builds block designs to match the model.

Completion of Drawings: The child uses a pencil to draw in the missing details in drawings of common objects.

Setting and Equipment

The standard testing environment is required. The examiner must supply a stopwatch and large quantities of 6- by 6-in. paper for the paper folding subtest.

Administration Procedures

Directions can be given either through pantomime (not sign language) or speech; standardized procedures for both are given in the manual. The Hiskey-Nebraska is not particularly difficult to administer, although many examiners might be uncomfortable with the lack of verbal interactions with clients.

Scoring

Within each subtest, each item is scored according to criteria outlined in the manual. When pantomime is used, the child's performance is compared with norms for deaf children; if speech is used, the hearing norms must also be used. Each subtest yields a total raw score, which is then compared with test norms in two stages. First, the norms indicate the age at which approximately 50 percent of children in the standardization group obtained a particular score; thus, a "learning age" equivalent for performance on each subtest can be obtained. Next the median of all the learning ages is computed. The test was designed to use the median score so that deaf children would not be unduly penalized for a low score on a subtest on which they may not have understood the directions. For children with whom spoken directions were used, the median learning age is then compared in the norms tables with the child's chronological age

to yield a deviation IQ (mean = 100; standard deviation = 16). No such norms have been developed for deaf children. Dr. Hiskey cautioned against computing a quotient of learning age divided by chronological age × 100, which would in effect be a ratio IQ, but at the same time provided a table to help test users in doing so.

Psychometric Properties

Standardization

The Hiskey-Nebraska was standardized on 1079 deaf and 1074 hearing children ranging in age from 2 years 6 months to 17 years 5 months. Most of the deaf children came from schools for the deaf in 10 states across the country. No information is presented in the manual about their status on standard demographic variables, but Dr. Hiskey stated that since most children of a particular age at the school were tested, the sample was probably quite representative of the total population of deaf children. The sample of hearing children was stratified, using the occupational level of their parents, according to the 1960 census. This sample included minority group children on a random basis.

Reliability

Both reliability and validity data from the Hiskey-Nebraska are somewhat incomplete, as they are for most tests of its era. High (.90s) split-half reliabilities are reported in the manual, but there was no information about test-retest or interrater reliability. Subsequent reviewers have pointed to the lack of information about these types of reliability as a weakness of the test [3, 6].

Validity

Several reviewers [1, 7] have described good correlations with other intelligence tests and with academic achievement (criterion validity). For example, Anastasi [1] reported correlations of Hiskey-Nebraska and Stanford-Binet or WISC-R scores with hearing children ranging from .78 to .86. However, Graham and Lilly [4] criticized the small sample sizes and heterogeneous populations on which criterion validity studies have been performed, and Newland described the research on the Hiskey-Nebraska as characterized by "impreciseness," although he thought the test was "the most promising one available for assessing the 'book learning' capability of deaf children" [6].

Guidelines for Use in a Clinical Setting

The primary group for whom the Hiskey-Nebraska is appropriate is hearing-impaired children. For hearing-impaired children functioning in the range of 4 years through middle childhood, this test is often the instrument of choice. Older and brighter hearing-impaired children can often be evaluated with the Performance Scale of the WISC-R, using the norms that are now available for the deaf [2]. Younger or more retarded hearing-impaired children might be better evaluated with the Smith-Johnson Nonverbal Performance Scale [8], which was developed at the John Tracy Clinic as a measure of nonverbal cognitive skills for children aged 2 to 4 years. The Smith-Johnson enables the examiner to describe a child's skills as below average (below the twenty-fifth percentile), average (twenty-fifth–seventy-fifth percentile), or above average (above the seventy-fifth percentile), but unlike the Hiskey-Nebraska does not yield a standard score. Thus, the Hiskey-Nebraska would be preferable when a more precise numerical representation of the child's functioning relative to chronological age peers is required.

The Hiskey-Nebraska may also be appropriate for children with normal hearing but severely impaired speech, if they have the motoric abilities to manipulate the test materials. For a child with multiple handicaps, it may not be possible to administer any test completely, so the fact that each subtest on the Hiskey-Nebraska yields an age equivalent would enable the examiner to administer only the items that a particular child could comprehend and perform. Of course, this procedure would yield only a general estimate of a limited sample of skills, rather than a global summary of cognitive ability.

Because there is no receptive or expressive language required on the Hiskey-Nebraska, it would be important to supplement the test with a measure of language in order to obtain a more complete picture of a child's skills. It is also interesting to observe the child's approach to several of the test tasks, particularly those involving memory, because the child's use of language symbols can often be inferred from the child's approach to the tasks.

Review

The Hiskey-Nebraska is a test of cognitive skills specifically designed for and standardized on deaf youngsters. The test is fairly popular among psychologists in the field of assessment of the deaf, but almost 20 years after its publication there is still limited information about its reliability and criterion-related and predictive validity.

REFERENCES

1. Anastasi, A. *Psychological Testing* (5th ed.). New York: Macmillan, 1982.
2. Anderson, R. D., and Sisco, F. H. *Standardization of the WISC-R for the Deaf* (Series T, No. 1). Washington, D.C.: Gallaudet College, Office of Demographic Studies, 1977.
3. Bolton, B. F. Review of the Hiskey-Nebraska Test of Learning Aptitude. In O. K. Buros (ed.), *The Eighth Mental Measurements Yearbook*. Highland Park, N.J.: Gryphon Press, 1978.
4. Graham, J. R., and Lilly, R. S. *Psychological Testing*. Englewood Cliffs, N.J.: Prentice-Hall, 1984.
5. Hiskey, M. S. The Development, Administration, Scoring, and Interpretation of the Hiskey-Nebraska Test of Learning Aptitude. In C. R. Reynolds and J. H. Clark (eds.), *Assessment and Programming for Young Children with Low-Incidence Handicaps*. New York: Plenum, 1983.
6. Newland, T. E. Review of the Hiskey-Nebraska Test of Learning Aptitude. In O. K. Buros (ed.), *The Seventh Mental Measurements Yearbook*. Highland Park, N.J.: Gryphon Press, 1972.
7. Rogers, J. S., and Soper, E. Assessment Considera-

tions with Hearing-Impaired Preschoolers. In G. Ulrey & S. J. Rogers (eds.), *Psychological Assessment of Handicapped Infants and Young Children.* New York: Thieme-Stratton, 1982.

8. Smith, A. J., and Johnson, R. E. *Manual for the Smith-Johnson Nonverbal Performance Scale.* Los Angeles: Western Psychological Services, 1977.

KAUFMAN ASSESSMENT BATTERY FOR CHILDREN

Descriptive Information

Test Identification

The title of this test is *Kaufman Assessment Battery for Children* (KABC), 1983. Its authors are Alan S. Kaufman, Ph.D., and Nadeen L. Kaufman, Ph.D. Both authors are psychologists with extensive backgrounds in school psychology, psychometrics, test construction, and clinical assessment. They have also coauthored interpretive books about the McCarthy Scales of Children's Abilities and the Wechsler Intelligence Scales for Children-Revised (WISC-R) (these tests are reviewed later in this chapter). American Guidance Service (Circle Pines, Minnesota 55014) publishes this test at a cost of $150–$200.

Age and Type of Client

The KABC was designed for children aged 2 years 6 months to 12 years 6 months and was intended for use with both normally developing children and those with learning problems, handicapping conditions, and minority group status.

Purpose

The purpose of the KABC is to measure intelligence and achievement in children.

Time Required to Administer and Score Test

The test takes from 1 to 1½ hours to administer, depending on the age and functioning level of the child. Scoring requires approximately 15 minutes.

Evaluator

The KABC should be administered only by a fully qualified psychologist.

Historical Perspective of Test Construction

Development and Source of Test Items

Some KABC items were newly developed, while others were variations of standard psychometric tasks (e.g., Number Recall, which is essentially the Digit Span task from the WISC-R). The authors developed and chose items in accordance with cognitive theories to which they adhere.

Review of Literature in Terms of Test Use

Since the KABC is a recent test, assessment of its utility by clinicians and researchers has not yet been summarized. The test is intended to be a test of cognitive abilities and achievement, to be used in the manner of the WISC-R, McCarthy, and Stanford-Binet. Because of the Kaufmans' background and because of changing views of what intelligence is, this new test is looked on with interest by many.

Theoretical Constructs and Implications for Intervention

The authors of the KABC define intelligence as both the style and the skill level of an individual's problem solving. They distinguish between two general modes of problem solving—sequential and simultaneous. *Sequential processing* entails perceiving and manipulating the order of stimuli, while *simultaneous processing* involves operating on numerous features at the same time, as formed into a whole. This distinction is the same as that resulting from numerous investigations of hemispheric specialization and factor analysis of other tests of cognitive abilities tests. The KABC also differentiates between intelligence and achievement testing; the set of subtests measuring reading, vocabulary, information, and arithmetic comprises the separate Achievement Scale.

A noteworthy feature of the test manual is the extensive discussion of remediation strategies based on test results. The concepts of sequential and simultaneous processing are reviewed, and remedial approaches and exercises to address specific areas of weakness are presented. There is also detailed discussion of remediation for reading, spelling, and mathematics deficits.

Content and Test Administration

Content

The KABC consists of three scales: Sequential Processing, Simultaneous Processing, and Achievement. The first two are referred to as the Mental Processing subtests. Individual subtests are as follows:

Sequential Processing Scale
  Hand Movements: The child performs a series of hand movements in the same sequence as the examiner performed them.
  Number Recall: The child repeats a series of digits in the same sequence as the examiner said them.
  Word Order: The child touches a series of silhouettes of common objects in the same sequence as the examiner said the names of the objects. More difficult items include an interference task between the stimulus and response.
Simultaneous Processing Scale
  Magic Window: The child identifies a picture that the examiner exposes by slowly moving it behind a narrow window, making the picture only partially visible at one time.
  Face Recognition: The child selects from a group photograph the one or two faces

that were exposed briefly on the preceding page.
  Gestalt Closure: The child names an object or scene pictured in a partially completed drawing.
  Triangles: The child assembles several blue and yellow triangles into a pattern to match a model.
  Matrix Analogies: The child selects the meaningful pictures or abstract design that best completes a visual analogy.
  Spatial Memory: The child recalls the placement of pictures on a page that was exposed briefly.
  Photo Series: The child places photographs of an event in chronological order.
Achievement Scale
  Expressive Vocabulary: The child names the object pictured in a photograph.
  Faces and Places: The child names the well-known person, fictional character, or place pictured in a photograph or drawing.
  Arithmetic: The child demonstrates knowledge of numbers and mathematical concepts, counting and computational skills, and other school-related arithmetic abilities.
  Riddles: The child infers the name of a concrete or abstract concept when given a list of its characteristics.
  Reading and Decoding: The child demonstrates reading comprehension by following commands that are given in sentences.

Setting and Equipment

The standard testing environment is required. The KABC consists of three easels, which contain the majority of the test stimuli, and four other pieces of equipment such as colored triangles and photo cards. The examiner does not supply any additional materials except for a stopwatch.

Administration Procedures

The easels function as both an administration manual and test materials. The page facing the examiner presents all relevant instructions and cues, while the page facing the child presents the individual item. Items are administered in a standardized order and manner. On several subtests, "teaching" the task is allowed for younger children or those who initially do not grasp the point of the task. Certain subtests are administered only to younger children. The guidelines for where to start and discontinue subtests are cued on the easel and the scoring form.

Scoring

The KABC yields a variety of scores. The scoring protocol provides places to record results of each item as well as a face sheet for recording summary and standard scores. Each of the Mental Processing subtests yields a scaled score and a national percentile rank based on age. Each of the Achievement subtests yields a standard score, a national percentile rank, and a sociocultural percentile rank (based on age, race, and parental educational level). The subtests are combined into four Global Scales: Sequential Processing, Simultaneous Processing, Mental Processing Composite (sum of Sequential and Simultaneous Processing), and Achievement. Performance levels on Global Scales are translated into standard scores and national and sociocultural percentile ranks. Mental Processing subtest scores have a mean of 10 and a standard deviation of 3. All other scores have a mean of 100 and a standard deviation of 15.

Psychometric Properties

Standardization

The national standardization program, conducted in 1981, included more than 2000 children at 34 test sites in 24 states. The sample was stratified within each age group by sex, geo-graphic region, socioeconomic status, race or ethnic groups, community size, and educational placement of the child.

Reliability

The average split-half reliability coefficients for the four global scales range from .86 to .97. The test-retest reliability coefficients for the global scales range from − .77 to .97.

Validity

Forty-three validity studies are reported in the KABC manual. Subtest scores correlate positively and significantly with age, with no significant effects of sex or race. Factor analysis offered strong support for three significant factors, which were then labeled *simultaneous processing, sequential processing,* and *achievement.* For normally developing children, Global Scales were correlated with Wechsler IQ scores in the following manner: low to moderate correlations were obtained with Sequential Processing scores (.30–.49), Simultaneous Processing scores (.28–.68), and with Mental Processing Composite (.37–.70), while slightly higher correlations were obtained with Achievement scores (.47–.78). Correlations between the KABC Global Scale and the Stanford-Binet were similar. These patterns of correlations demonstrate that the earlier IQ tests and the KABC are measuring somewhat different sets of abilities.

Literature further evaluating the test's validity is beginning to accumulate. The Fall 1984 issue of the *Journal of Special Education* was devoted to the KABC, and in it Mehrens [1] presented a critical analysis of the psychometric properties of the test. He concluded that "the psychometric properties are in line with what we would hope for in a newly constructed instrument" [1]. He described the KABC as a "good test," and indicated that although some shortcomings exist they are fewer and less serious than what are found in most new instruments.

Guidelines for Use in a Clinical Setting

Since the KABC is a relatively recent test, it should not be used alone for placement decisions or diagnostic purposes. Usually it is used as a supplementary or alternative test. The KABC appears to be useful when testing children with a variety of learning problems and handicapping conditions. For example, there is a separate Nonverbal Scale, made up of six subtests that can be administered in pantomime and require only motor responses, such as pointing, manipulating forms, and arranging a sequence of cards. The highest age at which the test can be used is 12 ½; therefore, other general intelligence tests must be used for adolescents.

It is imperative that test administrators study the manual for the purpose of interpretation as well as administration, and that reports contain common-sense translations of strengths and weaknesses. Too often a report written from KABC results is an unenlightening recitation of relative simultaneous and sequential processing abilities, without discussion of their relevance to school performance or general functioning.

Review

The KABC is a recently developed test of intelligence and achievement for children between the ages of 2 ½ and 12 ½ years. Its authors have extensive backgrounds in psychometrics, and thus standardization and validation is thorough. Two positive and unique features are that the test was generated from a theoretical base and that the manual gives detailed information on psychological interpretation of scores. The materials are colorful and interesting to children. A wide variety of children can be tested, including those with various handicaps.

The KABC must be used and researched extensively before general statements can be made about its clinical and research utility.

REFERENCE

1. Mehrens, W. A. A critical analysis of the psycho-

metric properties of the KABC. *J. Spec. Ed.* 18 : 297, 1984.

LEITER INTERNATIONAL PERFORMANCE SCALE

Descriptive Information

Test Identification

The title of this test is *Leiter International Performance Scale* (Leiter), 1948; in 1949, the *Arthur Adaptation* was developed. The author of the Leiter is Russell Leiter, Ph.D., and that of the Arthur Adaptation is Grace Arthur, Ph.D. Both authors were psychologists. The first version of the Leiter was designed in the 1920s as part of Dr. Leiter's master's thesis. His doctoral dissertation was based on research with a later version. Western Psychological Services (12031 Wilshire Blvd., Los Angeles, California 90029) publishes the Leiter at a cost of $595–$650, and the Arthur Adaptation at a cost of $435–$475.

Age and Type of Client

The Leiter can be used with individuals aged 2 years 0 months to adulthood. The Arthur Adaptation is designed for children aged 3 years 0 months to 7 years 11 months.

Purpose

The Leiter is intended to be a nonverbal intelligence test.

Time Required to Administer and Score Test

Both versions of the test require approximately 30 to 45 minutes to administer, with an additional 10 minutes to score.

Evaluator

The Leiter should be administered only by a fully qualified psychologist.

Historical Perspective of Test Construction

Development and Source of Test Items

Leiter's intent was to develop an instrument that could be used in cross-cultural research on intelligence. The development and revision of items took place over a long period of time. After the original 1920 version, revisions were made in 1936, 1938, 1940 (first commercially available version), and 1948 (present version). In 1949, Dr. Arthur published an adaptation of Leiter's scale, in which some administration and scoring procedures were modified, while the materials were left intact. She made her changes in part because the norms for children aged 3 through 8 had been found to be too high, so that the average score for that age group was now 95 rather than 100. Dr. Leiter's response to this problem, however, was not to adopt Arthur's system, but to revise his scoring system by computing the IQ and then adding 5 points. Thus, since 1949 there have been two sets of instructions for use with the same test kit.

Review of Literature in Terms of Test Use

The Leiter today is widely thought of as a test of intelligence particularly suited to the hearing-impaired [8, 10, 11]. However, as will be seen in the technical information to be presented under Psychometric Properties, the test is inadequate for this purpose, and probably does not deserve its prominent status.

The research literature does not indicate which version of the test (Leiter or Arthur) is preferable. In 1982, *The Leiter International Performance Scale: A Handbook* [6] was published by Western Psychological Services (the test publisher). This volume contains both sets of directions and scoring procedures, but no recommendations as to which to use. Although differences in administration between the two versions are minor and involve only a few subtests, scoring differences are somewhat more substantial. It is unfor-

tunate that the relative merits of the two editions are not more fully discussed in the literature.

Theoretical Constructs and Implications for Intervention

The number of items in the test is quite small while item content is extremely varied; thus, there did not appear to be a theory of cognitive development of children guiding the choice of items. The original theories underlying the development of the Leiter dealt with the nature of intelligence across cultures. Leiter viewed intelligence as the ability to cope with new situations [2]. He contended that cross-cultural differences on intelligence tests were due to language factors rather than to innate abilities; thus, his test was completely nonverbal, requiring neither speech nor hearing. Arthur described her version and uses of the test as being, in principle, a nonverbal Binet scale for young children [3], implying that item choice was based on discrimination between age groups, rather than on theoretical constructs of cognitive development.

Content and Test Administration

Content

The Leiter kit is a large, heavy, canvas suitcase containing three trays of wooden blocks required for the complete test; for preschool children only the first tray is needed, and most school-aged children can be tested with only two trays. The task on each subtest is to place between four and eight blocks into a wooden frame, in the order implied by a sample strip of paper placed by the examiner into the frame.

The Leiter is arranged as an age scale, with four subtests at each age level between year II and year XVI (however, there are no subtests at years XI, XIII, or XV). Types of items at each age level differ greatly, but the rationale for item choice and placement is not specified in the current manuals. Early subtests involve direct matching of colors or simple pictures. Most later items include a component of reasoning (e.g., smaller to larger, younger to older), although there are some color-matching tasks that simply involve smaller blocks, presumably requiring more mature fine motor coordination. There are no time limits on any items.

Setting and Equipment

Standard test conditions are required. No additional materials are needed.

Administration Procedures

The examiner places the sample in the frame and presents the blocks to the subject in the order specified in the manual. Early subtests allow the examiner to "teach" the task by correcting and demonstrating until the child displays independent mastery of the matching procedure. No verbal directions are allowed, however, and no communication techniques are suggested in the manual. Thus, the clarity of the directions and teaching provided by the examiner are not standardized, and probably vary greatly among examiners. The examiner must manipulate a large number of blocks fairly quickly to maintain the child's interest; it is also important to keep the blocks organized in the test kit. Although these factors may at first appear to make test administration difficult, it is actually a very simple test to learn and manage.

Scoring

The child should obtain a baseline of one age level completely passed, and a ceiling of two age levels completely failed. For each subtest, the examiner scores the child's arrangement of blocks as correct or incorrect. The test protocol is a small (5½ in. by 8½ in.) card, which does not provide adequate space for notes about the quality of the child's performance. A specified number of months of credit is given for each subtest passed. The child's cumulative mental age is then compared with the chronological age, thus yielding a ratio IQ (mean = 100; standard deviation, approximately 16). Under Leiter's system, this IQ is then increased by 5 points, for the reasons described previously. Under the Arthur adaptation, certain subtests are assigned additional months of mental age credit before the ratio IQ is computed.

Psychometric Properties

Standardization

The Arthur Adaptation of the Leiter was standardized in the late 1940s on 289 children with normal hearing. This small sample was not selected to be representative of the general population, and was in fact quite homogeneous with respect to geographic region and socioeconomic status. It is this extremely small and biased sample to which children are compared when the Arthur Adaptation norms are used. The sample used to develop the Leiter norms is essentially unknown to current users of the test. The only published description of this group is in an old and obscure psychological journal [4].

Reliability

Data on reliability are not included in the various test manuals and handbooks. However, because there are only four items at each age level, the child's score can be greatly affected by careless mistakes or lucky guesses [2, 9]. Anastasi [1] reported that split-half reliabilities ranged from .91–.94 in the studies she reviewed. Sattler [7] described several studies of handicapped children that found satisfactory test-retest reliabilities (.80s and .90s). However, he also described lack of information about the reliability of the scale at different age levels as one of the instrument's most serious problems.

Validity

Both Anastasi [1] and Sattler [7] cited the correlation of the Leiter with other IQ tests (Stanford-

Binet and WISC-R) as ranging from .56 to .92 (median, .83). Sattler commented, however, that in certain populations large differences between the Leiter and other tests may be observed, and cited a study of deaf children in which the average obtained Leiter IQ was 17 points lower than the WISC Performance IQ. Other reviewers [2, 9] have also commented that the Leiter, while correlating fairly well with other instruments, tends to yield lower scores. Predictive validity studies cannot be found in the current literature [1, 9].

Guidelines for Use in a Clinical Setting

The Leiter does not require the child to be able to hear, understand, or speak English. It thus can be useful at times with hearing- or speech-impaired children, or with youngsters who speak only other languages. Other tests that might be equally or more appropriate for these types of clients are the Hiskey-Nebraska Test of Learning Aptitude and the Columbia Mental Maturity Scale (CMMS) (test reviews are included in this chapter). The Leiter has the advantage of accommodating a wider age range, but both the Hiskey-Nebraska and the CMMS are superior in terms of the number and quality of items for children. Furthermore, the psychometric inadequacies of the Leiter make it suitable only as a rough screening measure of nonverbal reasoning.

Because children must manipulate small blocks, the Leiter is not appropriate for severely motorically impaired youngsters.

Review

The Leiter is a nonverbal test that can be used with clients with a wide range of ages and handicapping conditions. However, the instrument's psychometric properties are extremely weak. Sattler [7] described the Leiter as having serious limitations in content, standardization, norms, reliability, and the use of a ratio IQ. In spite of its many shortcomings, however, the Leiter contin-

ues to be available and familiar to clinicians and psychometricians.

REFERENCES

1. Anastasi, A. *Psychological Testing* (5th ed.). New York, Macmillan, 1982.
2. Arnold, G. Review of the Leiter International Performance Scale. In O. K. Buros (ed.), *The Fourth Mental Measurements Yearbook.* Highland Park, N.J.: Gryphon Press, 1953.
3. Arthur, G. *Manual for the Arthur Adaptation of the Leiter International Performance Scale.* Chicago: Stoelting, 1980.
4. Leiter, R. G. Part I of the Manual for the 1948 Revision of the Leiter International Performance Scale: Evidence of the reliability and validity of the Leiter tests. *Psychol. Serv. Cent. J.* 11 : 1, 1959.
5. Leiter, R. G. *General Instructions for the Leiter International Performance Scale.* Los Angeles: Western Psychological Services, 1969.
6. Levine, M. L. *Leiter International Performance Scale: A Handbook.* Los Angeles: Western Psychological Services, 1982.
7. Sattler, J. M. *Assessment of Children's Intelligence and Special Abilities* (2nd ed.). Boston: Allyn & Bacon, 1982.
8. Taylor, R. L. *The Assessment of Exceptional Students.* Englewood Cliffs, N. J.: Prentice-Hall, 1984.
9. Werner, E. Review of the Arthur Adaptation of The Leiter International Performance Scale. In O. K. Buros (ed.), *The Sixth Mental Measurements Yearbook.* Highland Park, N.J.: Gryphon Press, 1965.
10. Wodrich, D. L. *Children's Psychological Testing: A Guide for Nonpsychologists.* Baltimore: Paul H. Brookes, 1984.
11. Zieziula, F. R. *Assessment of Hearing-Impaired People: A Guide for Selecting Psychological, Educational, and Vocational Tests.* Washington, D.C.: Gallaudet College Press, 1982.

McCARTHY SCALES OF CHILDREN'S ABILITIES

Descriptive Information

Test Identification

The title of this test is *McCarthy Scales of Children's Abilities* (MSCA), 1972. Its author is Dorthea McCarthy (1905–1974). McCarthy was a clinical and developmental psychologist who taught in the Psychology Department at Fordham University (Bronx, New York). The Psychological Corporation (555 Academic Court, San Antonio, Texas 78204-0952) publishes the test at a cost of $225–$275.

Age and Type of Client

The MSCA was designed for children aged 2 years 6 months to 8 years 8 months. It was intended for use with both normally developing children and those with mental retardation and learning disabilities.

Purpose

The purpose of the MSCA is to determine general intellectual level as well as strengths and weaknesses over six cognitive and motor areas.

Time Required to Administer and Score Test

Testing time is from 1 to 1½ hours, depending on the level of cooperation and functioning of the child. An experienced examiner can score it in approximately 15 minutes.

Evaluator

The MSCA should be administered only by a fully qualified psychologist.

Historical Perspective of Test Construction

Development and Source of Test Items

McCarthy developed the pool of items over years of clinical and experimental work with children's abilities. Some items, such as Draw-A-Design and Digit Span, have been standard methods used since the earliest psychometric efforts. To determine the final selection, McCarthy used factor analysis of test results at three different age levels of subjects.

Review of Literature in Terms of Test Use

The MSCA was developed during the 1960s when interest in preschool readiness programs, and thus preschoolers' abilities, was at its highest. As an alternative to other preschool intelligence tests, the MSCA offered profile analysis across several broad skill areas (a feature that is absent from the Stanford-Binet) and assessment of gross motor skills, which is not possible using either the Stanford-Binet or the Wechsler tests (WPPSI, WISC, WISC-R). The MSCA subsequently has been the focus of a substantial body of research investigating its reliability and validity (see Psychometric Properties). The established method of combining subtests involves Global Scales of Memory, Motor, Verbal, Quantitative, and Perceptual-Performance; in addition, several alternative approaches to combining subtests for interpretation have been proposed. Tables of statistically extrapolated scores for gifted and mentally retarded children have been developed, although they may be of limited use with retarded children [1].

Theoretical Constructs and Implications for Intervention

Controversy exists over whether or not the main scaled score yielded by the MSCA, called the *general cognitive index* (GCI), is interchangeable with IQ scores. McCarthy deliberately avoided the term *intelligence quotient* because of the "many misinterpretations of that concept" (from page 5 of the test manual). Nonetheless, the MSCA aspires to measure general abilities that are enduring and that are related to achievement and abilities measured in other contexts, which is a functional definition of intelligence. Hesitation to use the GCI and IQ interchangeably stems from studies showing that with certain subject groups (e.g., educable mentally retarded, learning disabled), the GCI is significantly lower than Stanford-Binet and Wechsler IQ scores [1, 7]. Further research is needed to establish the meaning and predictive value of the MSCA scores.

Because the MSCA is reliable and shows evidence of construct validity, it does function well as a sample of behavior and thus can be used for planning remediation programming. Interpretations of a child's strengths and weaknesses as demonstrated on the test can yield recommendations about the modality (e.g., verbal, visual) and approach that might be most successful in teaching an individual child.

Content and Test Administration

Content

The MSCA kit is contained in a zippered carrying case. Eighteen subtests comprise the five scale indexes and the general cognitive index. The Verbal (V), Perceptual-Performance (P), and Quantitative (Q) Scales consist of mutually exclusive sets of subtests. The Motor Scale, however, includes subtests from the V, P, and Q Scales as well as three unique subtests, and the Memory Scale overlaps completely with the other scales. The general cognitive index combines all 15 tests on the V, P, and Q Scales. Individual subtests are as follows:

Verbal Scale
  Pictorial Memory: The child is shown pictures of six familiar objects and must remember as many as possible after they are taken away.
  Word Knowledge I: The child points to the picture named.
  Word Knowledge II: The child gives definition of words.
  Verbal Memory I: The child repeats series of words and sentences read to him or her.
  Verbal Memory I: The child answers questions about a story that was read to him or her.

Verbal Fluency: The child names objects that belong in a given class, e.g., animals or things to eat.
  Opposite Analogies: The child provides opposites for words, presented in analogy form.
Perceptual-Performance Scale
  Block Building: The child copies designs using 1-in. blocks.
  Puzzle Solving: The child assembles noninterlocking puzzles of familiar objects.
  Tapping Sequence: The child copies a simple note sequence that the examiner played on a toy xylophone.
  Right-Left Orientation: The child follows commands that demonstrate knowledge of right versus left.
  Draw-A-Design: The child draws geometric shapes from models.
  Draw-A-Child: The child draws a picture of a child of the same sex.
  Conceptual Grouping: The child groups colored plastic forms on the basis of shape, size, and color.
Quantitative Scale
  Number Questions: The child answers basic arithmetic questions.
  Numerical Memory I and II: The child repeats series of digits forward and then backward.
  Counting and Sorting: The child counts objects and demonstrates basic understanding of quantity concepts.
Memory Scale
  Subtests include Pictorial Memory, Tapping Sequence, Verbal Memory I and II, and Numerical Memory I and II.
Motor Scale
  Leg Coordination: The child walks a line, walks backward, skips, and so forth.
  Arm Coordination: The child bounces and throws a ball, throws a bean bag at a target, and so forth.
  Imitative Action: The child imitates the examiner's motor gestures.

Other subtests are Draw-A-Design and Draw-A-Child.
General Cognitive Index
Combines the subtests on the Verbal, Perceptual-Performance, and Quantitative Scales.

Setting and Equipment

The standard testing environment is required. For the motor subtests, an uncarpeted floor and 10 feet of clear floor space are needed. The child will need a pencil for drawing. The examiner will need a stopwatch and scotch tape to hold down a strip of cloth used for several Motor Scale items.

Administration Procedures

The MSCA is a standardized test, and thus the manual specifies the exact wording for all subtest directions. The items are to be given in the order presented in the manual, but some will be omitted depending on the age of the child.

The format of the subtests is quite variable. At times the child is asked questions; at other times the child is working with materials such as wooden colored blocks of different shapes or a toy xylophone; and at others the child is standing on one foot, skipping, or tossing a bean bag at a target. The directions for the subtests and for scoring the variety of responses and behaviors that will be forthcoming from young children is rather complex. Smooth administration requires considerable study of the manual as well as experience in giving the test with children of different ages.

Scoring

The scoring procedure entails a substantial amount of computation and transferring from one part of the test protocol to another, so scoring errors are possible. On the back of the protocol is a format for computing and recording subtest raw scores, which are then converted to scale indexes using the normative tables in the manual. The scale indexes have a mean of 50 and a standard deviation of 10. The GCI combines the Verbal, Perceptual-Performance, and Quantitative scales and has a mean of 100 with a standard deviation of 16.

Psychometric Properties

Standardization

The standardization testing took place in 1970 and 1971. Subjects were 1000 children (100 at each of 10 ages). They were evenly distributed throughout the geographic regions of the United States and were representative of the U.S. population in age, sex, race, and socioeconomic status.

Reliability

The internal consistency coefficients of the GCI averaged .93 across age groups; these coefficients for the five scale indexes ranged from .79 to .88. Test-retest reliability over a 1-month period averaged .90 for the GCI and .69 to .89 for the other scales. The Motor Scale has been shown to be the least stable of the scales [1]. More research is needed to determine longer-term stability of the MSCA Scales, particularly when exceptional children are subjects [5]. Importantly, stability of intellectual functioning of young children may prove to be elusive, since instability is a characteristic of developing abilities.

Validity

Complete reviews of validity of the MSCA are available [1, 3, 5, 6]. Validity of the MSCA has been evaluated in terms of factor analysis, relationship of the GCI to IQ, discrimination among groups, prediction of school achievement, and validity with minority populations [5]. All reviewing authors have concluded that the test is reasonably valid, although the validity issues examined across many studies yield very complex results that depend on the ages of the children being tested; their educational, racial, and socio-economic status; and the subscales being considered. Paget [5] concludes that the test has excellent psychometric properties, correlates strongly with school achievement, is racially unbiased, and differentiates learning-disabled from non-learning-disabled children well.

Guidelines for Use in a Clinical Setting

The MSCA scores can be used with the greatest confidence with children who are neither severely or moderately retarded nor gifted. Because the items at the beginning of the test are designed for normally developing toddlers, significantly delayed 2½ and 3 year olds will be unable to perform many tasks. Conversely, the highest items are easily passed by very bright 7 and 8 year olds. Although tables of extrapolated GCIs greater than 150 and lower than 50 are available [2], Kaufman [3] recommends that they be used only for research purposes until further empirical evidence exists supporting their validity. One reason for caution is that two studies have shown that the GCIs of mentally retarded children as a group were quite a bit lower than their IQs from the Stanford-Binet and WPPSI [6].

Caution is also required in interpreting the results of certain subscales for younger or relatively delayed children. In particular, Watkins and Weibe [8] suggested that the Memory and Motor scales not be used with younger children, and Naglieri, Kaufman, and Harrison [4] suggested that the Quantitative Scale not be used when the GCI is less than 84. Finally, studies of learning-disabled children have produced ambiguous results, so the test's applicability to learning-disabled children remains unclear [5]. Although the MSCA does discriminate between learning-disabled and normal children, on the MSCA learning-disabled children as a group score 1 standard deviation below their scores on other intelligence measures. The question of which test yields a more valid index of functioning remains an empirical question.

Normally developing children generally show considerable scatter over the scale indexes, so that scatter itself is not indicative of abnormality. Tables that show significance levels for inter-scale scatter are available [6]. In the manual, McCarthy suggests 15 points between pairs of subscales as a rule of thumb for determining noteworthy differences.

Because of the lack of equivalence of the GCI with IQ scores of certain groups, the MSCA is generally not recommended as the instrument of choice when school placement issues are present. For school-aged children who may need to be retested at multiple points in their academic program, the WISC-R is preferable for baseline-comparison purposes because the upper age limit for the MSCA is only 8½ years.

Review

The MSCA is a test of general cognitive and motor abilities for children 2½ to 8½ years of age. It was developed comparatively recently (1972), was standardized on a large, representative sample, and has been shown to be generally reliable and valid. The test scores yield a profile across five scale indexes (Verbal, Perceptual-Performance, Quantitative, Memory, and Motor), as well as a GCI, which has a mean of 100 and a standard deviation of 16. The advantages of the test are that it has good psychometric properties, children enjoy taking it (compared with the WPPSI, for example), it yields a profile for analysis of strengths and weaknesses, and it measures motor functioning and coordination. The main disadvantage is the relatively circumscribed group of children with whom the test can be used with confidence. It is best used with children who are in the middle range of abilities, i.e., those who are neither severely or moderately delayed nor gifted.

REFERENCES

1. Graham, J. R., and Lilly, R. S. *Psychological Testing.* Englewood Cliffs, N.J.: Prentice-Hall, 1984.
2. Harrison, P., and Naglieri, J. Extrapolated general

cognitive indexes on the McCarthy Scales for gifted and mentally retarded children. *Psychol. Rep.* 43 : 1291, 1978.

3. Kaufman, A. S., and Kaufman, N. L. *Clinical Evaluation of Young Children with the McCarthy Scales.* New York: Grune & Stratton, 1977.
4. Naglieri, J. A., Kaufman, A. S., and Harrison, P. L. Factor structure of the McCarthy Scales for school-age children with low GCIs. *J. Sch. Psychol.* 19 : 226, 1981.
5. Paget, K. D. Review of the McCarthy Scales of Children's Abilities: In O. K. Buros (ed.), *The Ninth Mental Measurements Yearbook.* Lincoln, Nebr.: University of Nebraska Press, 1985.
6. Sattler, J. M. *Assessment of Children's Intelligence and Special Abilities.* Boston: Allyn & Bacon, 1982.
7. Taylor, R. L. *Assessment of Exceptional Students.* Englewood Cliffs, N.J.: Prentice-Hall, 1984.
8. Watkins, E. O., and Weibe, M. J. Construct validity of the McCarthy Scales of Children's Abilities: Regression analysis with preschool children. *Ed. Psychol. Meas.* 40 : 1173, 1980.

THE MERRILL-PALMER SCALE OF MENTAL TESTS

Descriptive Information

Test Identification

The title of this test is *The Merrill-Palmer Scale of Mental Tests* (Merrill-Palmer), 1931. Its author is Rachel Stutsman, Ph.D. Dr. Stutsman was a psychologist at the Merrill-Palmer School, a laboratory school and center for the study of child development in Chicago. The development and refinement of the test was supervised by Dr. L. L. Thurstone, who was a famous and well-respected psychometrician. Western Psychological Services (12031 Wilshire Blvd., Los Angeles, California 90025) publishes the test at a cost of $395–$425.

Age and Type of Client

The Merrill-Palmer was intended for preschool children. Although items extend from 18 to 71 months, the author recommended its use primarily for children in the age range of 24 to 63 months.

Purpose

The Merrill-Palmer was designed to be a "mental test" for young children.

Time Required to Administer and Score Test

Administration requires approximately 30 to 45 minutes, with 15 additional minutes needed for scoring.

Evaluator

The examiner should be a fully qualified psychologist who is thoroughly familiar with the test administration, evaluation techniques with young children, and the psychometric limitations of this instrument.

Historical Perspective of Test Construction

Development and Source of Test Items

The Merrill-Palmer, now an old test, is a compilation of items developed by the author and other psychologists involved in what was at the time the new field of mental assessment of preschool children. The test manual is actually a reprint of a section of a book by Dr. Stutsman, *Mental Measurement of Preschool Children* [5], which was part of a series of assessment books edited by Lewis Terman, one of the authors of the Stanford-Binet Intelligence Scale. The Merrill-Palmer is a test in the Binet tradition of using an individual's performance on a wide variety of items to yield an age equivalent and standard score.

Review of Literature in Terms of Test Use

The Merrill-Palmer is no longer a commonly used instrument, because of its outdated norms.

However, it is still occasionally used with special populations of children, such as those with language delays [1] or autism [4].

Theoretical Constructs and Implications for Intervention

The Merrill-Palmer items were not designed or selected according to a theory of cognitive development, but were instead chosen for their ability to differentiate among nursery school children who were judged either "bright or dull" by their teachers and other observers [5]. Additional considerations in test development were traditional psychometric standards such as internal consistency and concurrent validity. During test construction a large number of potential items were evaluated, and the items that were psychometrically sound were retained. Thus, the test has an empirical rather than a theoretical base.

Content and Test Administration

Content

The Merrill-Palmer consists of approximately 90 items arranged in order of difficulty. Many items are nonverbal, and the suitcase-sized test kit consists of many colorful boxes containing test equipment such as interlocking puzzles, formboards, colored discs, blocks, and scissors. There are also some verbal items, for which directions are presented in the manual. Sixteen items are scored on a pass/fail basis, while 22 are credited at different age levels depending on factors such as the child's speed of performance or number of errors.

Setting and Equipment

The standard testing environment is required. The examiner must supply a stopwatch, plain paper, and instruments for writing. It is useful to supply a variety of writing instruments, such as a regular pencil, large pencil, and crayon.

The Merrill-Palmer manual contains directions for administration and scoring, along with guidelines for personality observations. However, background information about test construction is available only in Dr. Stutsman's book [5], which is not offered for sale along with the test kit by the publisher.

Administration Procedures

Items are grouped into 6-month levels. Testing begins with items at the child's chronological age, using materials that are of high interest to the child. The basal level is established as the age group at which the child passes all items. Testing continues until the child reaches a ceiling of an age group in which *fewer than half* of the items are passed; testing does *not* continue until the child fails *all* the items at a particular age group.

The manual contains standardized administration and scoring procedures, although some of them are incomplete or ambiguous. The format of the manual is extremely poor, since items are not presented in an order corresponding to test administration or scoring. This format makes administration of the test cumbersome, and undoubtedly increases examiner error.

Scoring

The test protocol is not designed to facilitate recording of all responses, but fortunately there is a great deal of blank space on the protocol, so notes can be made during the evaluation and transferred later to the appropriate spaces.

The child receives 1 point for each item passed, and credit is allowed for certain items that are omitted or that the child refuses to attempt. Several types of standard scores can be obtained using the Merrill-Palmer, although given the instrument's outdated norms, these standard scores are no longer meaningful. Based on the child's total number of points, a mental age can be determined from the norms tables in the manual. It is also possible to determine the standard deviation range within which the child's score falls (e.g., between -1.0 and -1.5 standard deviations). Standard deviations for mental ages can also be determined, and percentile values for each score at each age are also available. Finally, Stutsman described a procedure in which the examiner can compute a ratio IQ (i.e., mental age divided by chronological age) and then locate the standard deviation value of the ratio IQ. This curious two-step procedure was designed to overcome the problem with ratio IQs of different variability at different chronological ages. This problem, of course, has been dealt with in more modern tests with the use of deviation IQs.

Psychometric Properties

Standardization

The standardization sample of the Merrill-Palmer consisted of 631 children (331 boys, 300 girls). These children were located through a variety of agencies and probably represented a range of backgrounds and ability levels, but the sample was not stratified in a systematic fashion. As indicated by its publication date, the Merrill-Palmer was standardized many years ago, so that the applicability of its norms to today's children is highly questionable.

Reliability

Neither the manual nor Dr. Stutsman's book contains a discussion of reliability. Naglieri [2] reported the median test-retest reliability coefficient as .60 (range, .39–.92), which he compared unfavorably to the McCarthy Scales of Children's Abilities and the Wechsler Preschool and Primary Scale of Intelligence (both tests are reviewed in this chapter).

Validity

Sattler [3] reported a moderate median correlation (.51) between the Merrill-Palmer and the Stanford-Binet Intelligence Scale, and even higher correlations with other (unspecified) preschool tests. However, it must be remembered that correlations simply mean that scores on different instruments rise or fall in a similar fashion; the absolute value of scores may be quite different. It is highly likely that this would be the case with the Merrill-Palmer and other preschool tests given to children today, because young children are developing more skills at earlier ages than they did in the 1920s and 1930s when the Merrill-Palmer was normed [3]. Therefore, the Merrill-Palmer would be likely to yield scores that are too high.

Guidelines for Use in a Clinical Setting

Despite its psychometric limitations, the Merrill-Palmer can be a useful component of a larger test battery. The materials are sturdy and appealing to children, particularly because in their boxed form they resemble presents. It is often possible to use the Merrill-Palmer to engage shy, frightened, or very young children with the "toys," when more orthodox test equipment is overwhelming. The discrete format of one task per box can also be appealing to autistic children, who may be helped to cooperate in testing by the structure of "open a box, do the work, put away, finished."

Unfortunately, because of the mixed characteristics of the test items, there are many types of exceptional children to whom a complete Merrill-Palmer cannot be administered. For example, although the test is predominantly nonverbal, there are also verbal items, on which the total score depends, so that hearing-, language-, and speech-impaired children are penalized. In addition, a large number of items are timed, so that the cognitive skills of children with poor motor skills might be underestimated.

Review

The Merrill-Palmer, a test for young children, contains primarily nonverbal problem-solving and eye-hand coordination items, although there are some verbal items also. The test norms are seriously outdated, so scores are only gross estimates of a child's performance relative to chronological age peers. Another shortcoming is that because of the mixture of test content (e.g., verbal items, timed items) many categories of exceptional children would be improperly characterized by their total score on the test. Nevertheless, the test has the advantage of offering a variety of sturdy, attractive materials which may provide the clinician with a useful format in which to observe the skills and behaviors of young children.

REFERENCES

1. Hosking, K. E., and Ulrey, G. Overview of Assessment Techniques. In G. Ulrey and S. J. Rogers (eds.), *Psychological Assessment of Handicapped Infants and Young Children.* New York: Thieme-Stratton, 1982.
2. Naglieri, J. A. Review of the Merrill-Palmer Scale of Mental Tests. In O. K. Buros (ed.), *The Ninth Mental Measurements Yearbook.* Lincoln, Nebr.: University of Nebraska Press, 1985.
3. Sattler, J. M. *Assessment of Children's Intelligence and Special Abilities* (2nd ed.). Boston: Allyn & Bacon, 1982.
4. Schopler, E., and Reichler, R. J. *Individualized Assessment and Treatment for Autistic and Developmentally Disabled Children* (Vol. 1: *Psychoeducational Profile*). Baltimore: University Park Press, 1979.
5. Stutsman, R. *Mental Measurement of Preschool Children.* Yonkers, N.Y.: World Book, 1931.

PICTORIAL TEST OF INTELLIGENCE

Descriptive Information

Test Identification

The title of this test is *Pictorial Test of Intelligence* (PTI), 1964. Its author is Joseph L. French, Ph.D. In the early 1950s, Dr. French, a psychologist, became interested in developing a new test to measure the intelligence of young physically handicapped children because of the inadequa-

cies of the instruments that were being used for that purpose. He was particularly interested in identifying "appropriate readiness" for "educational programs" [2]. Riverside Publishing Company (1919 South Highland Ave., Lombard, Illinois 60148) publishes the test at a cost of $75–$100.

Age and Type of Client

The PTI was designed for children aged 3 to 8 years with motor impairments.

Purpose

According to Dr. French, the PTI was designed as an objective measure of "general intellectual level" in normal and physically handicapped children.

Time Required to Administer and Score Test

Administration of the PTI requires approximately 45 minutes, according to the manual; severely physically handicapped children may require much longer if individually adapted administration procedures are needed. Scoring requires 10 to 15 minutes.

Evaluator

The PTI should be administered only by a fully qualified psychologist.

Historical Perspective of Test Construction

Development and Source of Test Items

A preliminary version of the scale was developed and field tested on 400 children. After revisions, the test was standardized in 1962, this being the present version. Dr. French stated that he adapted some items from existing tests (not specified in the manual) and generated others by observing children and studying child behavior records.

Review of Literature in Terms of Test Use

The PTI (also called the *French*) is not a well-known test except among psychologists who work with motorically impaired children. It was not reviewed by Anastasi [1].

Theoretical Constructs and Implications for Intervention

The theoretical assumption underlying item selection was that intelligence is demonstrated through the perception and use of abstract symbols. Types of symbolic manipulation that French intended to measure were verbal comprehension, perceptual organization, reasoning, numerical computation, and memory. Since these abilities are difficult to define and operationalize in any population, the PTI represents an admirable attempt to evaluate these aspects of intelligence in young, physically handicapped children.

Content and Test Administration

Content

The materials for the PTI include 137 "response cards," which are large, square (11- by 11-in.) cards, each containing four line drawings. These four drawings are centered along the edges of the square. The cover of the test kit carrying case is designed to be propped at an angle to display the response cards, a procedure that provides many children with a better viewing angle than horizontal placement on a table.

The PTI contains 160 untimed items, divided into the following six subtests:

Picture Vocabulary: The child indicates which picture best exemplifies the single word spoken by the examiner.

Form Discrimination: The child selects geometric shapes to match the examiner's samples.

Information and Comprehension: The child selects pictures which best answer questions tapping general knowledge about the world.

Similarities: The child indicates which one out of a set of four items does not belong with the others.

Size and Number: The child demonstrates understanding of size concepts, number recognition, and arithmetic computation.

Immediate Recall: The child demonstrates memory for shapes.

Setting and Equipment

Standard testing conditions are required. For children with severe physical limitations, collaboration between a psychologist and physical therapist or occupational therapist may be needed to position the child correctly and facilitate the child's response selection (e.g., pointing, eye gaze). No additional test materials are needed.

Administration Procedures

Test directions are clearly worded in the manual. Test administration is fairly straightforward, although moving through the pile of response cards and keeping them organized can be cumbersome.

Testing with each subtest begins with item 1 and continues until the child has failed six consecutive items or is obviously making correct choices only by chance. After the test was standardized, however, the author recognized the need for a shorter version for young children; therefore, a "Short Form" is noted on the test protocol. The Short Form has earlier discontinuation rules and slightly different norms; the norms for this version are available only for 3- and 4-year-old children.

Scoring

The test protocol is clear and easy to use. Based on the child's total number of correct answers, summed across the six subtests, the manual provides a percentile rank and a deviation IQ (mean

= 100; standard deviation = 16). A mental age equivalent is also available for each subtest and for the total raw score.

Psychometric Properties

Standardization

The PTI was standardized on 1830 normally developing children. The sample was intended to be "representative of the United States population of children aged three through eight" [2], but the only variables controlled were geographic region, community size, and occupational level of fathers. There were unequal numbers of children at different ages, and sex distribution varied slightly at each age. Nonwhites were included in the sample on a random basis, except at two sites in the South where only black children were tested. In general, the standardization procedures appear to be adequate, although the 1962 norms may be outdated now.

Reliability

Split-half reliability studies cited in the manual are quite impressive (high .80s and .90s), although Sattler [5] described additional studies that reported lower reliabilities (.70s and .80s). Test-retest reliabilities were described by Himelstein as "woefully inadequate" [3]. Several reviewers [3, 4] cite the psychometric inadequacies of the test at the 8-year level.

Validity

The manual reports correlations ranging from .53 to .72 between the PTI and other intelligence tests (Stanford-Binet, WISC, and Columbia Mental Maturity Scale [CMMS]). Several studies of the correlation of the preliminary version of the PTI with later achievement tests are reported in the manual; these studies indicated quite strong relationships (.68–.82), but again Sattler [5] reported more moderate correlations (.23–.79; median,

.56). In addition, Himelstein [3] criticized the very small number of subjects (9–32) in the validity studies cited in the manual. None of the studies focused on the validity of the instrument for physically handicapped youngsters. Subsequent research cited by Himelstein [3] indicated that the PTI was useful and valid with mentally retarded children.

In the manual Dr. French made the point that as the PTI became more widely used, its predictive validity would be established. However, the test has remained a minor, though respectable instrument which few psychologists have actually administered.

Guidelines for Use in a Clinical Setting

There are a number of similarities between the PTI and the CMMS (test review is included in this chapter), so their clinical uses overlap. These two tests are among the few to which severely motorically impaired children can respond, and the range of cognitive skills covered by the PTI is superior to that of the CMMS. However, Dr. French and a subsequent reviewer [6] have cautioned that differences among subtests should be interpreted only with caution, because of the relative brevity and limited reliability of the individual subtests. The PTI is less appropriate than the CMMS for children with speech or hearing impairments or receptive language difficulties, since it requires comprehension of verbal directions. The PTI is also limited by its upper age level of 8 years. For clinical purposes, older retarded children with motor impairments can be assessed using the mental age equivalents of the PTI.

Review

The PTI is a motor-free test of cognitive abilities that does not require oral speech. Skills covered include receptive vocabulary, general information, numerical skills, form discrimination, and short-term visual memory. Reliability and validity data are quite good, but norms are old (early

1960s) and do not include handicapped children. However, the PTI can make useful contributions to the evaluation of motorically and speech-impaired children.

REFERENCES

1. Anastasi, A. *Psychological Testing* (5th ed.). New York: Macmillan, 1982.
2. French, J. L. *Manual for The Pictorial Test of Intelligence*. Lombard, Ill.: Riverside, 1964.
3. Himelstein, P. L. Review of the Pictorial Test of Intelligence. In O. K. Buros (ed.), *The Seventh Mental Measurements Yearbook*. Highland Park, N.J.: Gryphon Press, 1972.
4. Newland, T. E. Review of the Pictorial Test of Intelligence. In O. K. Buros (ed.), *The Seventh Mental Measurements Yearbook*. Highland Park, N.J.: Gryphon Press, 1972.
5. Sattler, J. M. *Assessment of Children's Intelligence and Special Abilities* (2nd ed.). Boston: Allyn & Bacon, 1982.
6. Smith, T. A. Review of the Pictorial Test of Intelligence. In O. K. Buros (ed.), *The Eighth Mental Measurements Yearbook*. Highland Park, N.J.: Gryphon Press, 1978.

SLOSSON INTELLIGENCE TEST

Descriptive Information

Test Identification

The title of this test is *Slosson Intelligence Test* (SIT). The first edition was published in 1961. The second edition was published in 1981, although the dates on the test manual and separate norms manual are confusing. Copyright dates for the second edition at different places on the documents range from 1981 to 1984. The author of the SIT is Richard L. Slosson, M.A. Background information on Slosson is not available from the manual or other easily accessible sources. Much of the recent work on the test, especially the normative tables, was done by a "research team" apparently employed by Slosson Educational Publications, Inc. Western Psychological Services (12031 Wilshire Blvd., Los Angeles, California 90025) publishes the test at a cost of $47–$65.

Age and Type of Client

The SIT has items that start at the 2-week level and extend up to the 27-year level. However, the norms tables for use in obtaining a deviation IQ start at a chronological age of 2 years and extend to 18 years. The manual suggests adaptations to use when testing children with a variety of handicapping conditions (e.g., deafness, blindness, learning disability).

Purpose

The SIT was designed to be a screening measure of the mental ability of children and adults. The manual states that it gives a reliable estimate of an IQ that would be obtained using the Stanford-Binet Intelligence Scale.

Time Required to Administer and Score Test

Administration and scoring combined take 20 to 35 minutes on the average.

Evaluator

The manual states that the test was "specifically designed for use by teachers, principals, guidance counselors . . . psychologists, psychometrists, social workers, and other responsible persons . . ." (see page 1 of the test manual). However, Reynolds [3] asserts that according to current professional standards [1], this statement is inappropriate, and that only persons specifically trained to administer and interpret intelligence test results should administer any test of cognitive ability.

Historical Perspective of Test Construction

Development and Source of Test Items

The majority of the SIT items were adapted from the Stanford-Binet and the Gesell Institute of Child Behavior Inventory.

Review of Literature in Terms of Test Use

The SIT was originally published in 1961. The ratio method for deriving an IQ used at that time was the focus of major criticism by subsequent reviewers. In 1977, a renorming was completed, yielding tables from which to obtain a deviation IQ. The 1981 manual presented the option of using ratio and/or deviation IQs. In the most recent printing of the manual and the accompanying norms tables, the ratio procedure is abandoned completely.

Pointed criticism of the SIT has been aimed at its psychometric properties, incompleteness of the manual, underlying suppositions, and intended use by nonpsychologists (e.g., Reynolds [3]). On the other hand, it has been described as a creditable screening measure, if in fact it is used only as such and not as a substitute for a full evaluation [4, 5]. From the reviewers' experience, the SIT is often used by physicians and other professionals who are not familiar with the psychometric shortcomings of the instrument.

Theoretical Constructs and Implications for Intervention

The manual states that the SIT can be considered a parallel form of the Stanford-Binet. Therefore, the interpretation given to the Stanford-Binet should apply to the SIT; that is, the SIT is a measurement of general comprehension, memory, reasoning, and so forth. The authors ("research team") of the SIT suggest that although the test can be substituted for a Stanford-Binet, in cases of a borderline SIT IQ, a longer test should be administered. However, others [3, 4] have stated clearly that the test should be used only as a screening measure.

Content and Test Administration

Content

The test materials consist basically of a manual, test blank, and accompanying norms tables. There are 194 items. The earliest items involve motor responses, attending and social responses, and preverbal skills. From the 2-year to the 4-year level, most items test receptive language. All items above age 4 require the child's verbal response. Examples (with year-month age levels in parentheses) are "Why do we have clocks?" (4-6); "What does destroy mean?" (8-10); "How is a clock different from a calendar?" (11-0); "What is a protozoa?" (18-9); "What is the cube root of 216?" (22-3).

Setting and Equipment

The standardized testing environment is required. Paper and pencil are needed for a few drawing tasks.

Administration Procedures

A standardized introductory paragraph is read and the questions are asked in the order presented in the manual. All items are untimed.

Scoring

A basal level is achieved when the examinee passes 10 consecutive items, and a ceiling is established when 10 consecutive items are failed. A mental age (MA) is obtained by totaling the month credit per item as indicated on the score sheet. A deviation IQ (mean = 100, standard deviation = 16) is then determined from the norms tables, which are contained in a separate booklet. The highest chronological age (CA) to be used is 18 years.

Psychometric Properties

Standardization

The SIT manuals (1961 and 1981) have been criticized for presenting insufficient information about its standardization sample and procedures [2, 4, 5]. The renorming sample for the 1981 revision consisted of 1109 persons from urban and rural New York state. Use of subjects from only one state obviously results in a nonrepresentative normative sample. The manual states that 4350 subjects have been tested subsequently, but it is not clear in what way these subjects were included in the normative data.

Reliability

A single study is reported in the manual, wherein a test-retest (2-month interval) reliability coefficient of .97 was obtained. Subjects were 139 children and adults aged 4 to 50.

Validity

Validity of the SIT has been tested almost exclusively through its correlations with the Stanford-Binet, the WISC (not the WISC-R), and, to a lesser degree, an assortment of other achievement and abilities tests, such as the Peabody Picture Vocabulary Test-Revised, Wide Range Achievement Test, and California Achievement Test. Correlations with the Stanford-Binet are particularly high (above .90), a result that is predictable due to the fact that many Slosson items were adapted from Stanford-Binet items. The SIT correlates more highly with the WISC Verbal IQ (.69, .82) than the Performance IQ (.58, .50) (data from the test manual, 1981). The magnitude of correlations with other tests is variable, ranging from low to quite high (.40–.90) [5].

Guidelines for Use in a Clinical Setting

The SIT should be used for screening only, and never for diagnostic or placement purposes. Because the test overestimates the IQs of preschool children and has low predictive validity for learning-disabled kindergarten children [5], it should be used with caution for these groups. Its highly verbal item content would also render it invalid for children with weaknesses in language reception or expression.

Review

The SIT is a 194-item untimed test that is best used only as a screening instrument for measuring intelligence. The items were adapted from the Stanford-Binet and the Gesell Inventory. The original version used ratio method for obtaining an IQ, but the current version relies completely on norms from which to derive deviation IQs for persons from 2 to 18 years of age. Standardization, reliability, and validity have been insufficiently addressed; however, it has been established that the SIT IQ correlates very highly with the Stanford-Binet and WISC Verbal IQs.

REFERENCES

1. American Psychological Association. Ethical principles of psychologists. *Am. Psychol.* 36 : 633, 1981.
2. Oakland, T. Review of the Slosson Intelligence Test. In O. K. Buros (ed.), *The Ninth Mental Measurements Yearbook.* Lincoln, Nebr.: University of Nebraska Press, 1985.
3. Reynolds, W. M. Review of the Slosson Intelligence Test. In O. K. Buros (ed.), *The Ninth Mental Measurements Yearbook.* Lincoln, Nebr.: University of Nebraska Press, 1985.
4. Sattler, J. M. *Assessment of Children's Intelligence and Special Abilities* (2nd ed.). Boston: Allyn & Bacon, 1982.
5. Taylor, R. L. *The Assessment of Exceptional Students.* Englewood Cliffs, N.J.: Prentice-Hall, 1984.

STANFORD-BINET INTELLIGENCE SCALE

Descriptive Information

Test Identification

The title of this test is *Stanford-Binet Intelligence Scale* (Stanford-Binet), Third Revision, 1973. Its authors are Lewis M. Terman, Ph.D., and Maud M. Merrill, Ph.D. Both authors were psychologists at Stanford University at the time the test was developed. Dr. Terman (1877–1956) was an academic researcher whose interest in the measurement of intelligence appeared to be purely scientific. Dr. Merrill (1888–1978), on the other hand, was a clinician and was particularly interested in disturbed and delinquent youth. Riverside Publishing Company (1919 South Highland Ave., Lombard, Illinois 60148) publishes the test at a cost of $100–$150.

Age and Type of Client

The Stanford-Binet can be used with individuals ranging in age from 2 years through adulthood, and ranging in intellectual level from severely mentally retarded through very superior.

Purpose

The Stanford-Binet is intended to be a test of general intelligence, rather than a measure of the separate components of cognitive ability.

Time Required to Administer and Score Test

Administration time is approximately 45 minutes with young children and 60 to 75 minutes with older children. Approximately 15 additional minutes is needed for scoring.

Evaluator

The Stanford-Binet should be administered only by a fully qualified psychologist.

Historical Perspective of Test Construction

Development and Source of Test Items

The 1973 edition of the Stanford-Binet represented the third American version of the scale of intelligence originally developed in France by Alfred Binet and Theodore Simon at the turn of the twentieth century. The impetus for the scale was the introduction in France of universal edu-

EDITORS' NOTE: The fourth edition of the Stanford-Binet was completed and available in early 1986. However, several years will probably be required for dissemination and general use of the fourth edition.

cation for children, which had led to a need for identification of mentally retarded children who required special class placements. Earlier versions of the Stanford-Binet, also developed by Terman and Merrill at Stanford University, were published in 1916 and 1937.

Review of Literature in Terms of Test Use

The Binet scales represented a breakthrough in the history of the psychological study of human behavior and abilities [5], and the Stanford-Binet stood for years as the classic intelligence test [1, 2]. The methodology devised to measure intelligence, such as the standardized administration of increasingly difficult items, has since been adapted to the measurement of numerous other human abilities in psychology and other fields. However, the Stanford-Binet, although recently revised, has not kept pace with methodological advances in test construction and standardization, and thus is no longer at the forefront of the field [2].

Theoretical Constructs and Implications for Intervention

Binet's original view of intelligence has been reflected in all of the subsequent revisions of his scale. He defined intelligence as the mental ability to adapt to new situations and solve novel problems. This conceptualization represented a change from an earlier focus on sensorimotor skills as a reflection of intellectual ability. Thus, a wide range of problem-solving abilities is sampled on the Stanford-Binet. However, no attempts have been made to evaluate different types of cognitive abilities separately. Instead, items that most clearly differentiated between age groups were chosen. Although it was recognized that there are different aspects of intelligence, the underlying assumption was that there is also a global factor of general intelligence that accounts for most of the differences in children's school performance.

Content and Test Administration

Content

The Stanford-Binet consists of a series of subtests placed at age levels which are identified by Roman numerals. Subtests are arranged at 6-month age levels from II–V, yearly age levels from VI–XIV, and four adult levels. At each level (except Average Adult) there are six subtests.

The content of the Stanford-Binet is sometimes criticized [5] for being exclusively verbal, but this is not the case at the lower age levels. At ages II, II-6, III, III-6, IV, IV-6, and V, there are a number of subtests of visual-motor and nonverbal reasoning abilities. Unfortunately, these subtests are not evenly distributed at each age level, which would have allowed the development of various skills to be evaluated systematically. Instead, some age levels (e.g., II-6, IV, IV-6) are heavily verbal, while others (III, V) are heavily motoric. Types of verbal items below the VI-year level include labeling pictures, following directions with objects and pictures, completing analogies, defining vocabulary words, and answering what/why questions. Nonverbal items include stringing beads, copying block patterns, matching and discriminating shapes, completing a drawing of a man, folding paper, and tying a knot. At the VI-year level and above, virtually all subtests are verbal (e.g., defining vocabulary words, analyzing verbal absurdities, repeating digits and sentences, and describing similarities and differences among words and concepts).

The Stanford-Binet materials are contained in a square, briefcase-sized kit. The kit is necessary because of the manipulable materials used at levels II through V. Above this level, the only materials needed are the questions contained in the manual, the individual test protocol (which has space for several drawing items) and printed material contained in one spiral-bound book.

Setting and Equipment

Standard testing conditions are required. The examiner should supply pencils, a stopwatch, and 6- by 6-in. paper for a paper folding task.

Administration Procedures

Test administration is closely standardized and requires careful study and training. Testing usually begins one age level below the child's chronological age, but with mentally retarded children testing may begin at a much lower level. Wherever testing begins, it continues downward until the child has obtained a basal level of one age level completely correct, and upward to a ceiling of one age level completely failed. For children with evenly developed skills, therefore, testing can be completed fairly quickly; children with scattered abilities may require much longer to obtain a basal level and a ceiling.

Scoring

The scoring protocol is a 14-page booklet. Once mastered, it provides a good format for recording the child's responses verbatim and making notes about the child's behavior. Scoring of some verbal responses is difficult and probably contributes to variability among examiners. Aside from decisions about the quality of verbal responses, the mechanics of scoring are straightforward. For each subtest passed, the child earns a specified number of months of mental age credit. Total mental age is then compared with the child's chronological age in the norms tables, and a deviation IQ is obtained.

It is imperative for child development professionals unfamiliar with the development of the Stanford-Binet to understand that the traditional relationship among chronological age, mental age, and IQ no longer exists. Dr. Terman was the first to use the term *Intelligence Quotient,* which is equal to the ratio of mental age divided by chronological age. However, this "ratio IQ" has since been replaced by a "deviation IQ," through which an individual child's deviation from the mean of his or her age group is expressed as a standard score with a mean of 100 and a standard deviation of 16. This change to a deviation IQ on the Stanford-Binet was made in 1960. In the 1973 normative population, however, it was found that young children were mastering more skills at younger ages than in the 1937 normative population [1]. Therefore, the total mental age score obtained on the Stanford-Binet was no longer representative of a child's developmental level of cognitive skills. For example, a child with a chronological age of 3 years 0 months and a mental age total of 3 years 0 months now obtains a Stanford-Binet IQ of 86, indicating that the child is almost 1 standard deviation below average. An "average" 3-year old (IQ = 100) obtains a Stanford-Binet mental age of 3 years 6 months. In effect, the obtained mental age on the Stanford-Binet is merely a raw score of subtests passed, rather than a meaningful mental age equivalent. Some psychologists now report a corrected or adjusted mental age, derived from the manual by locating the chronological age at which the child's obtained mental age equals an IQ of 100. Tables for obtaining corrected mental ages are also available in Sattler [5].

Another caution about the use of the mental age is in order. Frequently a developmentally delayed child will pass a subtest at or near his or her chronological age level. For example, a 3 year old may pass one or two subtests at the III-year level. Some nonpsychologists (and unfortunately some psychologists, too) may interpret this result as indicating that the child has some skills at age level. However, it must be remembered that all subtests at the III-year level would need to be passed for the child to obtain 3 years of mental age credit. So the III-year subtests actually reflect skills that are normally developed before the child reaches chronological age 3. In addition, as explained in the preceding paragraph, an average 3 year old obtains 3 years 6 months of mental age credit. Thus, for a 3 year old to pass only one or two items at the III-year level does not necessarily contradict a finding of developmental delay or mental retardation.

Psychometric Properties

Standardization

For the third revision (1973), the Stanford-Binet was standardized on approximately 2100 children located as part of a much larger normative study of a group intelligence test published by the same company. The larger sample had been stratified on the variables of community size, geographic region, and community economic status. It might be inferred that stratification was according to U.S. census data, but this fact was not explicitly stated in the Stanford-Binet manual. The variables of sex, race, and socioeconomic status were not specifically controlled, but were intended to be represented in a pattern characteristic of the total population of the United States.

Reliability

Reliability and validity data presented in the manual are remarkably sparse. The manual continues to rely on studies of older versions of the test, and even these studies are quite limited. Data are presented to show that the number of items passed increases with age, and that the mean correlation for individual items with total score was in the .60s. There is no discussion in the manual of test-retest, split-half, or interrater reliabilities. Anastasi [1], after an extensive literature review, described the Stanford-Binet as "highly reliable," with most studies reporting reliability coefficients above .90. Similar conclusions were reported by Graham and Lilly [3]. Interestingly, Sattler [5] did not subject the Stanford-Binet to the same psychometric analysis as he did with other intelligence tests. Waddell reported that for the 1973 revision "A search of the literature did not produce any reliability studies . . . A definite need exists for new reliability studies" [6].

Validity

Studies of the concurrent validity of the Stanford-Binet and various other intelligence tests abound in the literature and generally range from the mid-.50s to .90 [4]. Unfortunately these studies almost invariably use the Stanford-Binet as the criterion, rather than as the test under scrutiny. Although this finding does not invalidate the correlational relationships found, it does not represent rigorous study of the Stanford-Binet itself, since it is simply assumed to be the standard against which other, newer tests are evaluated [4]. Anastasi [1] reported that in most studies of the correlation of the Stanford-Binet and academic achievement, correlation coefficients range from .40 to .75, although according to a study cited by Helton, Workman, and Matuszek [4] such correlations are lower for black children.

Guidelines for Use in a Clinical Setting

In spite of limited psychometric data about the most recent revision of the Stanford-Binet, it remains the test of choice for certain populations when a norm-referenced evaluation of cognitive skills is desired. First, the Stanford-Binet is one of the few tests available for chronological ages 2 to 4 years. Although the Bayley Scales of Infant Development have norms through 2½ years, bright children at the top of the age range may not reach a ceiling on that test, while the Stanford-Binet can provide more developmentally advanced items. On the Wechsler Preschool and Primary Scale of Intelligence (WPPSI, reviewed in this chapter), there are no norms for children younger than 4, and some 4 year olds may be too developmentally delayed or uncooperative to take the WPPSI. Thus, the Stanford-Binet is a significant option for the evaluation of 3 and 4 year olds. Another option, of course, would be the McCarthy Scales of Children's Abilities (MSCA, reviewed in this chapter), but since that test does not yield an IQ, occasionally the Stanford-Binet is more appropriate for purposes such as diagnosis, educational classification, and insurance reimbursement.

The Stanford-Binet is often appropriate for older youngsters with significant degrees of mental retardation. The Wechsler Intelligence Scale for Children-Revised (WISC-R, reviewed in this chapter) does not yield a Full Scale IQ below 40, and is not recommended at the lower level of functioning. Therefore, moderately to severely mentally retarded children can often be more fully and confidently evaluated using the Stanford-Binet than the WISC-R.

For several groups of children, the Stanford-Binet is particularly inappropriate. As noted above, the Stanford-Binet has verbal items throughout the age levels, and is almost totally verbal from the VI-year tests upward. Therefore, it would not be a good test of overall cognitive abilities for speech- and language-impaired children. (However, it may offer a useful comparison of these children's abilities with those of normally developing age peers.) Below the VI-year level, there are so many items requiring visual-motor coordination that children with cerebral palsy or dyspraxia (motor planning difficulties) may be severely underestimated by this test.

Professionals should be aware that the Stanford-Binet overlaps significantly with the Preschool Language Scale (see Chap. 6), so there is no point in administering both instruments.

Review

The Stanford-Binet is one of the oldest and most widely known individual intelligence tests. Its psychometric properties are not as strong as those of newer tests such as the Wechsler scales. However, because of its long clinical history and acceptable psychometric base, it is still a useful test, especially with certain populations such as preschool children and older mentally retarded individuals.

REFERENCES

1. Anastasi, A. *Psychological Testing* (5th ed.). New York: Macmillan, 1982.

2. Freides, D. Review of the Stanford-Binet Intelligence Scale. In O. K. Buros (ed.), *The Seventh Mental Measurements Yearbook.* Highland Park, N.J.: Gryphon Press, 1972.
3. Graham, J. R., and Lilly, R. S. *Psychological Testing.* Englewood Cliffs, N.J.: Prentice-Hall, 1984.
4. Helton, G. B., Workman, E. A., and Matuszek, P. A. *Psychoeducational Assessment: Integrating Concepts and Techniques.* New York: Grune & Stratton, 1982.
5. Sattler, J. M. *Assessment of Children's Intelligence and Special Abilities* (2nd ed.). Boston: Allyn & Bacon, 1982.
6. Waddell, D. The Stanford-Binet: An evaluation of the technical data available since the 1972 restandardization. *J. Sch. Psychol.* 18 : 203, 1980.

WECHSLER INTELLIGENCE SCALE FOR CHILDREN-REVISED

Descriptive Information

Test Identification

The title of this test is *Wechsler Intelligence Scale for Children-Revised* (WISC-R), 1974. Its author is David Wechsler, Ph.D. (1896–1981). Dr. Wechsler was one of the leading psychologists in the field of assessment of mental abilities. His earliest work was in the area of adult assessment, but by the time of his death in 1981, he had developed three intelligence tests—Wechsler Preschool and Primary Scale of Intelligence (WPPSI), WISC-R, and Wechsler Adult Intelligence Scale-Revised (WAIS-R). These tests cover from age 4 through adulthood. The Psychological Corporation (555 Academic Court, San Antonio, Texas 78204-0952) publishes the test at a cost of $175–$250.

Age and Type of Client

The WISC-R was designed for children aged 6 years 0 months up to 17 years.

Purpose

The WISC-R was designed to be an individually administered intelligence test.

Time Required to Administer and Score Test

For most children, administration of the WISC-R requires 50 to 75 minutes. Scoring generally requires an additional 15 to 20 minutes.

Evaluator

The WISC-R should be administered only by a fully qualified psychologist.

Historical Perspective of Test Construction

Development and Source of Test Items

The WISC-R is the 1974 revision of the WISC, which was published in 1949. The WISC, in turn, represented a downward extension for children of Wechsler's scales for measuring adult intelligence. All of the Wechsler tests follow a similar format of having 10 to 12 subtests, divided into Verbal and Performance Scales. Similar or analogous items are used in all three tests. Item content was devised by Dr. Wechsler and extensively field tested during the development of the tests.

Review of Literature in Terms of Test Use

The WISC-R is generally regarded as the most commonly used intelligence test for school-aged children [4, 7]. This test and its predecessor, the WISC, have been the subjects of extensive research [5].

Theoretical Constructs and Implications for Intervention

Early in his career as a psychologist, Wechsler moved away from the study of intelligence as a developmental characteristic of childhood, and studied its measurement in adults. He rejected the concept of mental age as proposed and used by Binet, Terman, and Merrill (developers of the Stanford-Binet) and others, and instead based his measurement of intelligence on modern statistical methods. It was Wechsler who popularized the use of the deviation IQ, which precisely represents an individual's standing in relation to the normative group. Eventually, having developed his methodology, he came full circle to the measurement of intelligence in children, resulting in the development of the WISC. However, at least one reviewer has criticized the Wechsler tests for their limited theoretical base or definition of intelligence [3].

Content and Test Administration

Content

The WISC-R materials are contained in a zippered briefcase. The WISC-R consists of 12 subtests, divided into two scales, Verbal and Performance. Each subtest is described briefly below:

Verbal Tests
  Information: The child gives answers to questions of general factual information.
  Similarities: The child describes how pairs of objects or concepts are alike (e.g., plum and peach).
  Arithmetic: The child counts objects in pictures and answers oral arithmetic problems.
  Vocabulary: The child gives the definitions of words.
  Comprehension: The child answers hypothetical questions about social situations, and answers questions about the operation of societal agencies and organizations.
  Digit Span: The child repeats sequences of numbers, either forward or backward.
Performance Tests
  Picture Completion: The child names the missing part in a picture.
  Picture Arrangement: The child puts a series of pictures in order to tell a sensible story.
  Block Design: The child copies patterns with colored blocks.
  Object Assembly: The child completes non-interlocking puzzles of common objects.
  Coding: The child uses a pencil to copy a series of simple lines, following a sample code.
  Mazes: The child uses a pencil to indicate the correct paths out of a series of mazes.

Of these 12 subtests, 10 are administered as part of the standard battery, while one (Mazes) is an alternate that can be substituted for Coding, and one (Digit Span) is supplementary. Digit Span can yield valuable data and clinical observations, but is not used in computing the test scores.

Setting and Equipment

Standard, comfortable testing conditions are necessary. The examiner must supply red pencils without erasers (for Coding and/or Mazes) and a stopwatch.

Administration Procedures

Verbal and performance tasks are presented to the child in the standardized format described in the manual. Directions are clear and complete, but the variety of subtests and large number of items associated with each makes learning to administer the WISC-R a lengthy process. Examiners need careful instruction and supervised practice in order to master standardized administration.

Scoring

For the Verbal subtests the examiner records the child's responses verbatim, then scores them later based on scoring criteria contained in the manual. Several reviewers [3, 6] have indicated that scoring criteria for verbal items are ambiguous or incomplete. Performance items are much simpler to score, and the examiner can generally score each item as the child completes it. Most items can receive either complete or partial credit, and some performance items can also receive bonus points for rapid completion. The test protocol facilitates assigning points and obtaining a total raw score for each subtest. This raw score is then compared with the normative data for the child's chronological age group, yielding a standard or "scaled" score for each subtest. These scaled scores have a mean of 10 and a standard deviation of 3.

The norms tables also yield standardized scores for the total of scaled scores on the Verbal Tests, the Performance Tests, and all 10 subtests. These values are the verbal IQ, performance IQ, and full scale IQ, respectively. These three scores are deviation IQs with a mean of 100 and standard deviation of 15.

Contained in the manual is a table that allows the examiner to obtain a "test age" equivalent for raw score values on each subtest. Although Wechsler did not approve of the use of mental ages, he provided this table to enable WISC-R results to be compared with mental ages on other scales [9].

Psychometric Properties

Standardization

The WISC-R was standardized on 2200 children (200 at each year level from 6 years 6 months through 16 years 6 months). In addition, a small group of children aged 6 years 0 months was used to develop the norms for the lowest age level of the test. There were an equal number of boys and girls at each age level. The sample was stratified according to the 1970 U.S. census on the variables of race, geographic region, urban or rural status, and parental occupation. Bilingual children who could speak and understand English were included in the sample.

Reliability

Test-retest reliabilities reported in the manual for verbal, performance, and full scale IQs are .93, .90, and .95, respectively. On retesting, practice effects were noted, averaging 3½ points on the verbal scale IQ, 9½ points on the performance

scale IQ, and 7 points on the full scale IQ. The manual reports split-half reliabilities for each subtest at each age level, all of which are .70 or higher. Split-half reliabilities for the three IQ scores are even larger: across all ages the average verbal IQ, performance IQ, and full scale IQ reliability coefficients are .94, .90, and .96, respectively. Interexaminer reliability is not reported in the manual.

Validity

Very little information about validity is contained in the manual, a deficiency noted by many reviewers [1, 4, 8, 10]. Cited in the manual are three studies of WISC-R correlations with three other intelligence tests (Stanford-Binet, WPPSI, WAIS). The correlations obtained were quite high (.63–.80 with WPPSI IQs, .68–.95 with WAIS IQs, and .51–.82 with Stanford-Binet IQs). Both Graham and Lilly [4] and Sattler [6] reviewed numerous additional studies of concurrent validity, and concluded that the concurrent validity of the WISC-R is "satisfactory." In the literature there are very few studies of the predictive validity of the WISC-R; the studies that have been done tend to find correlations ranging from .35 to .72, with highest relationships between verbal IQ and language-related academic tasks [4].

Another valuable source of information about the validity of the WISC-R is research done using factor analysis to investigate the empirical relationships among the WISC-R subtests. Numerous studies, reviewed by Kaufman [5], have demonstrated that the WISC-R subtests cluster in factors essentially identical to the Verbal and Performance Scales designed by Wechsler. All of the Verbal subtests except Arithmetic and Digit Span generally load together into a factor Kaufman labeled *Verbal Comprehension,* while all of the Performance subtests except Coding comprise a factor called *Perceptual Organization.* For many groups of children at a variety of age levels, Arithmetic, Digit Span, and Coding cluster together in a third factor, labeled *Freedom from*

Distractability [5]. Thus, factor analytic research provides evidence for the construct validity of the WISC-R.

Guidelines for Use in a Clinical Setting

The WISC-R is usually the test of choice for children between the ages of 6½ and 16 years who have usable vision, hearing, and speech. In addition, some visually impaired and motorically impaired children can be tested with the Verbal Scale, while hearing-impaired children can be tested with the Performance Scale using modified directions [6] and/or special norms [2]. According to Sattler [6], the WISC-R is not as useful at the extremes of the age range or ability level. For 6 year olds the WPPSI is often preferable, while for 16 year olds the WAIS-R may be more appropriate. The range of IQs obtainable is 40 to 160; consequently, very retarded or very gifted students may be better assessed with the Stanford-Binet. The WISC-R is often particularly suitable for the evaluation of students with learning disabilities because it assesses a wide variety of cognitive skills that can be analyzed separately or grouped together. Many learning-disabled students demonstrate WISC-R patterns of widely scattered abilities within the Verbal or Performance Scales, or between those two scales. Kaufman's volume, *Intelligent Testing with the WISC-R* [5], includes an extensive discussion of various WISC-R profiles and their clinical significance.

Review

The WISC-R is a highly reliable, well-respected individual intelligence test for school-aged children. It is most useful for children without major handicapping conditions, although modified versions can be used with some categories of exceptional children.

REFERENCES

1. Anastasi, A. *Psychological Testing* (5th ed.). New York: Macmillan, 1982.

2. Anderson, R. D., and Sisco, F. H. *Standardization of the WISC-R for the Deaf* (Series T, No. 1). Washington, D.C.: Gallaudet College, Office of Demographic Studies, 1977.
3. Freides, D. Review of the Wechsler Intelligence Scale for Children-Revised. In O. K. Buros (ed.), *The Eighth Mental Measurements Yearbook*. Highland Park, N.J.: Gryphon Press, 1978.
4. Graham, J. R., and Lilly, R. S. *Psychological Testing*. Englewood Cliffs, N.J.: Prentice-Hall, 1984.
5. Kaufman, A. S. *Intelligent Testing with the WISC-R*. New York: Wiley, 1979.
6. Sattler, J. M. *Assessment of Children's Intelligence and Special Abilities* (2nd ed.). Boston: Allyn & Bacon, 1982.
7. Taylor, R. L. *Assessment of Exceptional Students: Educational and Psychological Procedures*. Englewood Cliffs, N.J.: Prentice-Hall, 1984.
8. Tittle, C. K. Review of the Wechsler Intelligence Scale for Children-Revised. In O. K. Buros (ed.), *The Eighth Mental Measurements Yearbook*. Highland Park, N.J.: Gryphon Press, 1978.
9. Wechsler, D. *Manual for the Wechsler Intelligence Scale for Children-Revised*. Cleveland: The Psychological Corporation, 1974.
10. Whitworth, R. H. Review of the Wechsler Intelligence Scale for Children-Revised. In O. K. Buros (ed.), *The Eighth Mental Measurements Yearbook*. Highland Park, N.J.: Gryphon Press, 1978.

WECHSLER PRESCHOOL AND PRIMARY SCALE OF INTELLIGENCE

Descriptive Information

Test Identification

The title of this test is *Wechsler Preschool and Primary Scale of Intelligence* (WPPSI), 1967. Its author is David Wechsler, Ph.D. (see Wechsler Intelligence Scale for Children-Revised for information about Dr. Wechsler). The Psychological Corporation (555 Academic Court, San Antonio, Texas 78204-0952) publishes the test at a cost of $155–$200.

Age and Type of Client

The WPPSI was designed for children aged 3 years 11 months to 6 years 7 months.

Purpose

The purpose of the test is to measure general intelligence using various tasks of verbal and nonverbal cognitive functioning.

Time Required to Administer and Score Test

Administration takes 1 to 1½ hours, and scoring takes approximately 15 minutes.

Evaluator

The WPPSI should be administered only by a fully qualified psychologist.

Historical Perspective of Test Construction

Development and Source of Test Items

Many of the WPPSI subtests are downward extensions of WISC-R subtests. Three WPPSI subtests were newly developed for the test—Sentences, Animal House, and Geometric Design. Each is similar in task and rationale either to a WISC-R subtest (e.g., Animal House parallels Coding on the WISC-R) or to a traditional psychometric task (e.g., Geometric Design involves copying designs; Sentences is a type of verbal Digit Span).

Review of Literature in Terms of Test Use

The WPPSI was developed by David Wechsler in the mid-1960s specifically as a downward extension of his other intelligence scales. Because of the test's good psychometric properties, it has been accepted as a criterion measure of intelligence in preschool children and is widely used. Compared with the Stanford-Binet, the WPPSI has the advantage of producing a profile of scores over several verbal and performance subtests. The McCarthy Scales of Children's Abilities (MSCA, reviewed in this chapter) has come to rival the WPPSI as a preschool test because some practitioners view the MSCA as more appealing

and interesting to children and because it includes assessment of gross motor functioning. The problems in interpreting the main scaled score of the MSCA (i.e., the General Cognitive Index), however, have kept the WPPSI from being supplanted by the MSCA.

Theoretical Constructs and Implications for Intervention

The WPPSI evaluates a child's performance over 11 subtests that sample a wide variety of behavior. The tests are divided into verbal and nonverbal scales, with subtests assessing functions such as memory, problem solving, sequencing, comprehension, and learned information. The child's average performance over the subtests is reflected in the IQ. The WPPSI can be used to address diagnostic and placement questions as long as it is supplemented with other appropriate tests and data about the child. Analyses of strengths and weaknesses in cognitive performance and detection of potential learning disabilities are the main uses of the test. Intervention usually involves reviewing the child's performance pattern and making recommendations for teaching strategies and educational placement based on that pattern.

Content and Test Administration

Content

The WPPSI materials are contained in a zippered carrying case. The test consists of eleven subtests, divided into the Verbal and Performance subscales. Eight of the subtests are the same as the WISC-R and are considered downward extensions of the WISC-R subtests. Each of the subtests is described below:

> Verbal Tests
> Information: The child gives short answers to questions of general factual information.
> Vocabulary: The child gives definitions of simple words.

Arithmetic: The child is asked about arithmetic concepts ranging from relative size, length, and quantity to simple addition.

Similarities: At the lower levels, the child supplies the last word of a sentence such as "you eat with a spoon and you also eat with a _____." At the upper levels, the child must describe how two objects are alike, e.g., a shoe and a glove, a horse and a sheep.

Comprehension: The child answers questions about social situations.

Sentences: The child repeats verbatim sentences read to him or her.

Performance Tests

Animal House: The child matches colored pegs to pictures of animals, according to the sample provided.

Picture Completion: The child names the missing part in a picture.

Block Design: The child copies patterns using colored blocks.

Mazes: The child draws a pencil line to work through a maze.

Geometric Designs: The child copies simple designs with a pencil.

Setting and Equipment

The standard testing environment is required. The test kit provides all materials needed except the scoring protocols and forms for the Mazes and Geometric Designs subtests, which can be purchased separately from the publisher. The child will need a pencil without eraser for drawing, and the examiner will need a stopwatch.

Administration Procedures

Test administration is standardized and requires extensive study and training. The rules for subtest start and discontinue levels are given in the manual and are cued on the scoring form.

Scoring

Using the tables provided, raw scores are con-

verted to scaled scores with a mean of 10 and standard deviation of 3 for each subtest. The sums of the scaled scores on the Verbal and Performance scales are then converted to verbal and performance deviation IQs, and the total sum of scaled scores to an overall deviation IQ (mean = 100, standard deviation = 15). The WPPSI protocol is similar to that of the WISC-R, with a format for recording responses, totaling scores, and a front sheet that summarizes background information, IQs, and a profile of subtest scaled scores.

Psychometric Properties

Standardization

A total of 1200 children, 100 boys and 100 girls at each of six age groups, made up the standardization population. The sample was representative of the U.S. population on the basis of race, socioeconomic status, rural versus urban, and geographic region, according to the 1960 census.

Reliability

The WPPSI has been shown to be highly reliable in terms of split-half reliability, with coefficients uniformly high (.77–.87) across six age groups (reported in manual). Test-retest reliability is high as well; correlations over 11 weeks ranged from .86 to .91 for the IQ scales. General practice effects were noted, with the greatest increase in points for the performance scale (average of 6.6), compared with the verbal scale (3.0) and the full scale IQ (3.6).

Validity

Validity information is thoroughly summarized in several sources [1–4]. After reviewing studies of concurrent validity (using the Stanford-Binet, WISC, and WISC-R as criteria), predictive validity (correlating WPPSI scores to achievement test scores), and construct validity (based on factor analytic studies), these authors conclude that the test demonstrates excellent validity.

Guidelines for Use in a Clinical Setting

The WPPSI has frequently been cited for requiring a long administration time, which may be taxing to young children. Special efforts at rapport building must be made, and sensitivity to the child's attention and fatigue levels is necessary. While two or more separate testing sessions are an option, research is lacking to evaluate the effect such a procedure would have on test performance. Another important feature—and drawback—of the WPPSI is that it measures abilities of children at the lowest and highest levels of functioning less accurately than at the middle levels. For example, the lowest IQ level calculable at age 4 is 51 for the full scale IQ. Sattler [4] presented evidence that the WPPSI may not yield accurate IQs for children functioning two or more standard deviations below the mean. The test has the same limitation for children in the very gifted range.

Some reviewers (e.g., Wodrich [5]) have found that the WPPSI items are of less interest to children than those of the McCarthy Scales, while others praise the test for its high interest [2, 4]. Apparently this is a matter of judgment among reviewers.

Review

The WPPSI is the Wechsler Scale designed to measure general intelligence in children aged 3 years 11 months to 6 years 7 months. It has the advantages of having excellent psychometric properties and providing a profile of scores for analysis of strengths and weaknesses. Disadvantages include its limited floor and ceiling, which may prevent severely to moderately retarded children as well as gifted children from being accurately assessed with this test. Some authors view the test items as intrinsically uninteresting to children and administration time as overly long.

REFERENCES

1. Eichorn, D. H. Review of the Wechsler Preschool and Primary Scale of Intelligence. In O. K. Buros (ed.), *The Seventh Mental Measurements Yearbook.* Highland Park, N.J.: Gryphon Press, 1972.
2. Freeman, B. J. Review of the Wechsler Preschool and Primary Scale of Intelligence. In O. K. Buros (ed.), *The Ninth Mental Measurements Yearbook.* Lincoln, Nebr.: University of Nebraska Press, 1985.
3. Graham, J. R., and Lilly, R. S. *Psychological Testing.* Englewood Cliffs, N.J.: Prentice-Hall, 1984.
4. Sattler, J. M. *Assessment of Children's Intelligence and Special Abilities* (2nd ed.). Boston: Allyn & Bacon, 1982.
5. Wodrich, D. L. *Children's Psychological Testing: A Guide for Nonpsychologists.* Baltimore: Paul H. Brookes, 1984.

TESTS OF EMOTIONAL FUNCTIONING

Although this chapter has focused on measures of intellectual functioning used in pediatric assessment, many psychological reports discuss the results of emotional and behavioral evaluations as well. Tests of emotional functioning fall into two broad categories: projective and objective. The following is a brief overview of each.

Projective tests use ambiguous stimuli onto which the child "projects" his or her needs, fears, and wishes. One of the best known is the Thematic Apperception Test (TAT), which consists of picture cards depicting human interactions. The child is shown the cards one at a time and asked to make up a story about what is happening in the picture. Responses are then analyzed for recurring emotional themes, such as anger, insecurity, optimism or hopelessness, specific feelings about various family members, and so forth. A version of the TAT often used with younger children is the Children's Apperception Test (CAT), which depicts animals engaged in humanlike interactions.

Other well-known projective tests are the Rorschach (the "inkblot test") and sentence completion methods. The Rorschach procedure consists of showing 10 inkblots to the child, who describes what each looks like. Several scoring systems are available (e.g., [3, 4]); however, many practitioners do not score the test but instead interpret the content of the child's verbalizations in somewhat the same manner as with the TAT. A sentence completion test consists of a series of sentence stems (e.g., I like . . . , Mothers should . . .) that the child completes in writing or verbally as the stems are read. Some scoring systems have been developed (e.g., [8]) but are used almost exclusively for research. Most psychologists analyze the child's answers based on clinical impressions.

Objective tests of personality or emotional and behavioral functioning can be further divided into two types. The first is self-report inventories, wherein the child reads each statement and indicates whether it is true for him or her. Examples are the Piers-Harris Children's Self-Concept Inventory [7] and the Children's Depression Inventory [5]. The child's score on self-report tests can be compared with reference groups (e.g., normal children, clinic samples).

The second type of objective test is a behavior checklist that lists several (often more than 100) behaviors or symptoms; the informant, most often a parent or teacher, endorses those that apply to the child being evaluated. Scores on different subscales, such as Aggression, Withdrawal, or Hyperactivity, are obtained and compared with national norms. Some of the most well-known behavior checklists are the Child Behavior Checklist [1], the Behavior Problem Checklist [6] and the Conners Teacher Rating Scale [2].

REFERENCES

1. Achenbach, T. M., and Edelbrock, C. S. *Manual for the Child Behavior Checklist and Revised Child Behavior Profile.* Burlington, Vt.: University of Vermont, Department of Psychiatry, 1983.
2. Conners, C. A teacher rating scale for use in drug studies with children. *Am. J. Psychiatr.* 126 : 152, 1969.
3. Exner, J. E. *The Rorschach: A Comprehensive System.* New York: Wiley, 1974.
4. Klopfer, B., and Kelly, D. *The Rorschach Technique.* Yonkers, N.Y.: World Books, 1942.
5. Kovacs, M., and Beck, A. T. An Empirical-Clinical Approach Toward a Definition of Childhood Depression. In J. G. Schulterbrandt and A. Raskin (eds.), *Depression in Childhood: Diagnosis, Treatment, and Conceptual Models.* New York: Raven Press, 1977.
6. Peterson, D., and Quay, H. *Behavior Problem Checklist,* unpublished manual, 1979.
7. Piers, E., and Harris, D. *The Piers-Harris Children's Self-Concept Scale.* Nashville: Counselor Recordings and Tests, 1969.
8. Rotter, J. B., and Rafferty, J. E. *Manual for the Rotter Incomplete Sentences Blank.* Cleveland: The Psychological Corporation, 1950.

CHAPTER REVIEW

The preceding reviews of psychological assessment instruments used with children have covered only a fraction of the total number of commercially available tests. The challenge to psychologists and to other professionals who read psychological test reports is to remain informed about the nature, psychometric properties, and clinical usefulness of the standard tests and the many new tests that are published each year.

Conclusion

Pediatric assessment is certainly one of the most important aspects of a therapist's role. Often therapists have little of the background knowledge and information that is required to select an appropriate test, administer it correctly, and then interpret the results based on a sound understanding of that test's particular characteristics and its place in the assessment process. This book has attempted to provide both information regarding evaluation of test instruments and an understanding of the strengths and weaknesses of many pediatric tests. The evaluation outline presented in Appendix B provides a format for the evaluation of test instruments not included in this book. It is expected that the years ahead will see the development of new tests, and the collection of more extensive statistical data for other tests. For example, the Southern California Sensory Integration Tests (SCSITs) has already been expanded and renormed to create the Sensory Integration and Praxis Tests (SIPTs), and it is expected to be available in the summer of 1987. Similar efforts are needed in other areas of assessment. While the clinical expertise of the therapist cannot be underestimated, the profound impact of pediatric assessment requires the development and use of valid, reliable standardized evaluation tools.

Appendix

SENSORIMOTOR HISTORY

Child's Name: _____ Date: _____

Play Skills: Please describe how your child plays. If you have any other observations of your child's play, please write them down.

1. Paper use
   a. Uses pencil or crayon? _____
      Draws what? Lines? _____ Circles? _____ People? _____ Other? _____
   b. Uses scissors? _____
2. Throwing and catching
   a. Throws towards target or person? _____ Poorly? _____ Well? _____
   b. Attempts to catch? _____ Catches adequately? _____
   c. Kicks balls appropriately? _____
3. Things to ride on or in (kiddie car, big wheel, tricycle, 2 wheel bike, sit 'n spin, roller skates)
   a. Will sit on voluntarily? _____
   b. Pushes or pedals self on what? _____
   _____
4. How does (or did when younger) your child play with these toys?
   a. Blocks _____
   b. Small cars or vehicles _____
   c. Small buildings, trees, animals, etc. used to create scenes _____
   _____
   d. Pegboards _____
   e. Toys involving putting together or taking apart _____
   _____
   f. Dolls _____
   g. Puzzles. How many pieces? _____
   h. Board games or cards _____
5. Outdoor play: how does he or she play with
   a. Sand or dirt _____
   b. Water _____
   c. Playground equipment (swings, climbs) _____
   d. Pool: Games? _____
              Swims? _____
6. Make believe
   a. Dresses up _____
   b. Helps around house or yard _____
   c. Other _____
7. When left alone, how does your child spend his time? _____
   _____
   _____

SENSORIMOTOR HISTORY—(continued)
8. Other observations of play or self-help _____
_____
_____

SENSORY HISTORY

                                                                YES   NO

Vestibular: Does your child:
Get carsick easily _____
Enjoy fast rides   _____
Spin or whirl more than most children _____
Like merry-go-rounds   _____
Seem fearful of space, i.e., going up and down stairs, riding teetertotters   _____
Has your child ever had seizures?   _____
Is your child on any seizure medication?   _____

Tactile: Does your child:
Dislike being cuddled or hugged _____
Dislike touch from others unexpectedly   _____
Dislike certain types of material in clothing   _____
Prefer long pants and long-sleeved shirts   _____
Prefer bland food_____
Avoid getting hands in paste, fingerpaint, or other "messy" material _____
Not like having face washed or wiped   _____
Not like to have hair washed or cut _____
Frequently bump or push other children   _____
As infant, resist solid food _____
Tend to feel pain less than others_____
Tend to feel pain more than others   _____

Visual: Do you observe:
Difficulty following a moving object (ball)   _____
Dislike of being blindfolded   _____
Poor eye contact _____
Reversals in letters   _____
Has your child had an eye examination? If so, give physician, results, and date_____
_____

Auditory: Does your child:
Respond negatively to unexpected or loud noises   _____
Have difficulty locating direction of sound   _____
Have trouble functioning if there is a lot of noise around _____
Not appear to hear all sounds _____
Has your child had a hearing test? If so, give date, results, and name of audiologist   _____
_____

COMMENTS:

MODIFIED FROM FORMS BY A. JEAN AYRES

SCHOOL QUESTIONNAIRE

Child's Name _____ *Date* _____
Birthdate _____ *Grade* _____
School _____ *Teacher* _____
Address _____ *Person completing*
_____ *form* _____

Classroom Concerns: _____
_____
_____

Is this child being seen by other specialists (P.T., Speech)? Please list by name and specialty: _____
_____

Please check appropriate box if applicable:

	Reading	Math	Spelling	Writing
Below grade level				
At grade level				
Above grade level				

Please complete the following observation checklist:

	Seldom	Sometimes	Often

Postural and Gross Motor
1. Unusual walking pattern (dragging feet, stiff, limps, falls often, runs rather than walks)
2. Poor posture (pot belly, round shoulders, forward curve of spine, works with head on desk)
3. Tires easily
4. Gross motor tasks (i.e., skipping, jumping, hopping, running) are awkward as compared to peers

Fine Motor
1. Difficulty manipulating small objects (pegs, beads)
2. Difficulty using scissors, coloring or fastening clothing
3. Abnormal pencil grip (_____ immature; _____ tight; _____ weak; _____ tires easily)
4. Jerky or tremorlike motions in hands when tracing
5. Difficulty staying on line when tracing

Basic Sensory Functioning
1. Pushes, shoves, kicks when standing in lines or crowds
2. Dislikes being touched, prefers touching
3. Difficulty identifying objects by touch alone
4. Fearful of movement
5. Craves spinning or rocking; does not get dizzy
6. Gets dizzy easily (avoids rolling/spinning)

Visual Perception
1. Poor understanding of spatial concepts (large, small and numbers)
2. Poor directional concepts (up, down, right, left, in, out, before, behind)
3. Bumps into chairs or desks often
4. Difficulty putting puzzles together which offer no problems to peers
5. Difficulty recognizing shapes

SCHOOL QUESTIONNAIRE—(continued)

	Seldom	Sometimes	Often
6. Difficulty sequencing			
7. Difficulty identifying relevant stimuli from distracting background			
8. Poor spacing of work on paper			
9. Reverses letters, numbers, words or phrases			
10. Omits words and phrases, skips lines and loses place while reading or copying			
Bilateral Integration			
1. Avoids or has difficulty performing tasks which require eyes or extremities to cross midline of body (e.g., tends to keep work on one side of midline, switches objects to opposite hand when working on that body side, pivots body to avoid crossing the midline)			
2. Doesn't stabilize paper while writing			
3. Inconsistent hand dominance			
4. Neglects or seems unaware of one side			
Learning Behavior			
1. Unable to attend to task as long as classmates			
2. Easily distracted			
3. Wiggles a lot; can't sit still			
4. Can't tolerate change in routine			
5. Disorganized, messy			
6. Slow worker			
7. Appears to have difficulty comprehending what's going on around him			
Social-Emotional			
1. Behavior annoys or bothers others			
2. Impulsive			
3. Lacks confidence (often says "I can't" or "too hard")			
4. Easily frustrated			
5. Happiest playing alone			
6. Fearful of new situations			
Self-help			
1. Difficulty with eating (chewing, drinking)			
2. Difficulty using utensils (knife, fork, spoon)			
3. Difficulty with dressing skills			
4. Difficult with toileting skills			

COMMENTS OR ADDITIONAL OBSERVATIONS: (Attach additional sheet if needed)

Modified from Patti Oetter, OTR

PARENT QUESTIONNAIRE

Date: _____

Child's Name: _____ Birthdate: _____ Sex: _____

Address: _____
   Street   City   State   Zip Code

Home Telephone: _____( )_____

Who referred child for evaluation?: _____

Insurance Coverage: _____

Family Data:

Father's Name: _____ Birthdate: _____

Occupation: _____ Business Telephone: (____)_____

Mother's Name: _____ Birthdate: _____

Occupation: _____ Business Telephone: (____)_____

With whom does child live? Biological Parents [   ]

                 Adoptive Parents [   ] (Adopted at Age _____)

                 Other [   ] (Specify: _____)

List all *other* persons living in home:

Name	Age	Relationship to Child	Present Health

Birth Information:

Any difficulties during pregnancy or delivery (specify): _____

_____

Length of Pregnancy: _____ Length of Labor: _____

Birth was: Normal [   ] Caesarian [   ] Breech [   ] Twins or More [   ]

Did baby need assistance in starting to breathe? _____

Birth Weight: _____

Any problems in newborn period (specify): _____

_____

Developmental Milestones: List the age at which your child accomplished each activity

Motor:	Sitting alone	_____	Reaching for objects	_____
	Pulling to stand	_____	Finger feeding	_____
	Walking	_____	Eating with spoon	_____
	Jumping	_____	Drawing a circle	_____
	Hopping on one foot	_____	Drawing a square	_____
	Riding tricycle	_____	Cutting with scissors	_____
	Riding bicycle	_____	Using a knife for cutting food	_____
	Skipping	_____		
Language:	Said first word	_____	Pointing to simple pictures	_____
	Combined words	_____	Following one-step commands	_____
	Spoke sentences	_____	Following several-step commands	_____

Self-Help:

Dressing: Pull off: socks _____ shirt _____ pants _____

           Put on: socks _____ shirt _____ pants _____ shoes _____

           zips _____ unzips _____ snaps _____ unsnaps _____

           buttons _____ unbuttons _____ ties_____

           Does your child dress independently? _____

Grooming: Bathing independently _____ Toileting independently _____

           Combing hair _____ Toilet trained _____

PARENT QUESTIONNAIRE—(continued)

School History:
Hand Preference:_____Familial Handedness:_____
Has child been enrolled in nursery or day care? _____ At what age? _____
Has child attended kindergarten?_____ At what age? _____
Has child begun elementary school?_____At what age (1st grade)? _____
What is present grade? _____ Have any grades been repeated? _____
What school does your child attend at this time? _____
Teacher's Name: _____
Is your child in a special class or receiving any support services (specify)? _____
_____
_____

Social History:
Does your child make friends easily? _____
How does your child play with other children (aggressive, picked on, loner, leader)? _____
_____
Does your child need to be in control of the group? _____
Does your child tend to play with friends of his or her own age, younger, or older? _____
Do you have any concerns about your child's social skills? _____
_____
Is your child difficult to discipline? _____

Professional and Medical Contacts:
Who is child's present physician? _____
    (Give name and address)   _____
                                   _____
Check any of the following with whom you have had contact concerning your child. (Give name and address)
[   ] Psychologist _____
[   ] Occupational therapist _____
[   ] Physical therapist _____
[   ] Speech therapist _____
[   ] Neurologist _____
[   ] Orthopedist _____
[   ] Others (please specify) _____
_____
Does your child use any specialized equipment?_____
_____

Parental Concerns:
What are your concerns about your child? _____
_____
_____
What have you been told by doctors, teachers, and/or others about your child's problem? _____
_____
_____
What do you see as your child's strengths? _____
_____
_____
Children with special needs sometimes act younger than their chronological age. What age do you feel best describes your child? _____
_____

TEST REVIEW OUTLINE

I. Descriptive Information
Test Identification
Age and Type of Client
Purpose
Time Required to Administer and Score Test
Evaluator
(Professional expertise; special training; appropriateness of use by nonprofessional)
II. Historical Perspective of Test Construction
Development and Source of Test Items
Review of Literature in Terms of Test Use
Theoretical Constructs and Implications for Intervention
III. Content and Test Administration
Content
(Areas the test covers, a list of test items, and equipment that is included in the test kit; charts, samples, and/or pictures of distinguishing features of the test)
Setting and Equipment
(Type of physical setting required; additional equipment that is required but not included in the test)
Administration Procedures
(Administration format; clarity of directions; complexity of procedures; ease of administration)
Scoring
(Clarity of directions; complexity of procedures; types of standard scores of information resulting from the tests)
IV. Psychometric Properties
Standardization
(Standardized procedure for test administration; demographic data; normative data)
Reliability
(Test-retest; interobserver [examiner]; split-half)
Validity
(Construct; criterion-referenced [predictive and concurrent]; content)
V. Guidelines for Use in a Clinical Setting
Review
VI. References

Index

Index